INTESTINAL STOMAS

PRINCIPLES, TECHNIQUES, AND MANAGEMENT

INTESTINAL STOMAS

PRINCIPLES, TECHNIQUES, AND MANAGEMENT

EDITED BY

John M. MacKeigan, M.D., F.R.C.S.(C), F.A.C.S.
Associate Clinical Professor, Department of Surgery,
Michigan State University School of Human Medicine, East Lansing;
Chief of Staff, Ferguson-Blodgett Hospital,
Grand Rapids, Michigan

Peter A. Cataldo, M.D.
Assistant Clinical Professor, Department of Surgery,
Wright State University School of Medicine, Dayton, Ohio;
Assistant Clinical Professor, Department of Surgery, Uniformed
Services University of the Health Sciences, Bethesda, Maryland;
Staff Colon and Rectal Surgeon and Director, Surgical
Research, United States Air Force Medical Center/SGHSG,
Wright-Patterson Air Force Base, Dayton, Ohio

ILLUSTRATORS

Scott Thorn Barrows, F.A.M.I. Craig L. Kiefer Kimberly A. Martens

with 242 illustrations, including 28 in color

QUALITY MEDICAL PUBLISHING, INC

ST. LOUIS, MISSOURI 1993

Every effort has been made to ensure the accuracy of the drug dosages listed in this book; however, the health care professional is legally responsible for verifying the indications and dosage requirements with the manufacturers' package inserts and is thus advised.

The opinions expressed in this book are those of the editors and the authors and do not reflect the opinions of the United States Air Force or the Department of Defense.

Printed in the United States of America.

PUBLISHER Karen Berger
EDITOR Beth Campbell
PROJECT MANAGER Carlotta Seely
PRODUCTION Judy Bamert
BOOK DESIGN Susan Trail
COVER DESIGN Diane M. Beasley

Quality Medical Publishing, Inc.
11970 Borman Dr., Suite 222
St. Louis, Missouri 63146

LIBRARY OF CONGRESS CATALOGING-IN-PUBLICATION DATA

Intestinal stomas: principles, techniques, and management / edited by John M. MacKeigan, Peter A. Cataldo.
p. cm.
Includes bibliographical references and index.
ISBN 0-942219-40-6 (casebound)
1. Enterostomy. I. MacKeigan, John M. II. Cataldo, Peter A., 1958-
[DNLM: 1. Colostomy. 2. Ileostomy. WI 520 I665 1993]
RD540.6.I59 1993
617.5′54—dc20
DNLM/DLC
for Library of Congress 93-7281
CIP

VT/WW/WW
5 4 3 2 1

CONTRIBUTORS

Herand Abcarian, M.D.
Professor of Surgery, Department of Surgery, University of Illinois at Chicago, Chicago, Illinois

H. Randolph Bailey, M.D.
Clinical Professor of Surgery and Chief, Division of Colon and Rectal Surgery, Department of Surgery, University of Texas Medical School at Houston, Houston, Texas

Joel J. Bauer, M.D.
Clinical Professor of Surgery, Department of Surgery, Mount Sinai School of Medicine, New York, New York

David E. Beck, M.D.
Staff Colon and Rectal Surgeon, Department of Colon and Rectal Surgery, Ochsner Clinic, New Orleans, Louisiana

W. Donald Buie, M.D.
Clinical Resident, Division of Colon and Rectal Surgery, Department of Surgery, University of Minnesota, Minneapolis, Minnesota

Peter A. Cataldo, M.D.
Assistant Clinical Professor, Department of Surgery, Wright State University School of Medicine, Dayton, Ohio; Assistant Clinical Professor, Department of Surgery, Uniformed Services University of the Health Sciences, Bethesda, Maryland; Staff Colon and Rectal Surgeon and Director, Surgical Research, United States Air Force Medical Center/SGHSG, Wright-Patterson Air Force Base, Dayton, Ohio

Zane Cohen, M.D.
Professor, Department of Surgery, University of Toronto; Surgeon in Chief, Mount Sinai Hospital, Toronto, Ontario, Canada

Marvin L. Corman, M.D., F.A.C.S.
Colon and Rectal Surgeon, Department of Surgery, Sansum Medical Clinic, Santa Barbara, California

Daniel P. Dalton, M.D.
Assistant Professor of Clinical Urology, Department of Urology, Northwestern Memorial Hospital and Northwestern University Medical School, Chicago, Illinois

Paula Erwin-Toth, R.N., M.S.N., C.E.T.N.
Manager, Enterostomal Therapy Nursing, and Director, Enterostomal Therapy Nursing Education, Department of Colorectal Surgery, The Cleveland Clinic Foundation, Cleveland, Ohio

Robert D. Fry, M.D.
Associate Professor of Surgery, Department of Surgery, Washington University School of Medicine, St. Louis, Missouri

Irwin M. Gelernt, M.D.
Clinical Professor of Surgery, Department of Surgery, Mount Sinai School of Medicine, New York, New York

Stephen R. Gorfine, M.D.
Assistant Clinical Professor, Department of Surgery, Mount Sinai School of Medicine, New York, New York

Richard L. Grotz, M.D.
Fellow in Colon and Rectal Surgery, Mayo Medical School, Rochester, Minnesota

Ian C. Lavery, M.D., F.R.A.C.S., F.A.C.S.
Staff Surgeon, Department of Colorectal Surgery, The Cleveland Clinic Foundation, Cleveland, Ohio

Donna L. Loehner, R.N., B.S.N., C.E.T.N.
Enterostomal Nurse, Department of Colon and Rectal Surgery, Lahey Clinic Medical Center, Burlington, Massachusetts

Martin A. Luchtefeld, M.D.
Assistant Clinical Professor, Department of Surgery, Michigan State University School of Human Medicine, East Lansing; Staff Surgeon, Ferguson-Blodgett Hospital, Grand Rapids, Michigan

John M. MacKeigan, M.D., F.R.C.S.(C), F.A.C.S.
Associate Clinical Professor, Department of Surgery, Michigan State University School of Human Medicine, East Lansing; Chief of Staff, Ferguson-Blodgett Hospital, Grand Rapids, Michigan

Robin S. McLeod, M.D., F.R.C.S.(C), F.A.C.S.
Associate Professor, Department of Surgery, University of Toronto, Toronto, Ontario, Canada

Amanda M. Metcalf, M.D.
Associate Professor of Surgery, Department of Surgery, University of Iowa Hospitals and Clinics, Iowa City, Iowa

Juan J. Nogueras, M.D.
Staff Surgeon, Department of Colorectal Surgery, Cleveland Clinic Florida, Fort Lauderdale, Florida

John R. Oakley, M.B., B.S., F.R.A.C.S.
Staff Surgeon, Department of Colorectal Surgery, The Cleveland Clinic Foundation, Cleveland, Ohio

Russell K. Pearl, M.D., M.S.(Surg.)
Associate Professor of Clinical Surgery and Biomedical Visualization, University of Illinois College of Medicine at Chicago; Attending Surgeon, Section of Colon and Rectal Surgery, Cook County Hospital, Chicago, Illinois

John H. Pemberton, M.D.
Associate Professor of Surgery, Mayo Medical School; Consultant in Colon, Rectal, and General Surgery, Mayo Clinic, Rochester, Minnesota

Bonnie Sue Rolstad, R.N., B.A., C.E.T.N.
Director, ET Nurse Consultants, P.A., Independent Nursing Specialty Practice, St. Paul; Editorial Advisory Board, Ostomy/Wound Management, and Lecturing Clinical Faculty Member, ET Nursing Education Program, Abbott Northwestern Hospital, Minneapolis, Minnesota

David A. Rothenberger, M.D.
Clinical Professor of Surgery and Chief, Division of Colon and Rectal Surgery, Department of Surgery, University of Minnesota, Minneapolis, Minnesota

Marc S. Rubin, M.D.
Instructor, Department of Surgery, Harvard Medical School and Beth Israel Hospital, Boston, Massachusetts

David J. Schoetz, Jr., M.D.
Chairman, Department of Colon and Rectal Surgery, Lahey Clinic Medical Center, Burlington; Associate Clinical Professor of Surgery, Boston University School of Medicine, Boston, Massachusetts

Anthony Senagore, M.D., M.S.
Assistant Professor, Department of Surgery, Michigan State University School of Human Medicine, East Lansing, Michigan

Michael P. Spencer, M.D.
Clinical Instructor, Department of Surgery, University of Minnesota, Minneapolis, Minnesota

Mary Ellen Swatske, R.N., C.E.T.N.
Department of Surgery, Washington University School of Medicine, St. Louis, Missouri

Steven D. Wexner, M.D., F.A.C.S., F.A.S.C.R.S.
Residency Program Director, Department of Colorectal Surgery, and Director, Anorectal Physiology Laboratory, Cleveland Clinic Florida, Fort Lauderdale, Florida

W. Douglas Wong, M.D., F.R.C.S.(C), F.A.C.S.
Clinical Assistant Professor, Division of Colon and Rectal Surgery, Department of Surgery, University of Minnesota, Minneapolis, Minnesota

To

our family,
friends, and teachers

FOREWORD

When asked to write the foreword for this book on intestinal stomas, I felt a curious mix of appreciation, pride, and fear. The first and second of these emotions arose for obvious reasons. The invitation was a gracious compliment. In addition, it offered me the opportunity to comment on the editors, Drs. MacKeigan and Cataldo, and to congratulate them on presenting a much needed, essentially North American, specialist-authored, superbly referenced and illustrated exposition of the state of the art and craft of ostomy surgery. The fear set in when I realized that I had never written a foreword or given much thought to its purpose. As I reviewed the forewords of prominent texts, it became apparent that there is no "correct" formula. The high quality of the book speaks for itself, and the editors and contributing authors—all experienced ostomy surgeons and therapists—have drawn from their wisdom and experience to produce their best efforts in succinct and clear terms.

Yet tradition compelled me to reflect on the evolution of the book's subject. I recalled the title of a presidential address given by Dr. Malcolm C. Veidenheimer, a former president of the American Society of Colon and Rectal Surgeons: "Who Dug Your Well?" Our "well diggers" have been numerous and distinguished. In many instances advances in the art of stoma surgery and care have come about through empiricism and serendipity as well as through scientific method and trial. The first chapter in this book is a masterful example of this fact. For example, all trainees of Rupert B. Turnbull, Jr., including myself, heard his recounting of the fortuitous discovery of the absorbent and adhesive quality of karaya powder, which became the first effective skin barrier for ileostomies. Yet Turnbull and his colleague, the late George W. Crile, Jr., in a series of elegant experiments, described and explained the nature of ileostomy dysfunction. To Brooke, Crile, and Turnbull belong the credit for changing, in the words of Peter Cataldo, "the ileostomy from a procedure of last resort to a well-tolerated solution for the treatment of ulcerative colitis."

As great an advance as primary maturation of the stoma was, the modern ostomy patient must be equally grateful for the establishment of the specialty of enterostomal therapy by Turnbull and his former patient, Norma Gill. Together, Turnbull and Gill founded the first school of enterostomal therapy at The Cleveland Clinic Foundation.

Currently, most fellows and trainees are often reminded that ostomy construction, done at the end of a difficult bowel resection, is an important phase of the procedure, one that should not be relegated to the unsupervised, inexperienced junior. In essence, an ostomy is an anastomosis to which the usual principles of good vascularity and freedom from tension apply. The conduct of the stoma construction has a direct and critical bearing on the future rehabilitation and quality of life for the patient. In his foreword to *Atlas of Intestinal Stomas* (Rupert B. Turnbull, Jr., and Frank L. Weakley), Leland S. McKittrick wrote: "If we, as surgeons, are to accept the responsibility of curing the patient of his disease . . . , then we must accept the additional responsibility of doing so in such a way that the patient will be in the best physical and emotional condition to face each hour of every day with a handicap we must not underestimate and from which there is no escape."

This theme—whether represented by exposition of surgical technique, physiology, and principles; meticulous attention to detail; or application of modern enterostomal therapy—is woven into the chapters of this book. I congratulate the editors and their contributors for having achieved this goal with clarity, skill, and compassion.

Victor W. Fazio, M.D., F.R.A.C.S., F.A.C.S.

Chairman, Department of Colorectal Surgery
The Cleveland Clinic Foundation
Cleveland, Ohio

PREFACE

The field of surgery is undergoing evolution. Surgical results can no longer be judged solely in terms of morbidity and mortality. Restoration of, or improvement in, preoperative form and function, reestablishment of a healthy self-image, and improvement in quality of life are parameters by which surgery must be judged. In no field are these aspects more important than in stoma surgery.

More than 200 years have passed since Pillore, a French country surgeon, created the first colostomy in the treatment of obstructing rectal cancer. This text follows the developments of stoma surgery from its origins, before the time of Pillore, to the present day. All aspects of stoma management, including preoperative and postoperative care, surgical techniques, complications, and enterostomal therapy are covered in detail. Individual chapters are dedicated to stoma physiology, dysfunction, and intestinal fistulas.

As gastrointestinal and genitourinary surgery have become increasingly complex, many procedures have been developed to achieve fecal and urinary diversion following resection for both benign and malignant disease. With these procedures the role of stomas—both temporary and permanent, continent and incontinent—has expanded. The proper timing of surgery, location of stomas, techniques of construction, and postoperative management are more difficult than ever before and are evolving. The body of knowledge in ostomy surgery is so large and so diverse that only a multiauthored text can address all the finer aspects of stoma construction and management. For the many hours that the contributing authors have dedicated to creating this book, we are truly thankful.

We must also acknowledge the contribution of the texts that preceded and inspired our efforts—in particular, the *Atlas of Intestinal Stomas* created by Rupert B. Turnbull, Jr., and Frank L. Weakley, which introduced the techniques of modern stoma surgery to physicians around the world. We can only hope that our text will add to the earlier contributions.

We would like to thank Sue Petty, Sally Bayne, and Sandy Sykes for their secretarial support. We are grateful to Sue Buffin and Joan Anderson in Enterostomal Therapy for their time in educating us and our patients. Beth Campbell, Cindy Lia, and Carlotta Seely of Quality Medical Publishing, Inc., have given valued assistance, direction, and encouragement. Scott Barrows and his associates are especially appreciated for their expertise and artistry. This book could not have been possible without their support and direction.

Finally, we would be truly remiss if we failed to acknowledge the efforts of our teachers and mentors. Knowledge comes in many forms and from many sources. It comes from the surgeons who have dedicated their lives to training us; from our coworkers, who have taught us many valuable lessons; from our students, who have learned but also have taught; from the enterostomal therapists, who have changed the lives of individuals with an ostomy more than any physician ever could; and finally, and possibly most important, from our patients, who have inspired us, learned with us, and taught us as no one else ever could. For the efforts of these individuals we are profoundly grateful.

John M. MacKeigan
Peter A. Cataldo

CONTENTS

PART THREE

SPECIAL PROBLEMS

APPENDIXES

INTESTINAL STOMAS

PRINCIPLES, TECHNIQUES, AND MANAGEMENT

PART ONE

OVERVIEW

1 HISTORY OF STOMAS

Peter A. Cataldo

Currently, there are approximately 1 million individuals with an ostomy living in the United States, and an industry has developed solely for the purpose of supplying ostomy products. These people live normal lives, and some of them even compete in the National Football League and play golf on the professional tour. However, this situation was not always the case. Great advances in both stoma surgery and the development of ostomy management systems have made it possible for individuals with an ostomy to lead a normally active life.

The history of stomas has its beginnings in biblical times, but the first purposeful creation of a stoma occurred only slightly more than 200 years ago. In a relatively short time, thanks to many of the great pioneers in surgery and enterostomal therapy, the stoma has evolved from a hastily constructed, foul-smelling, and unsightly artificial anus covered with only moss and leaves and held in place with a crude leather strap to an odorless, barely noticeable, and often continent opening that may require no device whatsoever.

NATURE'S STOMAS

The earliest stomas were not envisioned or created by imaginative surgeons but by the forces of nature (e.g., the result of a strangulated hernia in those individuals fortunate enough to survive) or by ancient warriors (e.g., survivors of abdominal wounds with visceral injury who occasionally lived with a permanent enterocutaneous fistula). One of the earliest accounts of visceral injury comes from the Old Testament, when Eglon was stabbed by Ehud: "He [Eglon] could not draw the dagger out of his belly and dirt came out."[1]

The first purposeful stomas were created for the treatment of abdominal trauma and bowel obstruction. A brief outline of the evolution of the medical

☐ The opinions expressed in this chapter are those of the author and do not reflect the opinions of the United States Air Force or the Department of Defense.

and surgical treatment of trauma and bowel obstruction will add insight into the origin of abdominal stomas.

One of the earliest accounts of the treatment of traumatic abdominal wounds is found in ancient Hindu writings. Susruta (600 BC) advocated the closing of traumatic intestinal wounds with the pincers of black ants, followed by emolument washings and reintroduction of the intestines into the abdominal cavity.[2] In the early sixteenth century, injuries of the gut followed one of three courses: the person died, the wound healed spontaneously, or an external fistula formed. The accepted surgical teaching involved supportive care only. Contrary to established principles, Von Hohenhiem, a German surgeon, began teaching his students to repair small intestinal wounds over silver cannulas.[3] However, he was not enthusiastic about this treatment. In the early sixteenth century, he was probably the first surgeon to suggest the creation of an artificial anus for penetrating gut injuries. However, there is no evidence that he actually performed this procedure.

In 1757 Lorenz Heister (1683-1758) (Fig. 1-1), after observing the spontaneous formation of stomas following abdominal trauma, recommended exteriorization of the injured intestine. He wrote: "that the lips of the intestines so wounded, would sometimes quite unexpectedly adhere to the wound of the

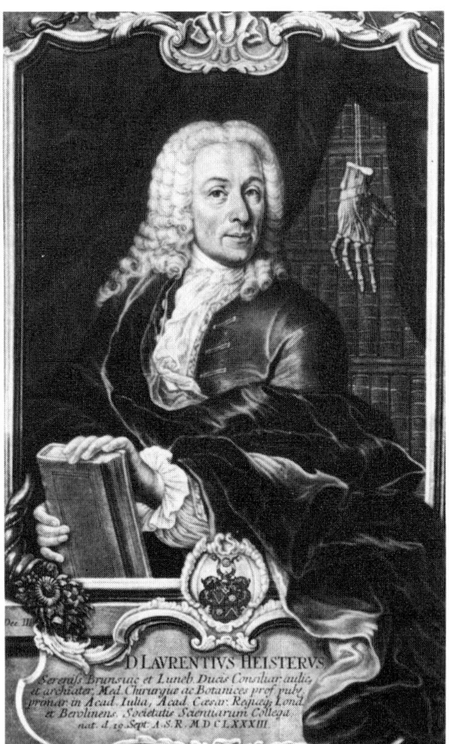

Fig. 1-1. Lorenz Heister. (Courtesy National Library of Medicine, Bethesda, Md.)

abdomen; and therefore there seemed no reason why we should not take hints from nature."[4] In response to criticisms related to the inconvenience of exteriorized intestine, Heister said: "It is surely far better to part with one of the conveniences of life than to part with life itself."[4] This philosophy was certainly not accepted by all surgeons. In the eighteenth century, Jean Palfin[5] and John Bell, both barber-surgeons, emphasized closing the wound of the abdominal wall while leaving the injured intestines alone. Exteriorization, however, grew more popular throughout the eighteenth century. Begny, Schafer, and François de la Peyronie[6] all used this technique in the treatment of abdominal wounds. In 1783 Benjamin Bell modified the exteriorization procedure by creating a double-barreled ostomy in order to prevent stomal stenosis.[7]

BOWEL OBSTRUCTION

Bowel obstruction and its treatments have been extensively reported throughout medical history. Incarcerated hernias and intestinal tumors were in the past, as they are now, the main causes of obstruction. The first surgical treatment of bowel obstruction was prescribed by the ancient Greeks. Praxagorus, a contemporary of Aristotle, wrote the following in 400 BC: "He [unidentified] seemed to be a very bold practitioner for in this distemper [bowel obstruction] if the remedies did not operate, he ordered an incision to be made into the belly and even into the gut itself and the excrements to be drawn out and the wound sewed up again."[8] However, no reports exist on the performance or results of such a procedure.

For the next 20 centuries, the treatment of bowel obstruction remained medical and centered around purgatives and enemas. Hippocrates (a cousin to Praxagorus) advocated a honey suppository anointed with the gall of a bull and followed by an enema. If this method failed, rectal insufflation with a smith's bellows was prescribed.[9] Dolaeus recommended drinking a concoction containing horse dung "because excrement expels excrement," whereas some physicians recommended rubbing the abdomen with slough of a snake seethed in oil or wine.[9] Other experts prescribed anal insufflation of tobacco smoke in the treatment of bowel obstruction.

Ambroïse Paré and many of his contemporaries treated bowel obstruction with large doses of crude mercury taken by mouth in the belief that the weight of the heavy metal would correct the blockage.[3] Application of heat to the abdominal wall was also a popular treatment. Willis and James covered the abdomen with calf's omentum while Thomas Sydenham preferred using a live puppy.[9] Even stimulation with galvanic current was tried. Opium, a popular treatment in the seventeenth century, often accompanied these ingenious remedies for the obstructed intestines.

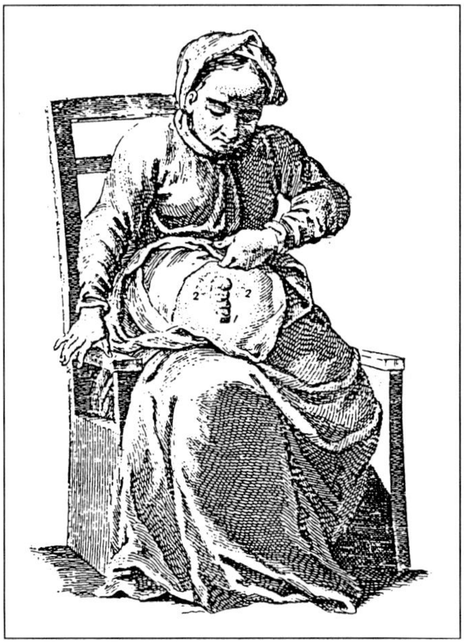

Fig. 1-2. In 1750 Margaret White developed a spontaneous colostomy as a result of a strangulated umbilical hernia. (From Devlin HB. Colostomy. Ann R Coll Surg Engl 52:393-395, 1973.)

As previously mentioned, physicians had observed relief of bowel obstruction as a consequence of spontaneous stoma formation (Fig. 1-2) and had exteriorized injured intestines, thus creating stomas. However, no one had yet proposed the purposeful creation of a stoma to relieve intestinal obstruction.

INTRODUCTION OF COLOSTOMY

In 1710 Alexis Littré (1658-1726) suggested the creation of an abdominal stoma for the treatment of imperforate anus after observations made during the autopsy of a 6-day-old infant. This event was reported by Fontanel, the historian to the Royal Academy of Sciences in Paris[10]:

> M. Littre saw in the dead body of an infant of six days a maldevelopment of the rectum. The rectum was divided into two portions both closed and connected by only a few threads of tissue about an inch long. The upper portion of the closed bowel was filled with meconium. The lower portion was entirely empty. M. Littre, wishing to render his observation useful, imagined and proposed a very delicate operation in the case where one would recognize a similar confirmation. It would be necessary to make an incision into the belly, open the two ends of the closed bowel, and stitch them together, or at least to bring the upper part of the bowel to the surface of the belly wall, where it would never close, but perform the function of an anus. Upon this slight suggestion a clever surgeon could imagine for himself details which we suppress. It often suffices to know in general that a thing may be possible and not to despair of it at first sight.[11]

Littré's idea remained untested for 66 years, until Pillore, a country surgeon from Rouen, France, performed a cecostomy for the treatment of an obstructing rectal cancer. Pillore's great achievement may have gone unnoticed if it had not been for Jean Amussat's inquiries. At the request of Amussat, who learned of the procedure through hearsay, Pillore's description of the first colostomy was found in his memoirs by his son many years later. Pillore's eloquent account was translated by Tilson Dinnick[10]:

> M. Morel, a wine merchant and posting master of Vert-Gallant in the district of Brai, was in the course of the year 1776 taken with difficulty in going to stool. He had first experienced some slight pain in the anal region. These pains became a little greater, without, however, becoming insupportable; but the difficulty in his motions increased to such a degree that he became anxious and determined to come to Rouen for consultation and the necessary remedies. He presented himself to M. Delaroche, a capable physician, who ordered him laxatives and gentle purgatives. These softened the bowel contents and relieved him for some time. But finally, as his difficulties increased daily, he was advised to make use of mercury (or quicksilver) in sufficiently large doses that by their mass would overcome the obstacle in the bowel. The patient indeed took 2 pounds of quicksilver. It was watched for every day but did not appear. The motions became totally suppressed and the belly increased in size from day to day, without, however, being tender or inflamed. In this state of affairs I was consulted. (It is now a month since the patient had taken the mercury without having passed a single drop of it.)
>
> I first examined the rectum, thinking indeed it was there the obstruction would be found, believing it was possibly formed by the hardened and incarcerated feces, as I had often seen to happen; but instead of the species of obstruction I found the upper part of the bowel fixed and scirrhous, forming a very large tumor which totally obstructed the rectum. I tried to pass sounds and cannulae of all shapes and sizes, continuing my efforts for several days, but uselessly. In this state, that is to say, the patient having passed nothing from the bowel for over a month, and his belly enlarging daily in spite of his most austere diet—I proposed to him that I should make him an artificial anus. He agreed with me and cited the case of a man in his village who for several years had had an artificial anus which nature had provided following a strangulated hernia. I knew of this case and also one of another woman in from the same cause.
>
> I was then indeed determined to perform the operation, but as the case was a very delicate one I first asked five or six of my colleagues to see the patient in consultation with me. No one was of my opinion and no one agreed with me. But the patient, a man of great sense, being present at our consultation, prayed my colleagues to show him another means by which he might be saved. They answered that they knew none. "Very well," he replied, "it is indeed imperative to operate since my illness is mortal and you know of no other means to save me."
>
> Encouraged by so strong an argument, I performed the operation in the presence of my confreres, and six pension pupils who were with me at the time. I chose the cecum as the part of the bowel most suited to our need, as much by its situation as because it would furnish a reservoir, and by its continual and involuntary action would hasten the evacuation of intestinal contents. A small plate furnished with a

sponge in the shape of a large button and held by an elastic bandage was devised in the place of a sphincter, so that the patient could at all times voluntarily remove it when he felt the need, and, by means of a small clyster, he could from time to time cleanse out the reservoir. My patient and I conferred together and thought of all these things before the operation. I then operated.

I commenced with a transverse incision a little above the groin which I deepened above and below to the depth of the cellular tissue. I arrived at the aponeurosis of the external oblique which I incised to the same extent a little above the fallopian ligament (Poupart's) in order to have at least a good inch of space from the integuments of the cecum. I made a transverse opening in the muscles in peritoneum almost to the same extent. The base of the cecum, easy to recognize by its appendix, presented itself—I did not have to search for it. I drew the cecum out as far as possible and without effort; there held by an assistant and myself, I opened it transversely and stitched it to the two lips of the wound by means of a thread on two needles which I passed from one side to the other. I passed them from within outward and pulled the thread in the middle, thus obtaining two ligatures which I tied above and below to compresses to press together the edges of the wound. The contents of the bowel came out in abundance. For a dressing I applied burnt charcoal and towels. I used no pressure in order that the issue of fecal matter might not be interrupted. In fact, it ran out in abundance for several days. And the belly diminished considerably in size. As the quicksilver was giving us anxiety and we had not seen a single drop of it appear, we caused the patient to be put in all possible positions that might give it an easy issue. There was not the slightest sign of it, however. Fourteen or fifteen days had passed since the operation, during which time the wound had separated and the bowel was glued to the skin. I had taken out the stitches and all appeared to be in the best possible state when the patient reported vague pains in different parts of the belly. We first attributed this to gasses shut in the intestines, but the patient, uneasy, always said the pains were due to the mercury and consequently continued to take positions that might help it to come out. On the 20th day the belly, which had been very flat, became swollen and painful. Emollient fermentations were applied, and through our artificial anus we threw some injections into the colon. It bled twice, but in spite of all our efforts the symptoms quickly augmented and the patient died on the 28th day after his operation.

I performed the autopsy in the presence of the same surgeons, colleagues, and pupils and found as follows:

The cecum and the whole colon were healthy and in good condition. The cecum was adherent to the lips of the wounds, except in one angle where there was a small area of suppuration in the neighboring cellular tissue, which did not, however, communicate within. The colon was opened to the whole of its extent, and only contained some glairy mucous. The cancerous obstruction which was the primary illness was 8 or 9 inches long, situated at the end of the colon in the beginning of the rectum, totally obliterating the intestinal canal. The tissues surrounding the rectum were hard and fixed. At the site of the rectum was an opening whose calloused edges announced it to be a species of chancre from which issued fecal and purulent material. The peritoneum in the neighborhood of the kidney was inflamed, without, however, being separated. The peritoneum was inflamed and inherent to the folds of the intestines. The quicksilver which the patient had taken was found in one of the last convolutions of the jejunum, which it had dragged down by its weight to the pelvis, behind the bladder. It was pocketed in that portion of the bowel which contained it. This bowel

> presented here and there gangrenous areas, and was inflamed, the inflammation extending to the loins. The mercury was all recovered and had not lost a bit of its weight. We believed that we could conclude that if the operation has not met our expectations for success it was because of the mercury. For it is very probable that when the intestines, which because of their greatest dilatation had lost the power of action, became empty of stercoral material, the peristaltic action was not sufficiently powerful to move the mercury. Then followed inverted retrograde movements, as announced by the nausea and colic which the patient experienced on the 20th day of his illness. Considering the pull on the mesentery in the intestines by the massive two pounds, one is not surprised that gangrenous inflammation occurred and produced the death of the patient.

In 1783 Dubois, a Parisian surgeon, performed an iliac colostomy on a 3-day-old child suffering from imperforate anus. Dubois was successful in relieving the obstruction but not in curing the patient. This child died on the tenth day following surgery.[10]

The colostomy had its true beginning with the surgery of Duret, a naval surgeon at the Military and Marine Hospital at Brest. In 1793 Duret performed the first successful left iliac colostomy in the treatment of imperforate anus in a 3-day-old infant. Tilson Dinnick[10] has provided us with a translation of Duret's original account:

> Friday, October 18, 1793, Marie Poulaouen, midwife of Brales, delivered the wife of Michael Ledreves, a laborer, of a child. She noticed that the infant had no anus and that the sexual parts were malformed; judging that in the best state of affairs the child had not long to live she advised the parents to bring the child to Brest to receive surgical aid. On Saturday at ten in the morning the father came to my house and I examined the child. The sexual organs were so formed that the scrotum was divided at the raphe into two equal parts, each containing a testicle. At first sight, one believed the child to be female. The glans penis lay upon the perineum pierced by the urinary meatus from which the urine issued freely. The region of the anus showed no sign of the existence of a rectum. The skin was natural consistency in color, and no tumor presented when the child strained. After making this examination I believed the case to merit the attention of those most skilled in the art of healing, and with this view I called a consultation of all the physicians and surgeons attached to the various hospitals in the city. The consultants advised opening the skin at the spot where the rectum should be present and searching for the bowel. The operation was not successful. I was able to appreciate by passing a sound through the wound into the pelvis that the lower portion of the big bowel was absolutely missing. It was now four in the afternoon; the infant appeared without resource. The vomiting, the extraordinary swelling of the belly, and the coldness of the lower limbs seemed signs of certain death. To my surprise, however, the next morning the child still lived. This decided me to call a second consultation, at which I proposed as a last resort, to prolong the life of the child, the performance of laparotomy and establishment of an artificial anus. To give me confidence in this most extraordinary procedure I performed it upon the dead body of a child of 15 days which I took from the poor house of the city. I made an incision on the left side between the last of the false ribs and the iliac crest about two inches long. I exposed the pole of the kidney and a portion of the left side of the colon;

this last was opened. I then injected some water by anus. A portion of the fluid came out through the opening of the colon and a portion escaped into the belly. I then recognized by opening the belly that in the fetus the lateral areas of the colon are not extra-peritoneal as in the adult, but that the colon has a mesocolon which renders it free and floating. This circumstance caused me to reject the operation in this region in the fear that it would give rise to an escape of meconium into the belly. Those assembled after witnessing this trial and after prolonging the discussion sufficiently to prove both its interest to humanity and to surgery, decided: (1) that without some extraordinary intervention the death of the child was inevitable; (2) that the axiom of Celsius, "that it is better to employ a doubtful remedy than to condemn the patient to certain death," here found its application; and finally (3) that the decisions of M. Hevin upon laparotomy were not transgressed by this operation, as a cause and course of the malady were, as here, recognized.

I opened the belly of the little patient in the left iliac region in the neighborhood where the sigmoid colon was forming a tumour a little apparent to the eye in where the meconium already imparted a slightly deeper colour to the skin. I made an opening about an inch and a half long which served for me to introduce the index finger into the belly, with which I lifted and pulled out the sigmoid colon. In the fear that it would immediately fall back into the belly I stitched it by two waxed threads passed through the mesocolon. I then opened the colon longitudinally. Gas and meconium came out in abundance. When the bowel had emptied itself to a certain extent I applied a dressing. It was simple and composed of a pierced compress. And the night between Sunday and Monday the baby slept well, the body heat returned, the vomiting ceased, and child took breast easily on several occasions. The day following the operation, all who had witnessed the operation the evening before expressed themselves satisfied with the advantageous changes they perceived. The bandages which had surrounded the child were filled with meconium, and his voice, which had previously hardly been distinguishable, was now heard lustily.

On the third day, as things were going from better to better, I charged the parents to bring the child twice daily to the hospital. Citizen Massac, Chief of the Administration, and Citizen Coulon, Physician in Chief, were charged to provide the necessary dressings. On the 4th day, the stools became yellow and less in quantity, so I ordered a washing out with simple water and 2 drops of serum of rhubarb. This produced a good effect and gave the patient several stools.

On the 5th day, the threads which held the bowel appeared useless, so I removed them, as they were already producing redness and irritation in the region of the artificial anus.

On the 6th day, about an inch of the internal coats of the bowel appeared through the opening, giving the wound the appearance of a chicken's egg. I attempted to reduce the prolapse by passing a lead cannula into the fistula, both to obstruct the further herniation and to keep a free passage of feces, but the child's cries made me defer this means. The instrument has, however, since been perfected by Citizen Morier, a clever cutler of this city. On the 7th day, the child was so well, both at the site of operation and in exercise of his functions, that I judged him no longer in need of care of supervision by a person of the art.

The child survived with an artificial anus until age 45. Duret was unaware of Littré's prior suggestions or Pillore's cecostomy. Duret's insight into colostomy surgery was remarkable. He antedated Callisen in the suggestion of lumbar colostomy. He used a mesenteric stitch to secure the colon to the abdominal wall (90 years prior to Allingham's famous mesenteric stitch). He noted and treated prolapse and used a colostomy for colonic washouts.[10]

In 1797 Professor Fine, Surgeon-in-Chief to the Hospital in Geneva, performed the first transverse loop colostomy in a 63-year-old woman suffering from rectal cancer.[10] Through a midline incision he drew out an inflamed loop of bowel, passed a stitch through its mesentery and sewed it to the skin. The patient's obstruction was relieved, and she lived another 3 months. Fine believed that he had created an artificial anus from the terminal ileum; however, autopsy revealed a successful transverse colostomy.

With the advent of colostomies, it became necessary to create a means for the collection of feces. The first mention of such a collecting device was reported by Daguesceau in 1795. He performed an inguinal colostomy in a farmer who impaled himself on a cart stake while unloading wheat. The farmer, then age 57, survived until the age of 81, and "conveniently collected his feces in a small leather pouch."[10] Daguesceau also performed the first colostomy for the treatment of intractable perianal fistulas. It is interesting to note that the fistulas healed and 2 years later the colostomy spontaneously closed.

INGUINAL vs. LUMBAR COLOSTOMY

By the 1800s the colostomy became an acceptable surgical solution to refractory intestinal obstruction. At that time debate centered on the technique of construction, and two distinct schools emerged, those favoring inguinal colostomy and those preferring lumbar colostomy.[12]

As mentioned earlier, lumbar colostomy was first suggested by Duret. Callisen, however, a professor of surgery at Copenhagen, is often cited as the first to perform a lumbar colostomy.[13] He performed a lumbar colostomy on the corpse of an infant who had died of imperforate anus. During the procedure he inadvertently entered the peritoneal cavity, yet was able to complete the lumbar colostomy through a second incision. Because of the difficulties he encountered, Callisen never became an advocate of the procedure.

Jean Zulema Amussat (1796-1856) (Fig. 1-3) can be considered the father of the lumbar colostomy. He began his medical career as a "medic" in the French army during the Napoleonic wars and became a studied anatomist as the result of many dissections performed on Russian corpses.[14] Amussat published manuscripts on hemorrhoidectomy, surgery for uterine fibroids, and experimental intestinal anastomosis. He is most famous, however, for his description of the lumbar colostomy.

After being called in consultation to see a 48-year-old woman with bowel

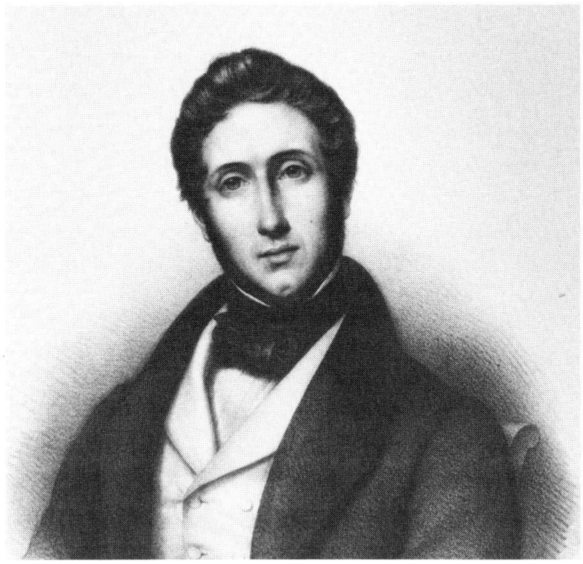

Fig. 1-3. Jean Zulema Amussat. (Courtesy National Library of Medicine, Bethesda, Md.)

obstruction, Amussat and his colleagues suggested enemas, uterine pessary, rectal sounds, aloe suppositories, and even galvanic current. When none of these standard remedies cured the intestinal obstruction, they recommended the creation of an artificial anus. Amussat, after hearing of Callisen's approach,[13] planned a lumbar operation and performed the procedure on a cadaver. The following day the patient underwent surgery. Amussat[12] described the procedure in the following way:

> The patient was placed on her abdomen leaning toward the right side, and two pillows were placed side by side under her abdomen. By this exposure the left side of the lumbar region was well exposed. There appeared, at this point, a round protuberance, indicating the point where the incision should be made.
>
> The skin incision was made two fingers above the iliac crest. I continued the incision deeper in a transverse fashion. An artery was twisted and after having incised the aponeurosis as well as after having gone through a considerable area of fat, I clearly recognized the intestine, which was very distended and outside the peritoneal cavity. Being at the point of perforating the bowel with the trocar, I thought that perhaps it could be decompressed, and then I decided to place two sutures into the bowel approximately one thumb's distance apart. The intestine was held by these two sutures by one of my assistants. I then punctured the point between the two sutures. Gas and fecal matter escaped through the trocar and cannula. Immediately after I passed a hernial probe adjacent to this cannula which permitted me to enlarge the opening I had created with the trocar. This allowed a copious amount of gas to escape as well as more fecal material.

> Two irrigations of the artificial anus were performed—one in the direction toward the lower part of the bowel and the other toward the upper bowel, which again resulted in more fecal material appearing. The quantity was so large that 3 buckets were quickly filled. The evacuation, as well as the gas which had previously distended the abdomen and created so much discomfort, caused the patient to state how much better she felt. The intestinal opening was then brought forward and anteriorly sutured to the skin in 4 points by everting the mucosa. The first suture was made of an ordinary curved needle. And the others were made with acupuncture needles which I usually employ, and were hardly felt at all. The posterior angle of the wound was reconstructed with sutures.
>
> The patient stoically withstood the operation. Immediately afterwards she was returned to her bed and a simple dressing of oiled cloth was applied. During the day the patient felt a great deal of relief. However, she slept very little that night.

The patient did well postoperatively and was discharged 39 days after surgery. At that time she was having one bowel movement every 24 hours. It is interesting that her lumbar colostomy was described as "continent" by Amussat.

Amussat collected and reported on 29 cases of artificial anus between 1776 (Pillore's cecostomy) and 1839 (his own first case).[10] Of the 29 cases, 20 patients died. Twenty-one operations were performed for imperforate anus, and there were only four survivors. (All four survivors were from Brest, the seaport town where Duret performed the first successful colostomy.) Of the eight adult cases, there were five survivors. All 29 patients had been operated on via the abdominal route. Amussat attributed the high mortality to peritonitis; therefore he considered the lumbar route to be the preferred approach for the creation of an artificial anus.

In 1820 Daniel Pring, a surgeon from Bath, performed a left iliac colostomy in the treatment of an obstructing rectal cancer, which made him the first English surgeon to successfully create an artificial anus. (Freer performed a similar procedure in 1815, but the patient died on postoperative day 9.) In his memoirs Pring made these comments concerning the artificial anus[10]:

> (1) The operation prolongs life in cancer of the rectum. (2) It is always acceptable in imperforate anus. (3) It would be useful in simple strictures of the bowel. (4) Peritonitis is a danger. (5) It is imperative to always open distended bowel. (6) Cecostomy is advocated for obstruction in the transverse colon. (7) The opening can be controlled to act once in 24 hours. (8) Prolapse can be prevented and the opening protected by means of a truss and a pad.

After Amussat's success with the lumbar approach, the debate between abdominal and retroperitoneal creation of an artificial anus swung in favor of the retroperitoneal route. The fear of peritonitis expressed by Amussat influenced many surgeons. Additional advantages attributed to the lumbar colostomy included the absence of a spur (then considered a disadvantage), less tendency to prolapse due to greater parietal fixation, a tendency toward constipation rather than incontinence, dependent drainage in the supine position, and absence of an offensive artificial anus on the abdominal wall. Until 1852 the debate continued based on personal preferences, not scientific evidence. However, in 1852 Caesar Hawkins, president of the Royal College of Surgeons in England, reported on a series of 44 patients treated surgically for intestinal obstruction.[13] Seventeen patients underwent transperitoneal colostomy, and 27 patients were operated on via the lumbar approach. The outcome was similar for both groups, and Hawkins concluded that neither approach was clearly better. With the advent of general anesthesia and improved surgical techniques, the abdominal approach gradually replaced the lumbar operation. However, in 1912 Paul of Liverpool emphasized that the lumbar colostomy was still a valued procedure. In his text *Personal Experiences With the Large Bowel,* Paul[15] advocated the right lumbar approach for obstructions beyond the cecum, because this approach would not complicate a subsequent abdominal procedure, and for inflammatory conditions of the colon. He recommended left lumbar colostomy for old or weakened patients with rectal obstructions, noting that it was safer than the transperitoneal route.

An interesting addition to the history of colostomy came from New Zealand. In 1876 de Lautour reported the case of a 37-year-old man with a carcinoma of the rectum so painful that he was afraid to have a bowel movement.[9] The patient, completely unaware of any previous achievements in colorectal surgery, placed his hand over his left groin and implored the surgeon to create an opening in his side through which his bowels might pass. Abiding by his patient's wishes, de Lautour created a left-sided colostomy, which successfully relieved the patient's pain.

In 1880 de Lautour presented to the Royal College of Surgeons Museum in London a specimen of a lumbar colostomy found in the loin of a sheep.[9] The case was remarkable not only for its occurrence but also for its method of creation. The colostomy had been made by the kea parrot *(Nestor notabilis).* Apparently this type of parrot feeds on sheep, most commonly dead ones but occasionally live ones. The birds hunt in pairs and tear through the wool of the sheep until they reach the meat on the sheep's sacral area. Most often this action results in the death of the sheep. However, in several instances it has resulted in a lumbar colostomy, as in the case of de Lautour's sheep.

END COLOSTOMY

Until this point in time, only loop stomas had been created, but they were prone to prolapse and often did not completely divert the fecal stream. In 1881

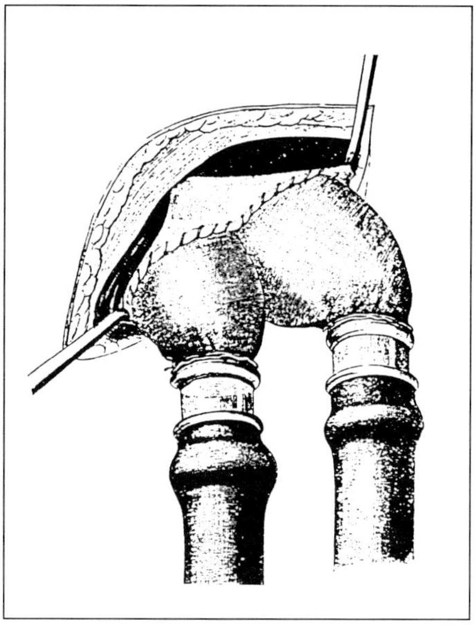

Fig. 1-4. Double-barreled colostomy with attached glass tubing to remove feces from the surgical wound, as described by F.T. Paul of Liverpool. (From Devlin HB. Colostomy. Ann R Coll Surg Engl 52:393-395, 1973.)

Schitzinger,[10] and in 1844 O.W. Madelung,[16] described a procedure of creating a proximal "single-barreled" stoma while returning the distal closed loop to the abdominal cavity. F.T. Paul[17] also advocated complete transection of the bowel in order to adequately defunctionalize the distal colorectum (Fig. 1-4). In conjunction with this procedure, he described the placement of a glass tube into the proximal colon to remove the intestinal contents from the wound and to prevent subsequent wound infection. These efforts represent the beginnings of the end colostomy.

COLONIC RESECTION AND ANASTOMOSIS (MIKULICZ PROCEDURE)

In most cases (i.e., imperforate anus or obstructing rectal carcinoma) a stoma is required for the remainder of the patient's life. However, in many cases only a temporary colostomy is needed, and the natural question is: How can the natural passage of feces per anum be resumed? The Mikulicz technique of intestinal anastomosis, described by Johann von Mikulicz-Radecki in 1903, solved that very problem.[18]

However, the idea had been alluded to by Schmalkalden[19] in 1798, over 100 years prior to Mikulicz. In his doctoral thesis, Schmalkalden described a 23-year-old man left with a double-barreled ostomy from a gangrenous inguinal hernia. Schmalkalden reported passage of a suture between the proximal and the distal intestinal ends and placement of a linen tent. He noted that this procedure eventually eliminated the ostomy spur and allowed the patient to pass feces normally per anum.

A brilliant paper entitled "Memoir on a New Method of Treating Accidental Anus," written by Baron Guillaume Dupuytren[20] in 1828, detailed the formation of a fecal fistula following a strangulated groin hernia. Dupuytren accurately described the proximal and distal intestinal ends appearing in the wound in the shape of a double-barreled gun, an analogy he ascribed to Sir Astley Cooper, and the intestinal spur. He also understood the importance of removing the obstruction between the proximal and distal limbs while creating a fibrous bond between the two limbs to prevent fecal peritonitis. After learning of the achievements of Schmalkalden[19] with the linen tent, Dupuytren performed a similar procedure in 1813 on a 36-year-old man with a fecal fistula resulting from a strangulated inguinal hernia. Eventually the patient passed feces via the normal route. However, during Dupuytren's attempts to cure the residual fistula (by dividing the deepest portion of the spur), the patient developed peritonitis and died. Dupuytren studied the effects of this procedure on dogs and realized that adhesive inflammation caused by the sutures prevented the escape of feces and prevented fatal peritonitis. Unhappy with the outcome with the linen tent, Dupuytren[20] experimented further and suggested a device called an enterotome. The enterotome contained a "male" and "female" limb, each having serrated edges. The male limb was fitted into a groove in the female limb, and both limbs were closed over the intestinal spur. The clamp was slowly tightened, which eventually resulted in the elimination of the intestinal spur.

Dupuytren studied the effects of his enterotome on animals and found well-formed fibrous adhesions between the proximal and the distal limbs in 2 to 3 days, long before the spur was divided (6 to 8 days). In 1815 Dupuytren first used this device in the treatment of a 26-year-old man with a strangulated hernia. The enterotome was induced into the double-barreled stoma and closed without producing any pain. Pressure was gradually increased. The patient passed some stool normally on day 6, and the clamp loosened and came away on day 8. Examination of the enterotome revealed two complete intestinal walls. The fecal fistula persisted, but eventually it closed with the help of silver nitrate, pressure dressings, and finally sutures.

Dupuytren[20] noted that he thought his method had received "the sanction of experience." He collected and reported on a series of 41 intestinal anastomoses performed with the help of his enterotome, 21 performed by him and 20 done by others. Thirty-eight of the 41 patients survived, and in 29 cases the fecal fistula had healed completely in 2 to 6 months. Of the remaining 9 patients, Dupuytren[20] said:

> It remains to find in all cases a means of producing the cicatrization in a useless opening. . . . I declare that without hesitation the discovery of a sure method of promptly achieving in all cases the healing of this disgusting malady would constitute one of the greatest steps of which the healing art was capable.

Soon after Dupuytren presented his work but before it was published, his pleas were answered. Because of the new developments in intestinal anastomosis, he added the following footnote to his paper just prior to publication. It concerns the methods of intestinal suture described by Lembert and Jobert: "Both of them [methods] seem to be perfect and, if I accord the preference to that of M. Lembert, I should fail not to say that he has been preceded by M. Jobert."[20]

Technical advances in the creation of ostomies continued throughout the nineteenth century, and "resection with exterioration" became the favored method of colonic resection. At this time, despite the work of Antoine Jobert de Lamballe and Antoine Lembert, primary intestinal anastomosis was considered too risky and therefore was not widely practiced. Paul, Morrison, Schede, Gussenbauer, Madyl, and von Volkmann all contributed to technical advances.[21] However, Mikulicz-Radecki was primarily responsible for the wide acceptance of resection with exteriorization in the surgical community.

Although Mikulicz popularized intestinal resection and the procedure that now bears his name, the first colonic resection was performed many years earlier. At Guys Hospital in London in 1832, Thomas Bryant[22] performed the first elective colonic resection followed by a double-barreled colostomy for a stricture of the descending colon.

Johann von Mikulicz-Radecki (1850-1905) (Fig. 1-5) was born in Cerno-

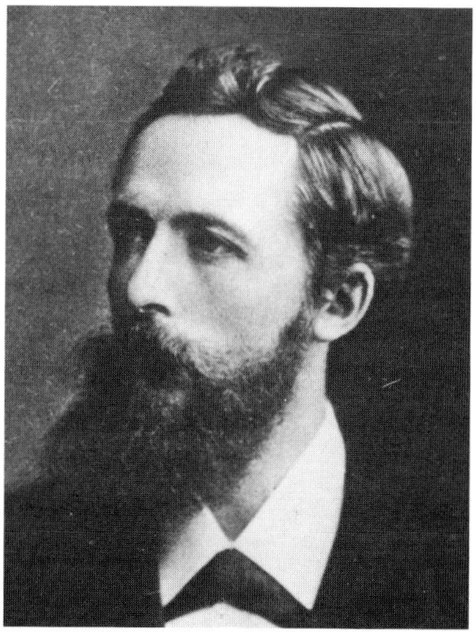

Fig. 1-5. Johann von Mikulicz-Radecki. (Courtesy National Library of Medicine, Bethesda, Md.)

wicz, Austria.[23] He earned his doctorate in medicine in Vienna and soon became assistant to C.A. Theodor Billroth. Mikulicz's titles included professor of surgery at Krakow, Konigsburg, and Berslaw. He died at the age of 55 of carcinoma of the stomach.[24]

Mikulicz[18] presented his technique of intestinal resection and anastomosis in a now famous article entitled "Surgical Experiences With Intestinal Carcinoma," first read before the Thirty-First Congress of the German Society of Surgery in 1903. He not only detailed his technique of intestinal resection but also included his personal experience in over 100 cases. Mikulicz eloquently described the presenting symptoms, anatomic distribution, microscopic pathology, surgical treatment, complications, and survival rate of 106 patients with intestinal (mainly colonic) carcinoma.

Mikulicz understood and explained the danger of primary anastomosis in the face of acute and chronic obstruction and in the malnourished, chronically ill patient. He appreciated the increased difficulty in colonic (vs. small intestinal) anastomosis: "The lessened strength of the wall of the large gut, the poor blood supply, the sluggish peristalsis as a result of which the firm feces stagnate at the site of suture, give far less assurance to the primary union than in the small intestine."[18]

Mikulicz realized, as did his contemporaries, the pathophysiologic and often fatal consequences of intestinal spillage, peritonitis, and sepsis; yet he showed unusual insight[18]:

> We can almost say as a rule a slight amount of bacterial invasion is overcome by the peritoneum; the effect produced is the circumscribed peritonitis observed in all stomach and intestinal operations. The capacity to overcome successfully an insignificant peritoneal infection of such a nature depends, in the first place, on the resistance of the entire organism.

He also appreciated the increased risk of bacterial seeding in the immunocomprised patients[18]:

> The patient [with intestinal cancer] is found in a state of chronic intoxication by which he is doubtless less resistant to intestinal bacilli. . . . I do not doubt that the frequent pneumonias following this operation in part at least are to be attributed to a bacterial infection of the peritoneum which is locally overcome but which leads to pneumonia by way of small pulmonary emboli.

Because of the aforementioned problems, Mikulicz considered primary anastomosis to be too risky in the treatment of intestinal carcinoma. He reviewed his peers' experience with primary suture and compared it to that of his two-stage procedure, citing a reduction in mortality from more than 50% to 12.5%. He described three main advantages of the two-stage resection: (1) the proximal dilated bowel is decompressed and the patient is detoxified, (2) the intestinal anastomoses are performed on normal intestine, and (3) the risk of peritonitis is minimized.

Mikulicz[18] described his technique in the following way:

> The intestinal tumor along with the diseased lymph glands in the corresponding portion of the mesentery are freed from all attachments as in the single stage resection, so the tumor is finally connected only with the gut leading to and from it. The mesentery must be loosened sufficiently to allow the section of bowel which is to be resected to be laid out on the surface of the abdomen without tension. When this is done the abdominal wall is closed off so that only the cleft necessary for passage of the afferent and efferent segments of the gut is left open; this cleft must not be so narrow that the afferent section is compressed. A series of serosal sutures is placed at the point where the parietal peritoneum comes into contact with the protruding portion of the bowel, these sutures also closing off the peritoneal cavity at this point. The outer skin is sutured carefully to the protruding bowel (with tamponades). Next a line of sutures as well as the surface of the contact between the exposed gut and the skin wound are thickly spread with zinc paste and over this a sterile dressing is placed. Over the bandage comes a large piece of waterproof material with a slit just large enough to allow the protruding gut to be drawn through. Thus the tumor which is to be resected is finally separated from the abdominal cavity not only by the secured abdominal wall but also by the protective dressing. Formally, I removed the tumor only after the passing of 12 to 48 hours, but now I usually do it at once. A thick glass tube is fastened into the discharging segment of gut and a thick rubber tube fastened to the glass one so that the intestinal contents flow off.
>
> The wound in the abdominal wall in this procedure heals, as far as it is sutured, by primary intention. After 2 to 3 weeks, by means of my spur-crusher, I transform the artificial anus resulting from the removal of the tumor first into a fecal fistula and then later make a closure by suture.
>
> The advantages of this procedure are evident. The main operation is shorter than by the single stage method, the peritoneal infection during the operation is absolutely avoided, and one can thus attempt it much earlier on a patient debilitated by disease. A further advantage is that the operation can be performed in cases of wide extension of the tumor or in deep locations as for example in the lower part of the sigmoid flexure, where it would be too dangerous to unite the intestines because of too forceful tension on the loops of gut. The method is not only less dangerous but also more easily performed. Of course, the procedure also has its drawbacks. The duration of the treatment is longer and the patient operated must bear with the unpleasantness of an artificial anus for a long time. But I think these disadvantages are greatly outweighed by the advantages of greater safety and increased ease of performance.

Mikulicz recommended his two-stage technique for all resections and anastomoses of the large bowel and for the small bowel when ileus (obstruction) was present. For resections of the small intestine without obstruction, he advocated primary anastomosis. For cecal resections in healthy patients, Mikulicz recommended primary anastomosis with simple resections; for patients in ill health or with large tumors requiring extensive dissection, he recommended a two-stage procedure.

Of the 106 patients who comprised his report, Mikulicz performed a two-stage resection in 16 cases. Two patients died, one from marasmus 7 weeks following surgery and one from injury to the descending colon, which was infiltrated with cancer and accidentally torn during the procedure. No patients died as a result of anastomotic leakage. It is interesting that also included in Mikulicz's report were 21 patients who underwent resection and primary anastomosis, nine of whom died (mortality, 42.9%). Mikulicz's "Surgical Experiences With Intestinal Carcinoma" received much attention because Mikulicz was a well-respected surgeon and an eloquent speaker. Following his presentation, the two-stage resection with exteriorization, a procedure that still bears his name, became the preferred technique for the treatment of carcinomas of the intestine. Mikulicz never acknowledged the contributions of Schmalkalden, Bryant, or Dupuytren to this procedure.

While Mikulicz was refining the two-stage resection, several other inventive surgeons were contributing technical advances of their own. Raybard of Lyon, in a report in the memoirs of the Paris Academy for Surgery in 1844, described the successful resection of an "orange-sized" tumor of the sigmoid colon with primary intestinal anastomosis by means of a "furrier's suture" in 1833.[25] However, the specimen was disposed of, and an autopsy was not performed after the patient's death 10 months later. The Paris commission found the report insufficient and lacking in precision.

In 1879 Martini of Hamburg may have been the first surgeon to perform what was later to become the Hartmann procedure.[25] After removing a large tumor in the sigmoid colon, he was unable to approximate the intestinal ends. Instead he closed the distal end and returned it to the abdominal cavity while creating an end colostomy with the proximal colon.

As previously mentioned, Schitzinger and Madelung advocated complete transection of the bowel with reintroduction of the closed distal end into the peritoneal cavity, even when a simple colostomy without resection was being performed. This idea was not widely accepted. In general, surgeons had two main concerns: (1) the fate of the undrained distal loop returned to the abdominal cavity, and (2) the possibility that the proximal loop would be inadvertently closed, thus creating an intestinal obstruction. Polloson championed this procedure, however, and after his presentation at the German Surgical Society, its popularity grew. As explained by Madelung, the advantages of complete fecal diversion included[25]: (1) no feces came in contact with the obstructing region, and therefore the patient experienced less irritation; (2) feces could no longer reflux from the distal end into the stoma; and (3) the accumulation of feces in the distal segment was avoided.

Polloson suggested, although he never received credit for, another important use for the completely diverting colostomy. He was first to recommend its use prior to transanal resection for rectal tumors in order to prevent the dreaded complication of pelvic sepsis, a use that is still occasionally employed today.

In 1886 Sonnenburg developed a method of avoiding the undrained distal loop. Operating through a lower midline incision, he implanted the closed lower loop just below the incision so that if infection and perforation did occur, a harmless intestinal fistula would develop.[25] In fact, Sonnenburg observed this occurrence in one of his patients who was thus treated.

COLOSTOMY SPUR

Sir Charles Ballance first used a rubber tube passed under the loop of bowel to lengthen the colostomy spur and to completely divert the fecal stream.[9] After using this method, however, he thought that it caused obstruction of the proximal loop and led to the death of his patient, and therefore he abandoned this technique.

Madyl is credited with being the true father of the colostomy rod. He described the use of a rigid rod covered with iodoform gauze. The rod was passed beneath the loop colostomy and left to rest on the abdominal wall, thereby preventing retraction of the bowel. The proximal and distal loops were further approximated by two sutures, one anterior and one posterior, in order to ensure proper spur formation and complete diversion of the fecal stream.

Bryant in England and Kelsey of New York described similar methods of creating a colostomy spur.[9,25] A harelip pin was passed through the skin and peritoneum, through the intestinal mesentery at the junction of its middle and lower two thirds and back through the peritoneum and skin on the opposite side (Fig. 1-6). This technique produced a protuberant stoma with a large spur that completely diverted the fecal stream.

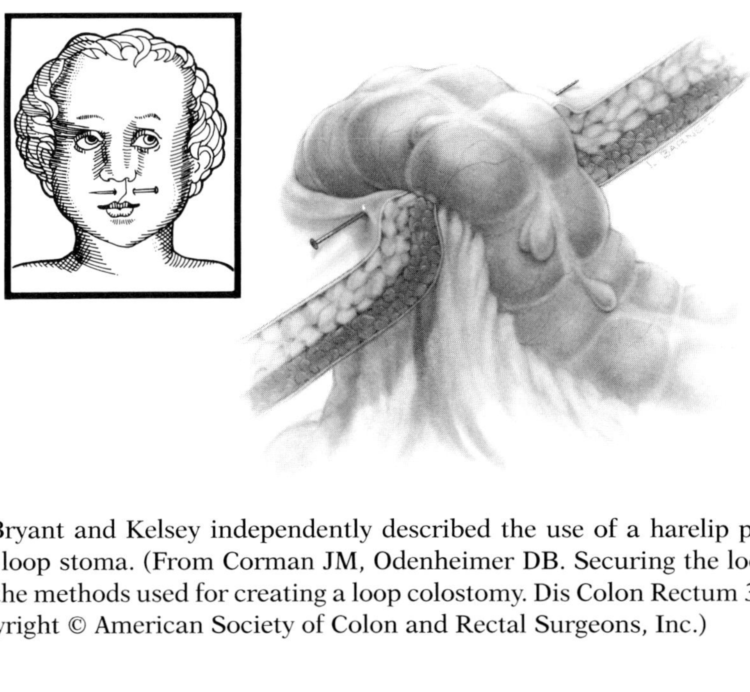

Fig. 1-6. Bryant and Kelsey independently described the use of a harelip pin (inset) to support a loop stoma. (From Corman JM, Odenheimer DB. Securing the loop—Historic review of the methods used for creating a loop colostomy. Dis Colon Rectum 34:1014-1021, 1991. Copyright © American Society of Colon and Rectal Surgeons, Inc.)

Allingham considered Madyl's technique to be too dangerous, and he subsequently developed "Allingham's mesocolic suture," a mattress suture placed through the mesentery to secure the bowel and create an adequate spur. To this suture application, Paul of Liverpool added his glass tube, which diverted feces away from the wound and thereby prevented infection.

While these modifications were being introduced and confusion surrounded the proper method of creating the colostomy spur, Reeves published "Sigmoidostomy Simplified" in the *British Medical Journal.*[25] He stated that an adequate colostomy spur could be created by passing a vulcanite rod through the mesentery of the exteriorized intestine and that sutures were generally unnecessary. Reeves thought that the bowel should be left unopened for 3 to 4 days and that the rod should be left in place for approximately 1 week. Reeves believed that many of the other modifications were unnecessary and considered simplicity to be always advantageous, as illustrated by the following quote: "The simplification of operative procedures should in the interest of the patients be the aim of the surgeon, and experience abundantly proves that the simpler the operation is the better are its results."[25]

RECTAL RESECTION

While stoma surgery progressed, other important advances were occurring in the surgical world. Rectal excision was particularly important in the development of intestinal stomas. In 1793 Faget performed the first rectal resection for extensive ischiorectal suppuration.[26] In 1826 Lisfrancz reported the first rectal extirpation for cancer, and 5 years later he reported a personal series of nine cases (six of which were successful).[27]

Early excisions were performed through the anal canal or the perineum, but exposure was limited and only lesions confined to the lower half of the rectum were amenable to excision. In 1873 Verneuil, at the suggestion of Amussat, excised the coccyx to extend the limits of resection.[28] This approach was also adopted by Kocher.[29] However, it was Paul Kraske who popularized the transsacral approach. After witnessing the removal of a sacral sarcoma, Kraske realized that the lower sacrum could be removed with minimum morbidity and that its removal provided excellent exposure to the upper rectum. Following Kraske's presentation to the Fourteenth Congress of German Surgeons in Berlin, transsacral excisions of the rectum flourished.[30] Other approaches also were attempted. A.T. Norton,[31] in 1889, described a transvaginal resection with the reestablishment of continuity and postoperative continence.

H.T. Byford[32] replaced the excised rectum with a vaginal segment in which both the proximal and distal ends were sutured to the vagina and the

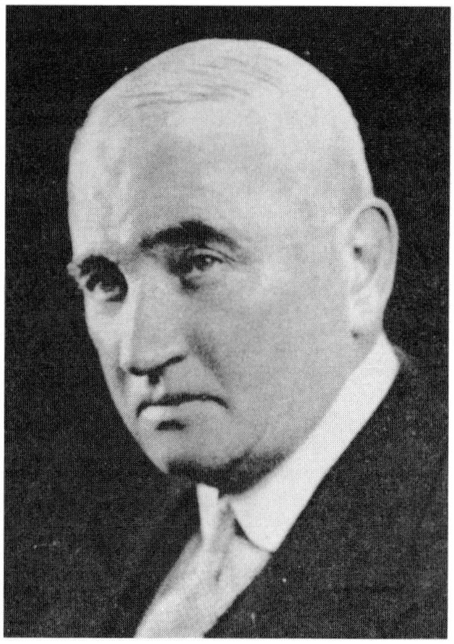

Fig. 1-7. Sir Ernest Miles. (Courtesy Marvin L. Corman, M.D.)

vaginal introitus was closed. L.L. McArthur,[33] after resecting recurrent rectal cancer, was unable to attach the rectum to the anus, and therefore he sutured it to the upper vagina and claimed that his patient (with a surgically created rectovaginal fistula) had good postoperative continence.

In 1883 Vincent Czerny performed the first combined procedure for rectal cancer. Unable to complete a transsacral resection of a high rectal lesion, Czerny turned the patient and completed the procedure transabdominally.[34] Unfortunately, the patient died.

As mentioned earlier, Polloson advocated a diverting colostomy prior to transanal rectal excision to prevent sepsis. Quénu, Hartmann, Juillard, Bishop, and Jaboulay also favored this approach. Ball and Edwards recommended preliminary colostomies on selected patients, but Kraske and Czerny thought that such colostomies were unnecessary except in unusual cases. Although pelvic sepsis was a concern in the early postoperative period, tumor recurrence was a major worry of surgeons. Allingham reported a 100% recurrence in 18 personal cases, whereas Cripps reported only a 38% survival in 85 cases. Vogel reviewed 1500 cases of rectal cancer treated by 12 prominent surgeons prior to 1900 and found an astonishing recurrence rate of 80%.

Charles Mayo and Sir Ernest Miles (Fig. 1-7) had similar experiences and believed recurrence was caused by the failure to resect perirectal lymphatics. Charles Mayo[35] in 1904 and Miles[36] in 1908 described their techniques of abdominoperineal resection. In the early period the perioperative mortality was high (20%), but the long-term survival was much improved. Colostomy had found a secure place in the management of rectal cancer.

HARTMANN PROCEDURE

During the nineteenth century the colostomy was extensively used in the treatment of rectal cancer. First, it was important for its palliative role in treating obstructing rectal lesions; second, for its protective role prior to transanal rectal excisions; and finally, for its curative role in association with abdominoperineal resections. However, colostomy is often used in the treatment of other diseases of the colon and rectum. In 1907 Mayo et al.[37] first described the use of the right transverse colostomy to "defunction" the sigmoid colon in the treatment of diverticulitis. The colostomy was often permanent, but it was occasionally closed after the acute episode has subsided. In the 1930s a three-stage approach, consisting of (1) diverting transverse colostomy and drainage, (2) sigmoid resection with anastomosis, and (3) closure of transverse colostomy, was independently described by Mayo[38] and by Rankin and Brown.[39] These procedures, however, are rarely, if ever, used today, having been replaced by the Hartmann procedure in the surgical treatment of complicated diverticular disease.

Henri Hartmann (1860-1952) (Fig. 1-8) was born in France and was graduated from the University of Paris medical school in 1887. He became the professor of surgery at Hotel Dieu in Paris in 1909.[40] During his medical career Hartmann performed over 30,000 operative procedures, and on his retirement he turned over to his successor his personally kept records for each patient. Sometime between 1909 and 1923, he devised what is now called

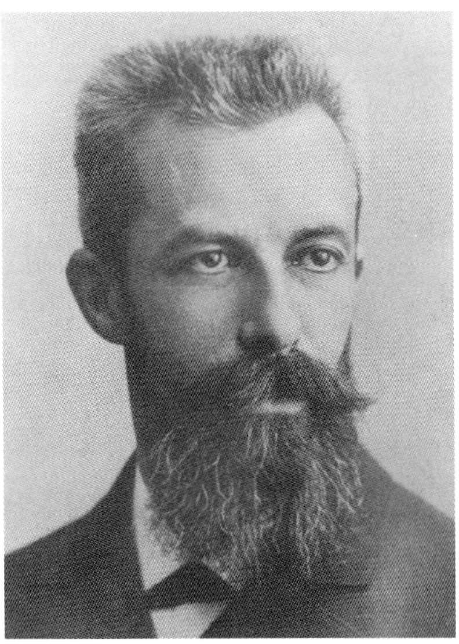

Fig. 1-8. Henri Hartmann. (Courtesy Marvin L. Corman, M.D.)

the Hartmann operation. The details of this procedure were published in his text *Chirurgie du Rectum* in 1931.[41] Hartmann described resection of the sigmoid colon and upper rectum, oversewing of the distal rectal stump, and creation of an end descending colostomy. However, he advocated this procedure for the treatment of carcinoma of the sigmoid colon. He even mentioned reanastomosis as a second procedure but thought it a very difficult undertaking. It is unknown whether Hartmann ever performed his procedure in the treatment of diverticulitis. It is believed that sometime in the 1930s an unknown surgeon first performed this two-stage resection and anastomosis for diverticulitis. Possibly, that surgeon was the first to call it the Hartmann procedure.[40] Albeit through a circuitous route, sigmoid resection with creation of a descending colostomy has become the most popular procedure for the treatment of complicated diverticulitis and is known as the Hartmann procedure.

CECOSTOMY AND APPENDICOSTOMY

In the late 1800s colostomy was first employed in the treatment of ulcerative colitis. Ulcerative colitis was first described by Sir Samuel Wilks[42] in 1875. In 1895 Keetley[43] of London described appendicostomy, and in 1902 Weir[44] of New York described appendicostomy with colonic irrigation in the treatment of severe ulcerative colitis. In 1895 Hale White reported the use of cecostomy and colonic irrigation with boric acid for severe "membranous colitis"[45]:

> It has been suggested that in a very intractable case it might be justifiable to open the colon high up and by allowing the feces for some time to pass out through the artificial anus to give it a rest and at the same time to flush it from the artificial anus to the natural anus with boric acid lotion.

Bolton in 1901, Braun in 1913, and Cattell of the Lahey Clinic in 1935 all used cecostomy and colonic irrigation in the treatment of severe ulcerative colitis.

Cecostomy and appendicostomy also were described in the treatment of chronic constipation. Keetley, a true champion of appendicostomy, Murray, and Sir William Bennett advocated appendicostomy in the treatment of intractable constipation.

ATTEMPTS AT CONTINENT COLOSTOMY

Shortly following the acceptance of abdominal colostomy, surgeons began to focus their attention on the establishment of a continent stoma. Cromar[25] classified the early attempts into three main categories: (1) obturation, (2) external pressure, and (3) sphincterization.

Obturation

In 1901 Payer created a skin flap to cover the colostomy outlet. Apparently he met with little success, and his technique never gained any popularity.

External Pressure

In 1889 Witzel directed a colostomy through the subcutaneous tissue over the crest of the ileum. With use of an external bandage, he compressed the colon to maintain continence. Lenkinheld and Borchardt used this method with success but found the external bandage unnecessary. Roux cut a V-shaped defect in the symphysis pubis and brought the sigmoid colostomy between it and the rectus muscle to maintain continence. Bailey, Tuttle, Braun, Andrea, and Burrows all used modifications of a subcutaneous tunnel combined with external pressure to maintain colostomy continence. Goldschmidt and many other surgeons maintained continence by means of a colostomy clip held in place with a tubular skin graft. Lambert created "anus en trompe," a 10 cm spout covered with skin grafts that was compressed against the abdominal wall by means of an adhesive strap. This technique was later modified by Hayem and Briscoe.

Sphincterization

In 1888 Maydl, the creator of the colostomy rod, and Hartmann advocated a muscle-splitting incision similar to McBurney's to create an artificial colostomy sphincter. Gersuny and Lilenthal both brought the colostomy through the rectus muscle and twisted the proximal end 180 to 360 degrees and claimed perfect continence within 1 month of the procedure. Bernays attempted a "sphincteropoiesis" by placating the circular muscle fibers of the terminal sigmoid colon without much success. Ryall attempted to create a sphincter by using fibers of the rectus muscle, again without success. Failure of both of these methods was attributed to the lack of autonomic nerve supply. In 1932 Spivack attempted to create an artificial sphincter with a reversed ileocecal valve. None of these methods met with any long-term success, and therefore all have been abandoned.

LOOP STOMAS

In 1888 Maydl first suggested the use of an external appliance to support a loop stoma and to facilitate creation of a spur. Since that time, hundreds of modifications have been used, but all are based on Maydl's idea. Maydl[46] described the use of an Indian rubber rod or goose quill passed through the mesentery and left to rest on the skin. Reeves used a vulcanite rod for the same purpose. In 1900 Hartmann[47] advocated rolled iodoform gauze passed through the colonic mesentery. He also covered the peristomal skin with iodoform gauze. These two maneuvers prevented stomal retraction while protecting the peristomal skin. Greig Smith devised a glass rod for stomal support, to which Makins added a piece of rubber tubing to prevent slippage. Mouat further modified the glass rod by adding a metal cap to prevent dislodgment and called it a "colostomy fixation pin."[25]

In the 1960s the glass rod was replaced by rubber tubing sewn to the abdominal skin, which facilitated the placement of an ostomy pouch. Wangensteen[48] developed a colostomy support device consisting of two glass rods connected to a belt with rubber tubing. With this device, the two ends of the bowel were pulled apart in order to better divert the fecal stream. Plastic devices created by Greene[49] and Aries[50] and in the 1970s by Hollister, Inc. (Libertyville, Ill.) involved the development of a butterfly-shaped stoma bridge, which is most commonly used today.

ILEOSTOMY

Although the history of colostomy dates back to the early 1700s, the ileostomy is a much more recent event. The first reported creation of an ileostomy was by Baum[51] in Germany in 1879. Baum performed a diverting ileostomy in the treatment of an obstructing right colon cancer. Eight weeks following the first surgery, he resected a tumor and performed an ileocolostomy. Unfortunately, the patient died on postoperative day 9, after an anastomotic leak. In 1883 Maydl[52] of Vienna, the inventor of the colostomy rod, performed the first successful ileostomy in combination with colonic resection. Six years later, J.M.T. Finney described the flush-loop ileostomy for the treatment of small bowel obstruction in association with appendiceal abscess.[53] Severe skin irritation resulted, and the procedure never gained any popularity.

The widespread use of ileostomy was a result of the work of John Young Brown (1865-1919) (Fig. 1-9), a St. Louis surgeon. In 1912 Brown[54] reported his experience with 10 patients. All 10 patients underwent ileostomy after failure of colonic irrigation following either a cecostomy or appendicostomy. These patients suffered from colon cancer, bowel obstruction, tuberculous colitis, amebic dysentery, and ulcerative colitis. Brown brought the end ileostomy through the lower pole of a midline laparotomy incision. This stoma protruded 2 to 3 inches beyond the abdominal wall and was emptied by means of a catheter sewn in place (Fig. 1-10). Eventually the catheter was removed, and, as a result of serositis caused by the ileal effluent, the mucosa everted to reach the abdominal wall. Brown was the first to advocate diversion of the fecal stream in the treatment of ulcerative colitis, and his technique was used for the next 40 years. However, ileostomy still remained a procedure of last resort, and most ileostomy patients were almost chronic

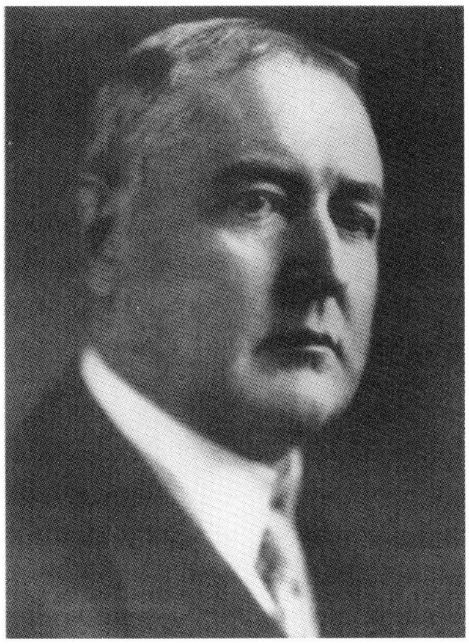

Fig. 1-9. John Young Brown. (From Royster HA, ed. Transactions of the Southern Surgical Association 32:526, 1919.)

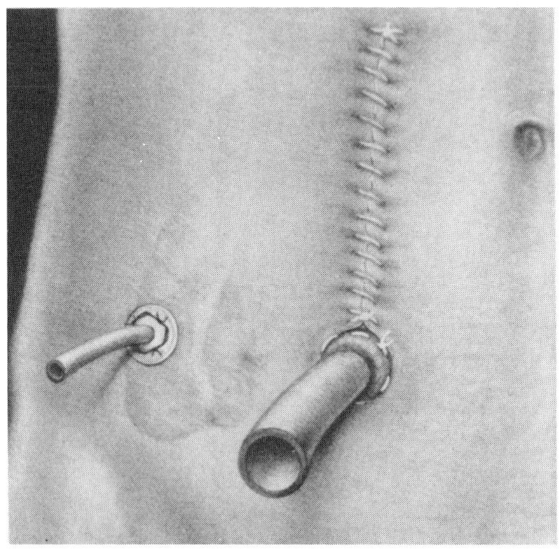

Fig. 1-10. Brown ileostomy. (From Brown JY. The value of complete physiological rest of the large bowel in the treatment of certain ulcerative and obstructive lesions of this organ. Surg Gynecol Obstet 16:613, 1913. By permission of Surgery, Gynecology, and Obstetrics.)

invalids. In 1932 the mortality of ileostomy for the treatment of ulcerative colitis at the Mayo Clinic was an astounding 32%.[55]

Minor improvements occurred in the 1930s and 1940s. Rankin[56] of the Mayo Clinic described creating an ileostomy in a separate wound in the right lower quadrant. The use of skin grafting around the stoma to prevent serositis gained some brief popularity[57] (Fig. 1-11). However, subsequent stenosis of the grafted skin led to ileostomy obstruction and dysfunction, and therefore the idea was abandoned. No significant advances occurred until the 1950s, when Crile and Turnbull[58] of the Cleveland Clinic described ileostomy dys-

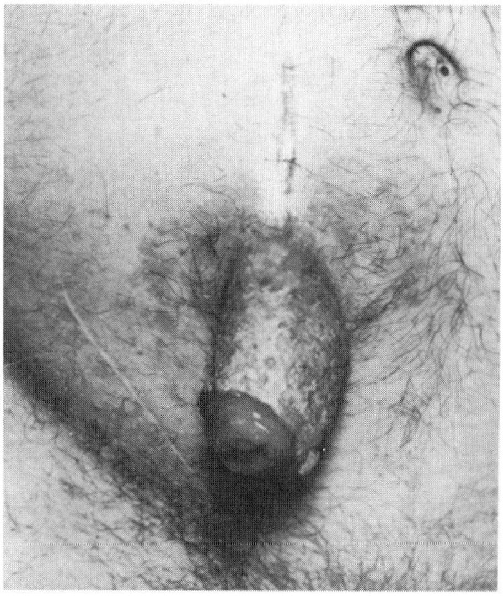

Fig. 1-11. Skin-grafted ileostomy as described by Lester Dragstedt. (From Dragstedt LR, Dack GM, Kirsner JB. Chronic ulcerative colitis: A summary of evidence implicating *Bacterium neocrophorum* as an etiologic agent. Ann Surg 114:655, 1941.)

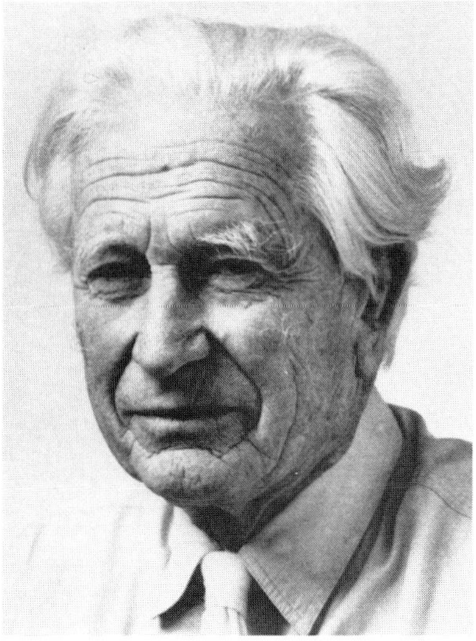

Fig. 1-12. Bryan N. Brooke. (Courtesy W.C. McGarity, M.D.)

function and Bryan Brooke of the University of Birmingham in London described the now famous Brooke ileostomy.[59]

In a 1952 paper entitled "Management of the Ileostomy and its Complications," Brooke (Fig. 1-12) described the ileostomy that remains in use today. One sentence, "A more simple device is to evaginate the ileal end at the time of operation and suture the mucosa to the skin; no complications have occurred from this,"[59] accompanied by a single illustration changed the ileostomy from a chronically inflamed and ulcerative stoma, frequently associated with dysfunction, to the functional "rosebud" we know today. In his article Brooke described the classic technique of primary eversion and maturation of the ileostomy, which eliminated ileoserositis and stomal dysfunction.

However, Crile and Turnbull were the first to fully understand and describe ileostomy dysfunction. Ileostomy dysfunction consisted of partial stomal obstruction manifest by watery diarrhea, abdominal pain and distention, and dehydration. They attributed this obstruction to serositis of the "naked" ileal serosa now exposed to ileal effluent.[58] The serositis led to a rigid stoma without peristalsis, which caused a functional intestinal obstruction and resolved only when the ileostomy had matured. Maturation, as described by Crile and Turnbull, was the natural process of eversion of the ileal mucosa to reach the abdominal wall. For the treatment of ileostomy dysfunction, they recommended catheter drainage of the ileostomy as having good results.

Unaware of Brooke's work in London, Crile in 1952 suggested "mucosal grafted ileostomy" to prevent ileostomy dysfunction. He described removing the distal 3 to 4 cm of serosa and muscle from the ileostomy and folding over and suturing the redundant mucosa to the abdominal skin in order to "mature" the ileostomy at the time of surgery.[58] Through the work of Brooke, Turnbull, and Crile, we now have an easily matured ileostomy rarely associated with dysfunction.

CONTINENT STOMAS

Even when functioning well, the Brooke ileostomy drained constantly and required the full-time use of a pouch. Many patients were disturbed by this feature, which led Nils Kock (Fig. 1-13) to begin work on a continent ileos-

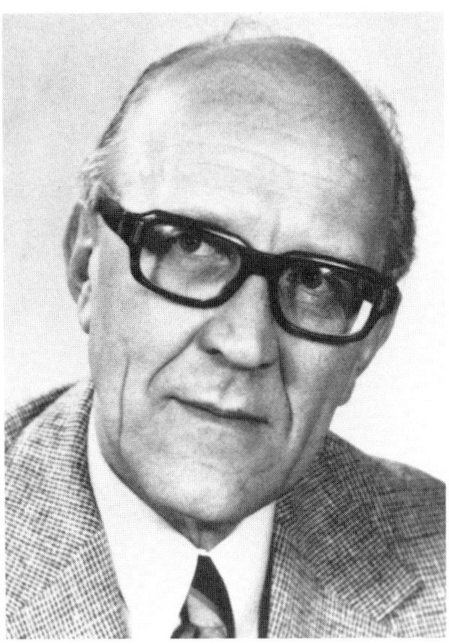

Fig. 1-13. Nils G. Kock. (Courtesy W.C. McGarity, M.D.)

tomy. In 1969 Kock[59] described the creation of an ileal reservoir drained by a tiny stoma brought through the rectus muscle. This method, however, did not lead to complete continence. Therefore in 1972 he added a nipple valve of intussuscepted ileum. Dozois et al.,[60] at the Mayo Clinic, followed a series of patients and found that most were fully continent, their stomas requiring only intermittent catheter drainage. Initially, valve spillage rates were high, but they were later reduced to less than 20%.

More recently, Barnett has developed a new continent ileostomy. A reservoir of ileum similar to the Kock pouch is created; to this is added a collar of functioning ileum. This collar functions similarly to a Nissen wrap, generating higher pressures (and therefore preventing leakage) when the intestine is distended with fluid. Early results with this method were encouraging. However, since the advent of J, S, and W pouches combined with ileoanal anastomosis, continent ileostomies are rarely required.

ENTEROSTOMAL THERAPY

In the 1950s Brooke in England and Turnbull and Crile at the Cleveland Clinic changed the ileostomy from a procedure of last resort to a well-tolerated solution for the treatment of ulcerative colitis. As the Brooke ileostomy gained popularity, the number of patients with long-term ileostomies increased dramatically. These patients required specialized care that needed to be continued long after hospital discharge. Because of this need, the field of enterostomal therapy developed. Rupert Turnbull had a special interest in intestinal stomas and realized the need for trained professionals dedicated to stoma care.

In 1954 Turnbull operated on a young mother of three, Norma Gill (Fig. 1-14), for ulcerative colitis, leaving her with a permanent ileostomy.[61] Since

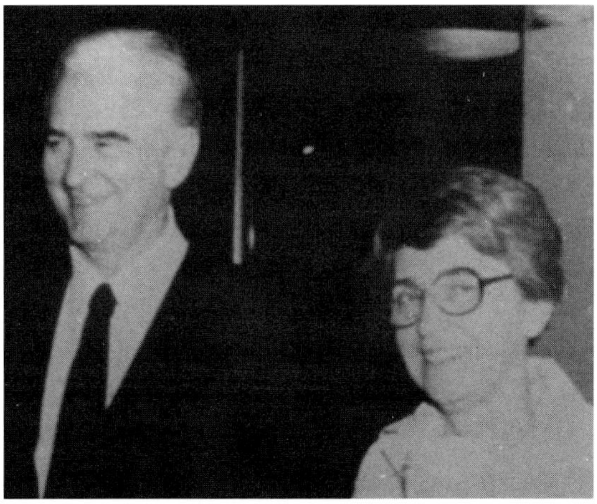

Fig. 1-14. Rupert Turnbull and Norma Gill. (Courtesy W.C. McGarity, M.D.)

Gill's mother had a colostomy, Gill was well aware of the problems of living with a stoma. During her own recovery period she became interested in helping other ostomy patients. When Gill returned to her home in Akron, Ohio, she began to volunteer her services to individuals with stomas in her local area. In 1958 Turnbull hired Gill as an ostomy technician. Together they later coined the term "enterostomal therapist." As the word spread, other hospitals became interested in sending personnel for specialized training with Turnbull and Gill.

In 1961 Turnbull opened the first school of enterostomal therapy because of increasing demand for trained enterostomal therapists. Only people with stomas were accepted as students, but many were also trained nurses. Joy Richey, a registered nurse from California, was the first graduate of the school in 1961. Similar schools opened in Grand Rapids, Michigan (Ferguson-Droste-Ferguson Hospital) and in Harrisburg, Pennsylvania.

At the United Ostomy Association (UOA) national meeting in Phoenix, Arizona, in 1968, the American Association of Enterostomal Therapists (AAET) was born. The first national meeting of the AAET was held at the Cleveland Clinic in 1969. Edith Lenneberg, who had had an ileostomy and was instrumental in the development of the UOA, was elected president, and Norma Gill was named as secretary. In 1969 the name of the organization was changed to the North American Association of Enterostomal Therapists (NAAET) and in 1971 to the International Association of Enterostomal Therapists (IAET).

OSTOMY MANAGEMENT SYSTEMS

Although spontaneous stomas had occurred for centuries, the first mention of an ostomy pouching device was not until 1795. In France, Dageusceau created an inguinal colostomy in a 57-year-old farmer who had impaled himself on the stake of a wheat cart. For the following 24 years, the farmer "collected his feces in a small leather pouch."[10] In 1824 Martland of Blackburn, England, created an ostomy device from a self-adjusting truss containing a tin box in the center for the collection of feces.[62] However, the advances in stoma surgery were not accompanied by advances in stoma management. As late as the early twentieth century, patients were using Model-T innertubes, tuna fish cans, and bread bags with talcum powder, cornstarch, or aluminum gel to prevent leakage. Vanilla and peppermint extracts, mouthwash, perfume, parsley, and bicarbonate of soda were used to diminish odors.[61]

Despite the fact that the colostomy irrigation had been reported in the early 1800s, it did not gain popularity until the 1920s. In 1924 Dudley Smith, a California surgeon, and John Greer, who worked for a surgical supply company, developed the Colostogator.[63] This device, which consisted of a metal

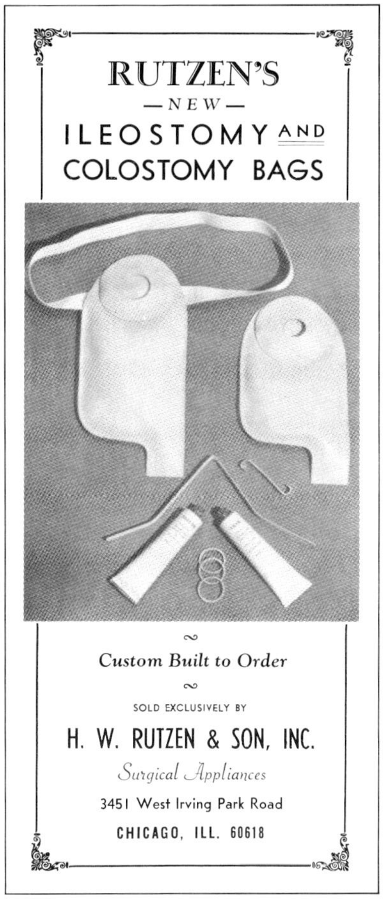

Fig. 1-15. Rutzen bag, 1944. (Courtesy H.W. Rutzen & Son, Inc., Chicago, Ill.)

cup held around the colostomy by means of a belt, was the first commercially available irrigation system. Attached to the cup was a long rubber sleeve that ran into a bucket placed at the patient's feet. The colostomy was irrigated by a rubber catheter placed through a hole in the sleeve. With this device patients were able to irrigate once every 24 hours, between which they wore a "simple belt of plastic webbing . . . [with] several pieces of absorbent paper."[61] The John R. Greer Company also developed a device for people who did not wish to irrigate. It consisted of a canvas bag lined with several thicknesses of toilet paper and a single sheet of oiled paper attached to a stoma ring in a belt.

In 1944 Henry Koenig of Chicago, who had undergone an ileostomy, was encouraged by his surgeon to create a pouching device. The revolutionary result was a rubber bag attached to a circular faceplate that was fixed to the skin with rubber-based cement (Fig. 1-15). This instrument was the first pouching device that could be drained while still in place. Eventually, Koenig recruited H.W. Rutzen, who had also had an ileostomy, to market his invention. The H.W. Rutzen & Son Co. remains in business today.

Another person who had an ostomy, Murle Perry, at the urging of his surgeon, developed a line of stoma management devices. The Perry Model 51, which was introduced in 1951, consisted of a plastic pouch with absorbent papers combined with a close-fitting rubber gasket designed to keep irritating stoma output away from the surrounding skin.[61]

Despite these advances, skin irritation continued to be a significant problem, particularly for ileostomy patients. Just as had happened with Alexander Graham Bell and the telephone many years earlier, an accidental discovery led to a great advance in stoma surgery by Rupert Turnbull.

> In 1952, he [Turnbull] was cleaning out the desk of his former chief, Tom Jones, and accidentally knocked over a small canister of Jones dental powder into spilled coffee on the desk. The karaya immediately absorbed the coffee and stuck to Turnbull's wet hand. He thought the powder might also absorb ileostomy effluent and protect the skin from excoriating effects of the liquid stool.[61]

Thus the use of karaya was introduced. Karaya powder (and later wafers) was a major advance in peristomal skin care.

Another dental product was found to be useful in stoma care. In 1964 Squibb (Princeton, N.J.) developed Orahesive paste and powder for use as a paste and dental fixative. E.S.R. Hughes, an Australian surgeon, realized the usefulness of this product in stoma care and conveyed his experiences to Turnbull, a close personal friend. The result was the Stomahesive wafer, introduced in 1972, a product that was particularly useful for patients with watery ileal effluent (which diluted the karaya) or those with an allergy to karaya. Recently, stoma adhesive wafers have been combined with a flange apparatus (Sur-Fit; ConvaTec, Princeton, N.J.) to create a two-piece ostomy management system. This system allows for easy stoma access since the pouches can be removed and the faceplate can be left intact. In addition, the pouches can be washed and reused.

CONCLUSION

Over the past 200 years intestinal stomas have developed from "last chance," life-saving efforts to well-planned, technically refined artificial anuses. Colostomies can be "trained" to function once every 24 to 48 hours. Ileostomies and urostomies can be made "continent" if the patient so desires. Although stomas formerly were foul-smelling and offensive, today they are rarely noticeable, even to the patient's closest contacts.

These advances in stoma management are the result of an increased understanding of intestinal physiology, refinements in surgical techniques, advances in ostomy management products, and the development of enterostomal therapy. It is hoped that the overview of these developments provided by this chapter will add perspective to the information found in the following chapters.

REFERENCES

1. Bible. Judges 2:3:22.
2. Graney MJ, Graney CM. Colorectal surgery from antiquity to the modern era. Dis Colon Rectum 23:432-441, 1980.
3. Malgaigne JF. Surgery and Ambröise Paré [1840]. Trans. W.B. Hamby. Norman, Okla.: University of Oklahoma Press, 1965, p 224.
4. Heister LA. A General System of Surgery, vol 1, 1739, pp 71-73.
5. Palfin J. Anatomie Chirurgicale, vol 2. Paris, 1743, p 76.
6. de la Peyronie F. Mémoire de l'Académie de Chirurgie, vol 3. 1793, p 1.
7. Hardy KJ. Evolution of the stoma. Aust N Z J Surg 59:71-77, 1989.
8. Le Clerc D. History of Physick. London: D. Brown, 1699, p 406.
9. Cromar CDL. The evolution of colostomy. Dis Colon Rectum 11:256-280, 1968.
10. Dinnick T. The origins and evolution of colostomy. Br J Surg 22:142-153, 1934.
11. Littré A. Diverses observations anatomiques. II. Histoire de l'Académie Royale des Sciences: Paris for the Year 1710 [1732 ed.], pp 36-37.
12. Amussat JZ. Mémoire sur la Possibilité d'Établir un Anus Artificiel dans la Région Lombaire sans Pénétrer dans le Péritoine. Paris: Baillière, 1839.
13. Systema Chirurqoe Hodierne, 1800, p 688.
14. Biography—Obituary, Jean Zulema Amussat. Bull Acad Med 1855-1856, Paris, p 21.
15. Paul FT. Personal experiences with the large bowel, 1912.
16. Madelung OW. Extirpation eines vom Mesenterium ausgehenden Lipoma oedematosum myxomatodes mit partellier Resection des Dünndarmes-Heilung 11. Berl King Woschr 18:75, 1881.
17. Paul FT. A method of performing inguinal colostomy, with cases. Br Med J 2:118, 1891.
18. von Mikulicz J. Surgical experience with intestinal carcinoma. Med Classics 1937-1938, 2:210-239 [trans. from Arch Klin Chir 69:28-47, 1903.]
19. Schmalkalden CD. Novum methodum intestina continui solutione facta uniendi et anum artificialem persanandi. Wittenberg: Tzschiedrich, 1798.
20. Dupuytren G. Memoir on a new method of treating accidental anus. Mem Acad Roy Med, 1828, p 259.
21. Ravitch MM. Dupuytren's invention of the Mikulicz enterotome with a note on eponyms. Perspect Biol Med, Winter 1979, pp 170-184.
22. Bryant T. A case of excision of a stricture of the descending colon through an incision made for a left lumbar colotomy. Proc Med Chir 9:149, 1882.
23. Biography. Professor Johann von Mikulicz-Radecki. Med Classics 1937-1938,2:107-109.
24. Obituary. Professor Johann von Mikulicz-Radecki. Boston Med Surg J 153:64, 1905.
25. Cromar CDL. The evolution of colostomy. Dis Colon Rectum 11:367-390, 1968.
26. Meade RH. An Introduction to the History of General Surgery. Philadelphia: WB Saunders, 1968, pp 277-314.
27. Rankin FW. How surgery of the colon and rectum developed. Surg Gynecol Obstet 64:705-710, 1937.

28. Colcock BP. Surgical progress in the treatment of rectal cancer. Surg Gynecol Obstet 121:997-1003, 1965.
29. Bacon HE. Anus, Rectum, Sigmoid Colon: Diagnosis and Treatment. Philadelphia: JB Lippincott, 1949.
30. Bacon HE. Evolution of sphincter muscle preservation and reestablishment of continuity in the operative treatment of rectal and sigmoidal cancer. Surg Gynecol Obstet 81:113-127, 1945.
31. Norton AT. A case of epithelioma of the rectum: Excision—restoration of function. Trans Clin Soc 23:222-223, 1890.
32. Byford HT. Extirpation of the rectum per vaginam, with utilization of the vagina to replace the lost rectal tissue. Ann Surg 24:631-633, 1896.
33. McArthur LL. Cancer of the rectum. J Obstet 24:567-573, 1891.
34. Morgan CN. Carcinoma of the rectum. Ann R Coll Surg 36:73-97, 1965.
35. Mayo CH. Cancer of the large bowel. Med Sentinel 12:466-473, 1904.
36. Miles WE. A method of performing abdominoperineal excision for carcinoma of the rectum and terminal portion of the pelvic colon. Lancet 2:1812-1813, 1908.
37. Mayo WJ, Wilson LA, Griffin MZ. Acquired diverticulitis of the large colon. Surg Gynecol Obstet 5:8-15, 1907.
38. Mayo WJ. Diverticulitis of the large colon. Ann Surg 92:739-743, 1930.
39. Rankin FW, Brown PW. Diverticulitis of the colon. Surg Gynecol Obstet 30:836-847, 1930.
40. Sanderson ER. Henri Hartmann and the Hartmann operation. Arch Surg 115:792-793, 1980.
41. Hartmann H. Chirurgie du Rectum. Paris: Masson et Cie. 1931.
42. Wilks S, Moxon W. Lectures on pathologic anatomy, 2nd ed. London: Churchill, 1875.
43. Keetley. Quoted in Brooke BN. Ulcerative colitis and its surgical treatment. Edinburgh: E&S Livingston, 1954.
44. Weir RF. A new use for the useless appendix in surgical treatment of obstinate colitis. MRCC 62:201, 1902.
45. Cromar CDL. The evolution of colostomy. Dis Colon Rectum 11:423-446, 1968.
46. Maydl K. Zur Technik der Kolotomie. Centralblatt Chirg 15:433-440, 1888.
47. Hartmann H. Technique de la colostomie dans le traitement de certaines tumeurs inopérables du rectum. Rev Chir 22:613-620, 1900.
48. Wangensteen OH. Complete fecal diversion achieved by a simple loop colostomy. Surg Gynecol Obstet 84:409-414, 1947.
49. Greene HG. Loop colostomy—Bar versus rod. Dis Colon Rectum 14:308-309, 1971.
50. Aries L. Colostomy and ileostomy retainer. Int Surg 58:490, 1973.
51. Baum WG. Resection eines carcinomatösen Dickdarmstuckes. Centralblatt fur Chirurgie 6:169-176, 1879.
52. Maydl C. Ein Beitrag zur Darmchirurgie. Wiener Med Presse 5:500-503, 1883.
53. Lund FB. The valve of enterostomy in selected cases of peritonitis. JAMA 41:74-80, 1903.
54. Brown JY. The value of complete physiological rest of the large bowel in the treatment of certain ulcerative and obstructive lesions of this organ. Surg Gynecol Obstet 16: 610-613, 1913.
55. Bargen JA, Brown PW, Rankin FW. Indications for and technique of ileostomy in chronic ulcerative colitis. Surg Gynecol Obstet 55:196-202, 1932.
56. Rankin FW. Total colectomy: Its indication and technic. Trans Am Surg Assoc 49: 263-290, 1931.

57. Dragstedt LR, Dack GM, Kisner JB. Chronic ulcerative colitis: A summary of evidence implicating *Bacterium neocrophorum* as an etiologic agent. Ann Surg 114:654, 1941.
58. Turnbull RB Jr. Management of the ileostomy. Am J Surg 86:617-624, 1953.
59. Kock NG. Continent ileostomy. Progr Surg 12:180-201, 1973.
60. Dozois RR, Kelly KA, Beart RW Jr, Beahrs OH. Improved results with continent ileostomy. Ann Surg 192:319-324, 1980.
61. Turnbull RW, Turnbull GB. The history and current status of paramedical support for the ostomy patient. Semin Colon Rectal Surg 2:131-140, 1991.
62. Brooke BN. Historical Perspectives: Alternatives to Ileostomy. Chicago: Year Book, 1985, p 21.
63. Smith D. Status of colostomy. JAMA 99:1129-1130, 1932.

2 STOMA PHYSIOLOGY

Richard L. Grotz and John H. Pemberton

Patients with well-functioning stomas differ little physiologically from healthy persons. Stomal physiology studies have elucidated the importance of changes in fluid and electrolyte homeostasis that occur as a result of diversion of the fecal stream. Furthermore, modern techniques of stomal construction and postoperative care have minimized the metabolic complications resulting from creation of a stoma. Thus understanding the normal physiologic and systemic response to an ileostomy or colostomy has enabled physicians to improve the life-style of individuals with a stoma.

CONVENTIONAL ILEOSTOMY

Ileostomy Output

In the early postoperative period the ileostomy effluent is bilious and liquid in nature. Once solid food has been ingested, the effluent thickens. The daily stomal output increases gradually until a plateau is achieved, usually by 10 days.[1] Subsequently, when the ileostomy has become well established, a relatively constant stool volume, ranging from 200 to 700 ml/day, is expected. This process of adaptation by the small intestine allows conservation of most of the 1500 to 2000 ml/day that enters the colon in a normal subject. Moreover, little daily variation occurs in an individual irrespective of dietary changes. Hill[2] classified individuals with ileostomies into two groups: patients with low stomal volume (<700 ml/day) and patients with output >1000 ml/day. Higher stool volumes are characteristic of patients with Crohn's disease.

High ileostomy output soon after operation is considerably less common since the eversion technique of ileostomy construction was described by Brooke[3] in 1952. Prior to that development, a serositis of the exposed ileostomy developed and led to partial small bowel obstruction, increased intestinal secretion, and, consequently, high stomal output. Partial small intestinal obstruction is suggested if the fecal content is either scant in volume or is light green or clear and large in volume. Such obstructions usually resolve with conservative management.

By 6 months postoperatively the volume of ileostomy effluent varies little. The consistency of the effluent is porridge-like with a yellow-brown color and food particles present. Formed feces are extremely unusual since normal ileostomy effluent is 90% water (Fig. 2-1). Variations in consistency and volume are governed by the amount of water in the stool. Gas and stool are expelled intermittently throughout the day and night. Larger volumes are ejected more rapidly after meals. Infectious episodes, dietary indiscretions, and disease recurrence (i.e., Crohn's disease) often result in sudden dramatic

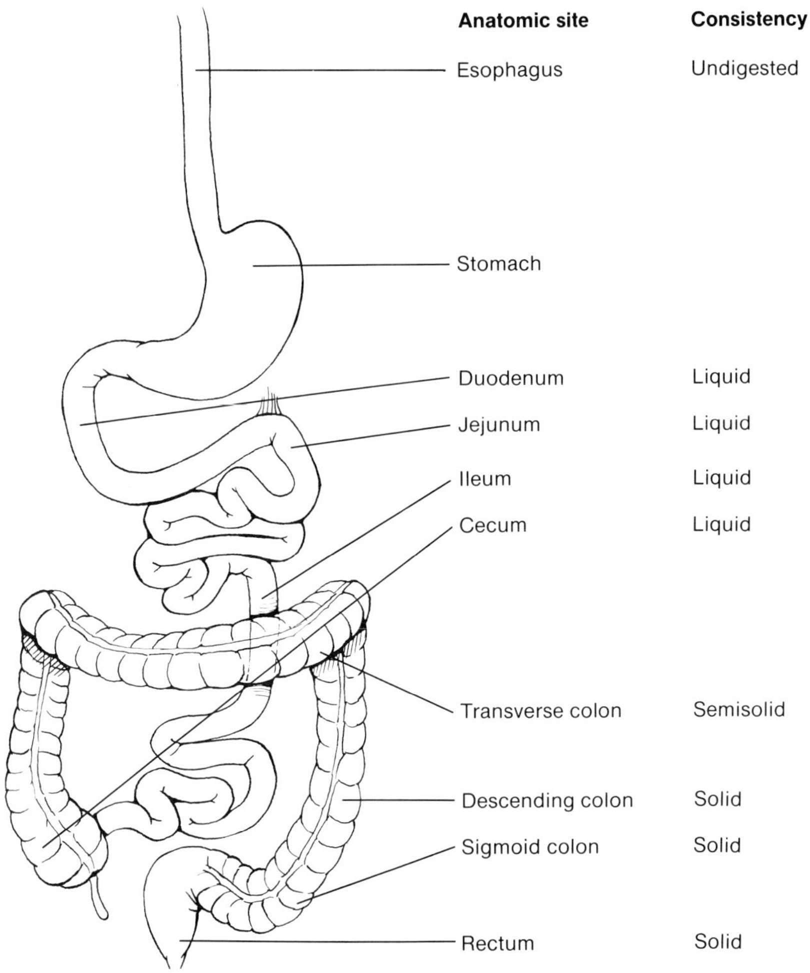

Fig. 2-1. Consistency of stool becomes more solid as it progresses through the gastrointestinal tract. (Redrawn from Zuidema GD, ed. Shackelford's Surgery of the Alimentary Tract, vol 4. Philadelphia: WB Saunders, 1991, p 161.)

increases in volume. Hill[2] observed that the normal output from an ileostomy is directly related to the size of the patient.

Effects of Oral Intake

The influence of diet and fluid intake on the consistency and volume of ileal effluent is well known. Consumption of large quantities of water, having no effect on the effluent volume, simply increases the urine output.[4] The quantity of sodium in the diet directly correlates with volume of stomal output without affecting the dry weight of stool. Grape juice or other fruit juices, however, do increase the wet weight of the stool. The wet and dry weights of the effluents are increased by ingestion of cooked cabbage. Dietary fiber increases the dry stool weight. Elemental diets reduce stomal effluents. Fasting also decreases the output of the ileostomy dramatically to between 50 and 100 ml/day.[5] Food impaction should be suspected if the ileostomy suddenly ceases to function in association with crampy abdominal pain and stomal swelling. The majority of patients report maintaining or gaining weight after construction of an ileostomy.

Nutritional Effects

It is clear that normal nutrition is the rule in patients with well-adapted ileostomies. Normally, nutrients are absorbed readily from the small intestine. However, when nutrient malabsorption occurs, osmotic diarrhea may result; this condition is suggested by malodorous floating stools. Fat malabsorption, from impaired bile salt absorption or reduced bile salt pool, is a common cause of osmotic diarrhea. Bile acid feeding also increases stomal effluents, most likely by interfering with water absorption. Other disorders of nutrient malabsorption occur with carbohydrates (lactase deficiency) and protein (enterokinase deficiency). Body composition is preserved if patients increase their dietary consumption of fluid, nutritious foodstuffs, and minerals. However, fat losses cannot be compensated for by dietary measures if the terminal ileum has been resected.

Malabsorption of vitamin B_{12} is unusual in individuals who have undergone ileostomy with only a limited ileal resection ($<$10 cm).[5,6] Transient malabsorption of vitamin B_{12} may be related to a temporary alteration in the ileal microflora, and vitamin B_{12} supplementation is unnecessary in such patients. However, resection of large portions of ileum and stagnation from distal obstruction or bacterial overgrowth predispose the patient to malabsorption of vitamin B_{12}.

Metabolic Effects

The well-adapted ileostomy excretes no substances in excess that would cause a clinically apparent deficiency. Intestinal water absorption is controlled by solute transport across the epithelium. Sodium transport is considered the major determinant of water absorption by the small intestine. The effluent of the well-adapted ileostomy has a low volume and a high potassium concentration to compensate for chronic salt depletion. An elevated aldosterone level has been proposed as a means of mediating ileal fluid composition.[7]

If dietary sodium is decreased, diuresis occurs with reduced renal sodium excretion and increased ileal potassium losses that maintain a normal plasma sodium concentration. It is important to note that this renal response may lead to hypovolemia in individuals with an ileostomy who are already at risk for dehydration because of fixed salt and water losses. The mechanism for this response is unknown, but it may be related to changes in secretion of arginine vasopressin. However, studies have failed to show significant changes in plasma arginine vasopressin levels.[8,9] Sutters et al.[10] have shown that diuresis resulting from sodium restriction in ileostomy patients is blunted by administration of synthetic vasopressin without renal sodium losses or the composition of ileal effluents being affected.

The normal amount of sodium lost in the ileostomy effluent is approximately 60 mEq daily, compared to 2 to 10 mEq daily in the normal individual. Stomal sodium losses average 1 mEq/hr in the fasting state but increase to 3 to 4 mEq/hr postprandially. However, symptomatic salt depletion in persons having well-established ileostomies is rare. Instead, urine output and sodium excretion are decreased because of enhanced renal conservation of salt and water.[11] Hill[2] showed that despite adaptation a decreased total volume of body water and exchangeable sodium exists in ileostomy patients compared to healthy persons. This obligatory ileal sodium loss is normally overcome with a standard diet. It is important to note, however, that the onset of volume depletion is rapid in patients who develop high volumes of effluents for any reason.

The adaptation process of an ileostomy is impaired in patients who have had extensive small bowel resection since the terminal ileum is an important region for resorption of water and sodium. Ileostomy output and electrolyte losses for these patients are higher during the early postoperative period in comparison to patients who have had preservation of the small bowel; furthermore, the volume and electrolyte composition are unchanged by 6 months.[1] In addition, fat and nitrogen losses are higher following small bowel resection.[12]

A proximally located loop ileostomy has an effect comparable to that of ileal resection. When the ileal pouch–anal anastomosis is performed, approximately 100 cm of terminal ileum is excluded from exposure to enteric contents. Patients with a loop ileostomy have higher volumes of fecal output that is more liquid in nature than that of stomas placed distally in the ileum. Poor weight gain and dehydration reverse once the loop ileostomy has been closed.

Total body potassium depletion is rare in patients with an uncomplicated ileostomy. Potassium losses from an ileostomy range from 6 to 12 mEq/day. A chronic state of salt depletion causes ileal potassium secretion to increase in exchange for maximization of ileal sodium absorption. Excess potassium and total body nitrogen losses reflect extensive resection of the small intestine. The well-adapted ileostomy excretes approximately 1.5 g of nitrogen daily. Cooper et al.[13] found patients to have a normal body weight with normal fat and water content if the ileal resection was limited to 4 cm. This state was associated with reduced total body nitrogen and potassium, which implies a decreased fat-free body mass. In patients requiring >50 cm of small intestinal resection, the total body weight was reduced from the decreased total fat content.

Calcium and magnesium losses are unaffected by ileostomy unless extensive ileal resection has been performed. In the latter situation malabsorption of dietary calcium is compounded by abnormal bile salt and vitamin D metabolism resulting from terminal ileal resection.

Intestinal Transit

Soper et al.[14] studied the gastrointestinal transit time in ileostomy patients (Table 2-1). Using a dual isotope technique, they noted that gastric emptying of liquids in ileostomy patients was not altered. However, gastrointestinal transit time was significantly longer in ileostomy patients compared to con-

Table 2-1. Gastrointestinal transit time (in minutes) after proctocolectomy*

	Group (mean ± SD)		
Parameter	Control (N = 8)	Ileostomy (N = 5)	*P*
Gastric emptying†	120 ± 22	109 ± 10	NS
Small bowel transit‡	243 ± 32	348 ± 12	<0.01

*Modified from Soper NJ, Orkin BA, Kelly KA, et al. Gastrointestinal transit after proctocolectomy with ileal pouch–anal anastomosis or ileostomy. J Surg Res 46:300, 1989.

†T 3/4 of gastric emptying of a liquid marker.

‡Interval for reaching cecum in controls and ileostomy bag in ileostomy subjects.

trols (348 min vs. 243 min, respectively [$P < 0.01$]). The authors concluded that proctocolectomy and ileostomy slowed small bowel transit. These observations confirmed those of an earlier study.[5] The reason for this finding is unclear, but it may be related to small bowel adaptation following colectomy facilitated by epithelial hypertrophy resulting in an increased absorptive surface.[15,16] Furthermore, an inverse relationship between electrolyte and nutrient absorption and intestinal transit has been demonstrated.[17]

Bacteriologic Environment

The bacterial flora of the ileum after ileostomy is both small intestinal and colonic in nature. Gorbach et al.[18] found an 80-fold increase in organisms in the terminal ileum; furthermore, coliforms were 2500 more common than in normal ileal fluid. Overall, the ileostomy effluent bacterial count was still considerably less than that of normal feces. Staphylococci, streptococci, and fungi were increased in number while *Bacteroides fragilis* was rarely found in the ileostomy effluent.

Systemic Effects

Urinary calculi occur more commonly in patients with ileostomies than in normal individuals. The reported incidence of 3% to 13% is related to dehydration and excess sodium losses. Uric acid stones comprise 60% of calculi. High-output ileostomies and extensive ileal resection predispose patients to stone formation. The etiology of this condition is likely related to a reduction in urinary volume and pH that facilitates stone precipitation. Prophylaxis is directed toward increasing daily fluid intake and urine output.

The association between ileostomy construction and increased gallstone formation is controversial. Well-adapted patients excrete bile acids in amounts similar to those of persons with an intact colon.[19,20] However, with extensive terminal ileal resection or inflammation, the enterohepatic circulation is disrupted. Subsequently bile acid malabsorption or depletion alters the saturation of bile, thus promoting precipitation and stone formation. Ritchie[21] found no difference in the number of ileostomy patients who required cholecystectomy as compared to those without an ileostomy. However, Kurchin et al.[22] urged consideration of prophylactic cholecystectomy in female patients undergoing proctocolectomy or small intestinal resection for inflammatory bowel disease because of a threefold increase in asymptomatic gallstones being found in women receiving an ileostomy. At the Mayo Clinic prophylactic cholecystectomy is performed infrequently. If gallstones are discovered during laparotomy and the resection of diseased intestine has gone smoothly, cholecystectomy is considered.

KOCK POUCH
Continent Ileostomy Output

The majority of patients appear to have no major sequelae from receiving a continent ileal reservoir. The physiologic consequences of creating a continent ileostomy have been well described. The initial postoperative fecal output is approximately 1500 ml/day. By 6 months the volume is between 400 and 600 ml/day. Well-established continent reservoirs and conventional ileostomies have similar stool volumes.[23] However, unlike the conventional ileostomy, the continent reservoir accommodates to increasing intraluminal volume passively, similarly to the rectum. The fecal volume may increase to over 1000 g/day if part of the small intestine is sacrificed at the time of operation, or if an exacerbation of Crohn's disease or pouchitis is present.[24]

Bacteriologic Environment

The ileal luminal environment changes when formed into a pouch. The flora resembles that of colonic bacteria both in quantity and ratio of anaerobic to aerobic bacteria.[23,25] The contents from the Kock pouch are more fecal than those of the conventional ileostomy. These changes in the flora occur shortly after the operation. It is presumed that adding a reservoir to the terminal ileum promotes stagnation of the fecal contents for prolonged periods, allowing the microbial population to be altered. Increased bacterial flora then compete with the host for nutrients, bile acids, and vitamin B_{12} for substrate. However, bacterial overgrowth tends not to be a significant clinical problem. Increased anaerobic bacteria in the pouch have been implicated as a cause of pouchitis, but data from the Mayo Clinic have not confirmed a correlation between stomal microbial effluent and pouch dysfunction.[25]

The bacterial counts in the proximal small bowel also increase in patients with a continent ileostomy. Qualitatively, the flora is similar to that of the normal jejunum. Kelly et al.[25] postulated that decreased jejunal motility and impaired clearance of swallowed bacteria are explanations for this finding.

Histologic Alterations

Histologically, the small intestinal villi in the pouch become blunted and undergo a metaplastic response resembling that of colonic epithelium.[23,26] The number of crypt cells and the mucosal volume increase while the neuroendocrine cell population remains unaltered. These changes occur within the first year of reservoir construction but stabilize by 6 to 10 years postoperatively.[27] The etiology of the altered mucosa is unknown, but it may be related to exposure to bacterial metabolites and toxins or to stagnation of stool in the pouch. However, oxidative enzymatic and secretory activities appear unaltered by the morphologic changes.[27] The long-term effects of these changes are uncertain, but dysplasia or malignant degeneration has not been reported in the continent ileostomy in patients with ulcerative colitis.[27,28] The metaplastic epithelium may normalize to small intestinal villi with time.[27] Furthermore, structural changes in the ileal mucosa have not correlated with pouch dysfunction.[25] It remains uncertain whether the histologic changes in the terminal ileum are a primary phenomenon or are secondarily related to the altered microbial environment.

Metabolic Effects

The metabolic consequences of constructing a continent ileostomy are minor despite the altered histology and bacterial environment in the pouch. The absorptive pattern of the continent ileostomy is similar to that of the conventional ileostomy. Absorption of fat, water, xylose, and phenylalanine as well as bicarbonate secretion are not different from absorption with standard ileostomies.[29] Mucosal transport of sodium, chloride, and water within the reservoir is also unaltered despite large concentration gradients.[30] Total body water and urinary excretion of sodium and potassium are also similar. Furthermore, Ojerskog et al.[31] found no evidence of depletion of potassium or water in conventional ileostomy patients who underwent conversion to a continent pouch. The pH of the reservoir contents is lower than that of the conventional ileostomy, presumably because of increased bacterial fermentation of polysaccharides and production of short-chain fatty acids within the reservoir.[32]

Bile acid excretion is not different from that associated with conventional ileostomies[29,33] (Table 2-2). Normal daily fecal bile acid loss is approximately 200 mg or 5% of the bile acid pool. Bile acid depletion of up to 20% is

Table 2-2. Bile acid excretion after proctocolectomy*

	N	Daily Fecal Bile Acid Loss (mg)	Comments
Brooke ileostomy	16	150-300	Some had ileal resection[19]
Brooke ileostomy	10	235-1070	Some had ileal resection[20]
Brooke ileostomy	5	Mean 400	mg/kg/day[32]
Continent ileostomy	5	Mean 550	mg/kg/day[32]
Continent ileostomy	5	Mean 1400	With ileal resection[32]
Healthy controls		<500	

*Modified from Phillips SF. Biological effects of a reservoir at the end of the small bowel. World J Surg 11:763, 1987.

Table 2-3. Fecal weight and excretion of fat after proctocolectomy*

	N	Fecal Weight (g/24 hr)	Fecal Fat (g/24 hr)
Continent ileostomy[24]			
Excellent results	29	616 ± 27	4.6 ± 0.5
Diarrhea/pouchitis	13	1405 ± 57	9.6 ± 2.1
Brooke ileostomy[24]	19	651 ± 44	3.4 ± 0.4
Healthy controls		<250	<7

*Modified from Phillips SF. Biological effects of a reservoir at the end of the small bowel. World J Surg 11:763, 1987.

balanced by the enhanced hepatic synthesis. Hence disruption of the enterohepatic circulation is uncommon unless bacterial overgrowth or ileal resection is present. Hylander et al.[34] reported that bile acid deconjugation may occur in the reservoir; however, this possibility has been disputed by others.[30,32] Furthermore, the incidence of cholelithiasis is similar with a continent or conventional stoma.[28] When the bile acid pool is preserved, the ability to absorb fat is retained in most patients with a continent ileostomy (Table 2-3).

Abnormal and borderline Schilling tests have been reported in patients with a continent ileostomy.[29,30] However, vitamin B_{12} absorption is generally unimpaired, and any defect in this absorption is often transient. Furthermore, serum plasma levels of vitamin B_{12} tend to be normal. Active absorption of vitamin B_{12} and intrinsic factor has been demonstrated by instillation of the complex into the reservoir of patients with intact ileal segments.[30] Gadacz et al.[30] postulated that the prolonged contact time between the intestinal contents and the ileal mucosa may enhance vitamin B_{12} absorption. Thus construction of a Kock pouch does not predispose the patient to vitamin B_{12} malabsorption unless the terminal ileum has been removed.

Schjonsby et al.[35] found increased concentrations of *Bacteroides* associated with vitamin B_{12} malabsorption in the continent ileostomy effluent compared to the conventional ileostomy. These patients with "stagnant loop syndrome" received oral lincomycin and had improvement of vitamin B_{12} absorption, decreased fecal fat excretion, and decreased concentrations of ileal *Bacteroides*.

Continent Ileostomy Motility

Patterns of small bowel motility within the pouch also have been studied.[36] Small intraluminal pressure waves (amplitude <10 cm H_2O; frequency 5 to 7 min) constituted the basal motor activity, which was similar to the normal terminal ileal motor pattern. However, with distention of the pouch to >60% of its maximum capacity, high-pressure waves (HPW; amplitude >25 cm H_2O; frequency 1 every 3 min) were superimposed on the basal motor pattern. These waves were associated with fullness and discomfort. The authors concluded that the ileum is able to accommodate large intraluminal volumes with only small incremental increases in intraluminal pressure.

COLOSTOMY

Approximately 1500 ml of fluid and 120 mEq of sodium are passed daily from the ileum to the colon. The colon secretes little fluid to add to this volume; rather, the colon stores the fecal content and slowly propels the stool in a caudad direction for eventual evacuation. During the passage of stool from the right to the left colon, absorption is so efficient that <200 ml of water and <25 mEq of sodium are expelled daily in the feces. To a lesser extent, bile acids not absorbed in the terminal ileum are absorbed by the colon. However, ileal resection predisposes the patient to excessive bile acids in the colon, which promotes colonic secretion of water and electrolytes.

When a colostomy first begins to function, the output is liquid; the liquid steadily increases in volume and is expelled on an irregular basis. After 10 to 14 days the consistency of the effluent becomes quite viscous. Slowly, a pattern of stool evacuation develops and the stool is expelled on a more predictable basis.

In general, the diet of a patient with a colostomy should be unrestricted. The patient soon recognizes specific foods that increase stomal output or flatulence. Similar to the situation with an ileostomy, high fiber foods increase fecal weight in patients with a colostomy. If sufficient colonic absorptive surface is preserved proximal to the colostomy, dehydration and electrolyte disturbances are rarely matters of concern.

Medications introduced through the stoma are readily absorbed. The exceptions are enteric-coated or time-release medications that may be expelled before adequate absorption has occurred. This situation is more of a problem with proximal colostomies in which excretion is common.

Proximal Colostomy

Ileal content that enters the right colon is predominantly liquid. The right colon is important for mixing the ileal effluent to facilitate water and electrolyte absorption through uniform exposure of the luminal contents to the mucosal surface. The cecum and the ascending colon store and knead the luminal contents through a series of antiperistaltic annular contractions. The proximal colon is the origin of giant migrating contractions responsible for mass movements of luminal contents distally.[37] Constructing an ascending or proximal transverse colostomy interferes with the storage and mixing of stool and reduces the absorptive capacity of the colon. Hence the output from these stomas is a high-volume liquid effluent with a high sodium concentration. Fecal material is expelled from the colostomy on a frequent and irregular basis, which allows little or no planned control of stomal output.

Middle Colostomy

The midcolon is responsible for transit and absorption of the luminal contents. The motor activity is characterized by annular contractions that divide the fecal mass and propel it distally and proximally in a to-and-fro manner. Constructing a distal transverse or descending colostomy increases the length of absorptive surface and allows enhanced colonic mixing of the fecal material. Sodium is actively absorbed, thereby generating osmotic gradients that facilitate passive absorption of water. Hence the effluent from distal transverse and descending colostomies is lower in volume and less liquid than that from proximal colostomies.

Distal Colostomy

The distal colon functions primarily as a storage area for fecal material until willful defecation occurs at an appropriate time. Infrequent strong contractions in the distal colon, which are occasionally sensed by the patient, facilitate caudal propagation of fecal material.[37] The consistency of fecal matter reaching the distal colon is ordinarily semisolid to solid in nature. After construction of an end sigmoid colostomy, the colonic contents, composed of unabsorbed food products and bacteria, are expelled usually no more than once or twice a day. Hence regulation of stool elimination from a distal colostomy through the use of irrigation techniques is often possible. Irrigation initiates colonic distention, which stimulates colonic peristalsis and mass contractions and facilitates stool evacuation.[38]

Fecal volumes in a well-adapted sigmoid colostomy approximate the losses from patients with an intact colon. Similarly to the small intestine, the colon adapts to increased fluid losses from the gastrointestinal tract via aldosterone-mediated fluid and sodium resorption by the colonic epithelium.[39] Thus fluid and metabolic homeostasis is facilitated by preservation of the colon proximal to the colostomy with active participation of the colon in correction of volume and salt depletion.

CONCLUSION

The small intestine and colon are critical organs that maintain fluid and electrolyte homeostasis. Nearly all patients adapt readily to the physiologic changes caused by an intestinal stoma if sufficient healthy intestine is preserved proximal to the stoma. Metabolic disturbances in patients with stomas are often subtle and develop gradually. Long-term careful attention to fluid and electrolyte balance is therefore necessary to preclude complications related to intestinal diversion. Nonetheless, the metabolic consequences of creating an intestinal stoma are minor and, by themselves, rarely alter the patient's life-style dramatically.

REFERENCES

1. Hill GT, Mair WSJ, Goligher JC. Impairment of "ileostomy" adaptation in patients after ileal resection. Gut 15:982, 1974.
2. Hill GT. Ileostomy: Surgery, Physiology, and Management. New York: Grune & Stratton, 1976, p 65.
3. Brooke BN. Management of ileostomy including its complications. Lancet 2:102, 1952.
4. Kramer P, Kearney MM, Inglefinger FJ. The effect of specific foods and water loading on the ileal excreta of ileostomized subjects. Gastroenterology 42:535, 1962.
5. Pemberton JH, van Heerden JA, Beart RW Jr, et al. A continent ileostomy device. Ann Surg 197:618, 1983.
6. Hulten L, Kewenter J, Persson E, et al. Vitamin B_{12} absorption in ileostomy patients after operation for ulcerative colitis. Scand J Gastroenterol 5:113, 1970.
7. Kennedy HJ, Al-Dujaili EAS, Edwards CRW, et al. Water and electrolyte balance in subjects with a permanent ileostomy. Gut 24:702, 1983.
8. Moss S, Gordon D, Forsling ML, et al. Water and electrolyte composition of urine and ileal fluid and its relationship to renin and aldosterone during dietary sodium deprivation in patients with ileostomies. Clin Sci 61:407, 1981.
9. Unwin RJ, Moss S, Peart WS, et al. Renal adaptation and gut hormone release during sodium restriction in ileostomized man. Clin Sci 69:299, 1985.
10. Sutters M, Carmichael DJS, Unwin RJ, et al. "Low sodium" diuresis and ileal loss in patients with ileostomies: Effect of desmopressin. Gut 32:649, 1991.
11. Gallagher ND, Harrison DD, Skyring AP. Fluid and electrolyte disturbances in patients with long-established ileostomies. Gut 3:219, 1962.
12. Neal DE, Williams NS, Barker M, et al. The effect of resection of the distal ileum on gastric emptying, and small bowel transit and absorption after proctocolectomy. Br J Surg 71:666, 1984.
13. Cooper JC, Laughland A, Gunning EJ, et al. Body composition in ileostomy patients with and without ileal resection. Gut 27:680, 1986.
14. Soper NJ, Orkin BA, Kelly KA, et al. Gastrointestinal transit after proctocolectomy with ileal pouch–anal anastomosis or ileostomy. J Surg Res 46:300, 1989.
15. Mibu R, Itoh H, Nakayama F. Effect of total colectomy and mucosal proctectomy on intestinal absorptive capacity in dogs. Dis Colon Rectum 30:47, 1987.

16. Wright HK, Cleveland JC, Tilson MD, et al. Morphology and absorptive capacity of the ileum after ileostomy in man. Am J Surg 117:242, 1967.
17. Holgate AM, Read NW. Relationship between small bowel transit time and absorption of a solid meal: Influence of metaclopramide, magnesium sulfate, and lactulose. Dig Dis Sci 28:812, 1983.
18. Gorbach SL, Nahas L, Weinstein L, et al. Studies of intestinal microflora. IV. The microflora of ileostomy effluent: A unique microbial ecology. Gastroenterology 53: 874, 1967.
19. Miettinen TA, Peltokallio P. Bile salt, fat, water, and vitamin B_{12} excretion after ileostomy. Scand J Gastroenterol 6:543, 1971.
20. Huibregtse K, Hoek F, Sanders GTB, et al. Bile acid metabolism in ileostomy patients. Eur J Clin Invest 7:137, 1977.
21. Ritchie JK. Ileostomy and excisional surgery for chronic inflammatory disease of the colon: A survey of one hospital region. I. Results of complications of surgery. Gut 12:528, 1971.
22. Kurchin A, Ray JE, Bluth EI, et al. Cholelithiasis in ileostomy patients. Dis Colon Rectum 27:585, 1984.
23. Phillips SF. Biological effects of a reservoir at the end of the small bowel. World J Surg 11:763, 1987.
24. Kelly DG, Branon ME, Phillips SF, et al. Diarrhea after continent ileostomy. Gut 21:711, 1980.
25. Kelly DG, Phillips SF, Kelly KA, et al. Dysfunction of the continent ileostomy: Clinical features and bacteriology. Gut 24:193, 1983.
26. Go PM, Lens J, Bosman FT. Mucosal alterations in the reservoir of patients with Kock's continent ileostomy. Scand J Gastroenterol 22:1076, 1987.
27. Nilsson LO, Kock NG, Lindgren I, et al. Morphological and histochemical changes in the mucosa of the continent ileostomy reservoir 6-10 years after its construction. Scand J Gastroenterol 15:737, 1980.
28. Ojerskog B, Kock NG, Philipson BM, et al. Long term follow-up of patients with continent ileostomies. Dis Colon Rectum 33:184, 1990.
29. Jagenburg R, Dotevall G, Kewenter J, et al. Absorption studies in patients with "intra-abdominal reservoirs" and in patients with conventional ileostomies. Gut 12:437, 1971.
30. Gadacz TR, Kelly KA, Phillips SF. The continent ileal pouch: Absorptive and motor features. Gastroenterology 72:1287, 1977.
31. Ojerskog B, Andersson H, Bosaeus I, et al. Total body water and total body potassium in ileostomy patients before and after conversion to the continent ileostomy. Gut 29:1198, 1988.
32. Kay RM, Cohen Z, Siu KP, et al. Ileal excretion and bacterial modification of bile acids and cholesterol in patients with continent ileostomy. Gut 21:128, 1979.
33. Nilsson LO, Andersson H, Hulten L, et al. Absorption studies in patients six to ten years after construction of ileostomy reservoirs. Gut 20:499, 1979.
34. Hylander E, Ladeford M, Nielsen ML, et al. Excretion, deconjugation and absorption of bile acids after colectomy for ulcerative colitis. Scand J Gastroenterol 21:1137, 1986.
35. Schjonsby H, Halvorsen JF, Hofstad T, et al. Stagnant loop syndrome in patients with continent ileostomy (intra-abdominal ileal reservoir). Gut 18:795, 1977.
36. Akwari OE, Kelly KA, Phillips SF. Myoelectric and motor patterns of continent pouch and conventional ileostomy. Surg Gynecol Obstet 150:363, 1980.
37. Sarna SK. Physiology and pathophysiology of colonic motor activity. Dig Dis Sci 36:827, 1991.

38. MacLeod JH. Colostomy irrigation—A transatlantic controversy. Dis Colon Rectum 15:357, 1972.
39. Elmslie RG, Mulholland AT, Shields R. Blocking by spironolactone [SC 9420] of the action of aldosterone upon intestinal transport of potassium, sodium and water. Gut 7:697, 1966.

SUGGESTED READINGS

Hill GL. Ileostomy: Surgery, Physiology and Management. New York: Grune & Stratton, 1976.

This comprehensive review of the original physiologic studies of conventional ileostomies is a required reference for stomal physiology.

Pemberton JH. Management of conventional ileostomies. World J Surg 12:203, 1988.

Provides an up-to-date review of the normal and abnormal physiologic effects of a conventional stoma.

Phillips SF. Biological effects of a reservoir at the end of the small bowel. World J Surg 11:763, 1987.

Offers an excellent review of normal terminal ileal physiology and the pathophysiologic effects of constructing a reservoir.

3 PREOPERATIVE CONSIDERATIONS

Marvin L. Corman

Once the surgeon has determined that the patient can be treated optimally through a procedure that involves the creation of an ostomy, an in-depth discussion between surgeon and patient becomes necessary. Such a discussion should focus on the nature of the procedure, the risks involved, and the alternatives to surgery.

Overcoming ignorance and fear is often the most important challenge for the surgeon who is preparing a patient for a stoma. Some patients may have somewhat negative feelings about ostomies because of the experiences and jeremiads of family and friends. Myths and misunderstandings may further prejudice the patient. The surgeon must help the patient to confront fear of the disease itself, the potential for complications, and, indeed, the possibility of death. These issues must be addressed as part of a comprehensive rehabilitative program.

It is often helpful to have teaching aids available during this preoperative discussion. Videotapes, anatomic models, photographs and drawings, and samples of ostomy management systems all can be used to help prepare the patient for his or her stoma. These aids often will alleviate the patient's misconceptions and fears, allowing the person to approach the surgery with a positive attitude.

PATIENT INTERVIEW

Consent

In today's litigious society jurists have opined that a surgeon must communicate to the patient whatever information a reasonable person would deem relevant for decision-making. It is not adequate simply to ask: "Are there any questions?" Specific issues need to be discussed in order to obtain a truly

☐ Portions of this chapter have been taken from Corman ML. Colon and Rectal Surgery, 3rd ed. Philadelphia: JB Lippincott, 1993, with permission.

informed consent. Although it is not necessary to summarize a textbook on the complications of colon and rectal surgery, several important complications merit a reasonably detailed review.

Potential Complications

It should be sufficient to touch briefly on the general concerns that every surgeon confronts on a daily basis. However, if the patient asks for more information, it should be given. The basic issues to be addressed are risk of death, possibility of infection, prolonged hospitalization because of various potential complications (associated with any major surgical procedure), and length of disability. Two possible complications demand specific attention: impotence and infertility. Although preoperative libido is probably the most important factor contributing to postoperative sexual functioning, removal of the rectum may be associated with subsequent impotence. Occasionally a man may elect to "bank" his sperm to ensure the potential for procreation. Infertility is less likely to be an issue in the older man or woman. However, retrograde ejaculation is a greater risk than impotence and needs to be addressed in the decision-making process. Other complications specific to stoma surgery include parastomal hernias, prolapse, ischemia, and local wound complications, and therefore the patient also should be made aware of these possibilities.

Counseling

It is often very helpful to provide the patient with literature concerning the nature of the surgery and the reasonableness of living with a colostomy or an ileostomy (see the Suggested Readings at the end of this chapter). In addition, it is often advisable to have someone of similar age, gender, and socioeconomic position serve to acquaint the patient with the concept of living and functioning normally with a stoma. Whenever possible, an enterostomal therapy (ET) nurse should be involved with preoperative counseling, not necessarily to provide detailed stomal care at that time but to offer information about the wide variety of ostomy products available. Information regarding local support organizations (e.g., United Ostomy Association, The Crohn's and Colitis Foundation, The International Association of Enterostomal Therapists) also will be beneficial.

PREOPERATIVE STOMA MARKING

The location of the stoma has a direct bearing on subsequent ostomy management. Establishment of the stoma site before surgery is usually the responsibility of the surgeon, but in many instances it may be delegated to a trained ET nurse. Proper location of the colostomy or ileostomy can prevent complications such as prolapse, hernia, and skin problems.

Groin, waistline, costal margins, umbilicus, skinfolds, and scars frequently interfere with the ostomy management system. It is advisable to leave a 5 cm margin of smooth skin around the stoma. Whenever possible, the stoma should be placed at the summit of the infraumbilical bulge and within the rectus muscle. When the site is being marked, it is helpful to have the patient lie in the supine position and tense the abdominal muscles. This posture allows the physician to feel the lateral border of the rectus muscle. A triangle is formed by drawing an imaginary line from the umbilicus to the pubis, one from the umbilicus to the anterosuperior iliac spine, and another from the pubis to the anterosuperior iliac spine (the inguinal ligament) (Fig. 3-1). The stoma usually should be in the center of the triangle. The faceplate should be taped over the site and the patient should stand, sit, and bend with

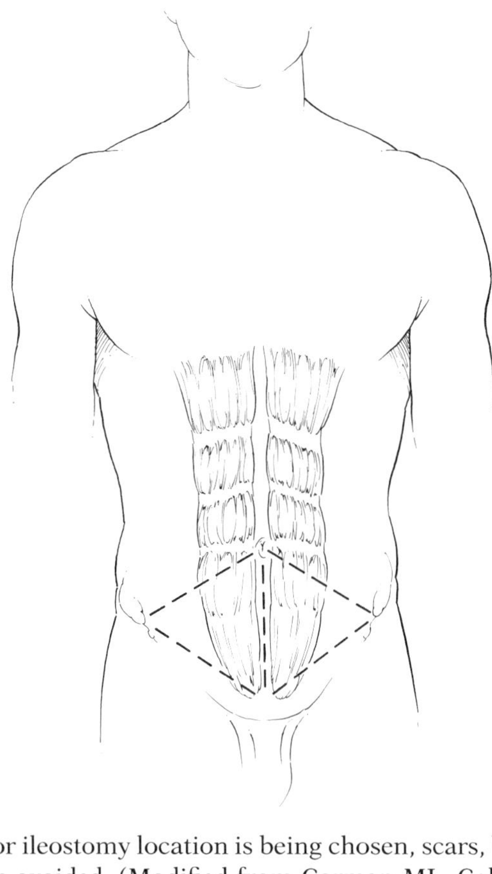

Fig. 3-1. When a site for ileostomy location is being chosen, scars, bony prominences, and the umbilicus must be avoided. (Modified from Corman ML. Colon and Rectal Surgery, 3rd ed. Philadelphia: JB Lippincott, 1993, p 939.)

the faceplate in place. Slight adjustments may be required because of interference from skin creases and adipose tissue.

Another factor to consider is the patient's preference for clothing style. For example, special attention should be given to where the belt is worn because stomas must be placed below the waist and preferably below the belt line. If an individual requires two stomas, the new opening must be placed either above or below the existing one (Fig. 3-2). Occasionally, it may be necessary to keep a faceplate in place for 24 hours to ensure the patient's subsequent comfort and ease of movement, especially when the abdomen contains multiple scars. The proper location is marked permanently by wiping the skin with alcohol, placing a drop of India ink on the spot, and pricking the skin with a fine hypodermic needle. An alternative method is simply to scratch a mark onto the proposed location. If the stoma site is marked in pen, indelible ink should be used to prevent obliteration of the mark during preoperative skin cleansing.

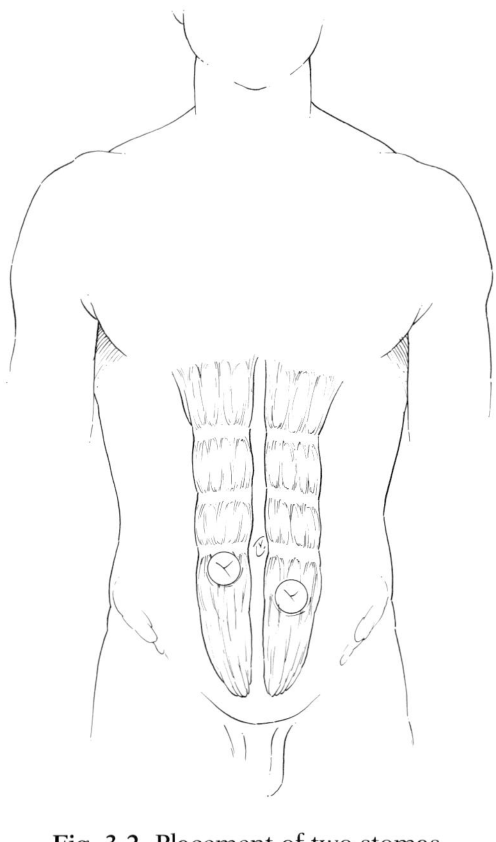

Fig. 3-2. Placement of two stomas.

INTRAOPERATIVE SELECTION OF STOMA SITE

If a site is not selected until the patient is in the operating room, what is perceived to be an ideal location may subsequently present a difficult management problem. The same principles that apply to preoperative stoma site selection are equally important in intraoperative selection. The stoma should pass through the rectus muscle. It should be situated at least 6 cm away from the umbilicus or bony prominences and placed away from skin creases or scars. The outer margin of the faceplate may appear at the waistline or in the groin. If the stoma is located on the undersurface of the infraumbilical bulge, it will be impossible for the patient to fit the skin barrier properly and to center the pouch. At the very least, a flange that corresponds to the diameter of the faceplate of the ostomy device can be used to identify the site and to give some degree of assurance to the patient. However, preoperative marking is always preferable. It takes only a few minutes and therefore should be done for any patient who requires a stoma.

The above considerations are applicable to all intestinal stomas—ileostomy, sigmoid colostomy, transverse colostomy, and urinary conduit.

ALTERNATE STOMA SITES

Although the right and left lower quadrants are the ideal sites for ileostomies and colostomies, respectively, these sites will not always be available. Prior stoma surgery, multiple surgical scars, nonhealing skin lesions, obesity, and other factors may make alternative siting necessary. In these difficult circumstances preoperative marking becomes even more important. Alternate sites include the left and right upper quadrants, the umbilicus, the midline above and below the umbilicus (particularly useful in infants) (Fig. 3-3, *A*), and even the left and right lumbar areas (a choice of last resort) (Fig. 3-3, *B*).

In selection of an alternate site, the general principles are followed as closely as possible. The stoma should pass through the rectus muscle (or the linea alba in the case of midline stomas). It should be positioned 6 cm away from the costal margin or iliac crest, and it should be placed to avoid prior scars or other stoma sites. Occasionally, a stoma may be brought through the surgical wound, but only when no other viable option exists. Such placement increases the chance of hernia formation and makes application of the pouch very difficult. After a stoma site has been selected, the patient should wear an ostomy management system for 24 to 28 hours preoperatively to assess the acceptability of its position.

Some patients may require two or more stomas, for example, after pelvic

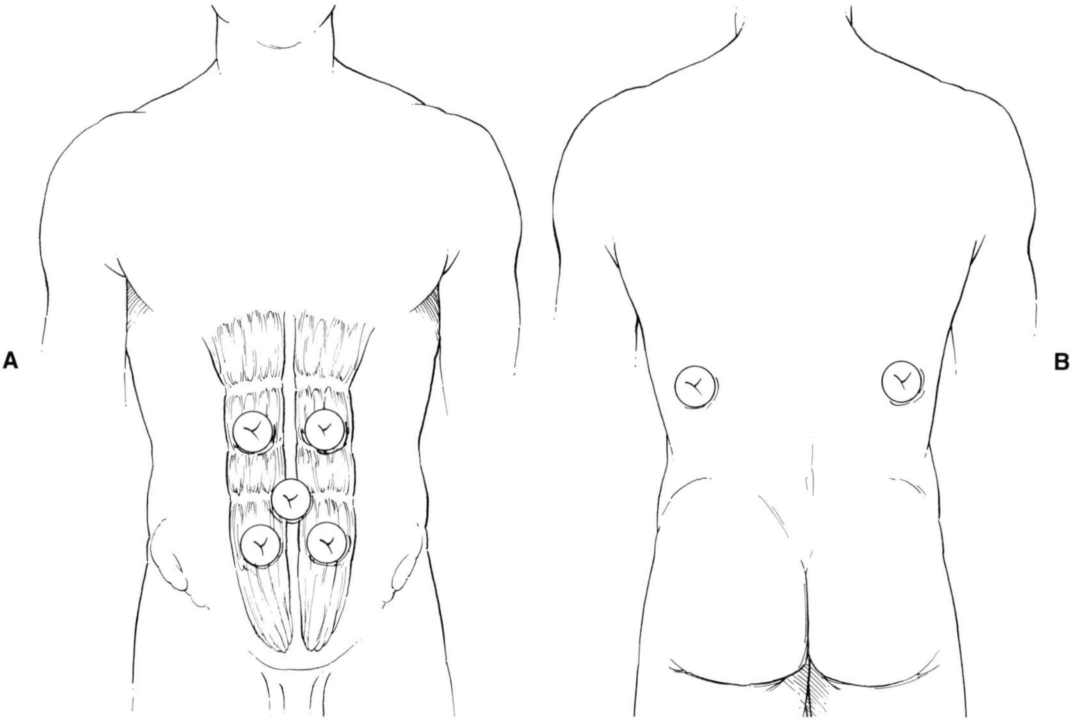

Fig. 3-3. A, Potential stoma sites. **B,** Lumbar sites for limited, rare circumstances.

exenteration or with combined distal rectal and genitourinary obstruction or trauma. When multiple stomas are needed, they should be created at different levels, if possible. When stoma belts were required, this approach was essential. However, with modern pouching techniques, belts are usually unnecessary. In general, the urinary conduit should be placed slightly higher than other stomas because this stoma will function continuously, unlike an end sigmoid colostomy, which may only require a stoma cap.

SPECIAL CIRCUMSTANCES

1. *Cirrhosis.* Since patients with cirrhosis are at high risk for the development of parastomal varices, alternate surgical options should be considered for such patients whenever possible.
2. *Extreme obesity.* Large panniculi make infraumbilical stomas difficult to create, awkward for the patient to see, and impossible to care for. Therefore upper abdominal stomas should be considered for extremely obese patients (Fig. 3-4).

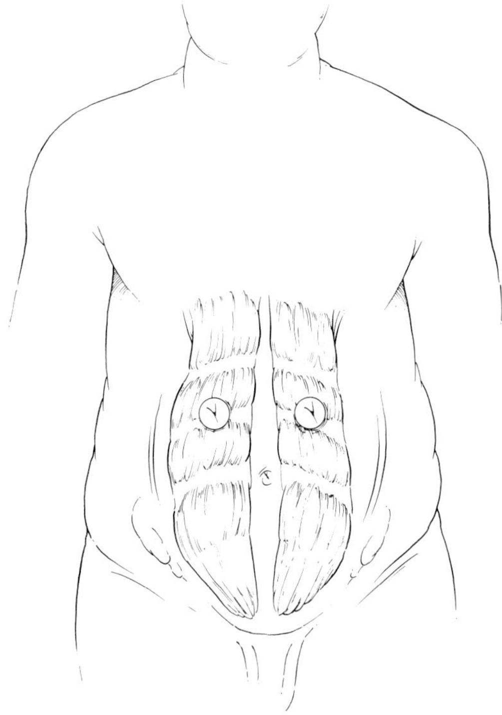

Fig. 3-4. Upper abdominal stoma sites for extremely obese patients.

3. *Physical disability.* Paraplegics may require stomas for control of bowel and bladder function. Since these individuals spend most of their time sitting, slightly higher than usual stoma placement may be necessary. Preoperative marking with the patient in his or her natural environment will help to avoid postoperative problems. Patients suffering from other physical disabilities, such as neurologic deficits, severe arthritis, or blindness, may lose their independence as the result of a stoma, possibly requiring long-term full-time care. Alternative surgical options should be explored. If such options are not practical, postoperative care arrangements should be planned prior to surgery.
4. *Radiation therapy.* Stoma sites should be placed away from areas of prior or future irradiation since severe skin and stomal complications may develop as the result of radiation therapy.
5. *Continent stomas.* Continent ileostomies and urostomies commonly require no external management device. Patients often cover their stomas with only a Band-aid and prefer sites below the bikini line.

SUGGESTED READINGS

Broadwell DC, Jackson BS, eds. Principles of Ostomy Care. St. Louis: CV Mosby, 1982.

Cox BG, Wentworth AE. The Ileal Pouch Procedure. Rochester, Minn.: Mayo Comprehensive Cancer Center, 1977.

Hampton B, ed. Ostomies and Continent Diversions. St. Louis: Mosby–Year Book, 1992.

Hill GL. Ileostomy: Surgery, Physiology, and Management. New York: Grune & Stratton, 1976.

Jeter KF. These Special Children. Palo Alto, Calif.: Bull Publishing, 1982.

Mullen BD, McGinn KA. The Ostomy Book: Living Comfortably With Colostomies, Ileostomies, and Urostomies. Palo Alto, Calif.: Bull Publishing, 1980.

Patient Education Booklets. Patient Education Press, 417 Cleveland Ave., Plainfield, NJ 07060.

Steiner T, Banks TA, Present DH, eds. People Not Patients: A Source Book for Living With Inflammatory Bowel Disease. New York: National Foundation for Ileitis and Colitis, 1985.

Walker FC, ed. Modern Stoma Care. London: Churchill Livingstone, 1976.

4 STOMA THERAPY

Ian C. Lavery and Paula Erwin-Toth

Optimum care of a patient with a stoma is achieved through active participation of both the surgeon and the ET nurse. This participation should begin in the preoperative period with physical examination and preoperative preparation of the patient.

The ET nurse who provides ostomy care should determine from the surgeon and staff nurse what information has been communicated to the patient and family and their level of understanding. This knowledge provides the basis for anticipatory care.

In addition, the patient needs counseling and psychologic preparation for surgery. The surgeon should not abdicate responsibility in this area because such preparation can influence the patient outcome appreciably.

The most common problems that may occur are related to placement of the stoma and parastomal sepsis. Incorrect placement of the stoma predisposes the patient to problems that cannot be managed conservatively (i.e., with a change in equipment). Although correct siting of the stoma is a fundamental consideration, it is often ignored or forgotten in the myriad of things that need to be accomplished in preparation for surgery. Discussion of the patient's concerns about activity, odor, diet, employment, and intimacy are topics that are commonly addressed during preoperative preparation.

The objective of stoma construction is to provide an anatomically stable opening that allows placement of an ostomy management system that will maintain a seal for stool and gas for 5 to 7 days. If every abdomen were flat, muscular, and unscarred, placement of the stoma would not be a major problem. In reality, many patients have a protuberant abdomen and lax musculature. Often they have incision lines that were placed in different directions and have created creases and weak muscles from neurovascular interruption. Under these circumstances the time taken to plan the site for a stoma is crucial because it can minimize the number of postoperative problems.

Siting of the stoma is done with the patient awake. An ostomy management system or a specially prepared disk of the same dimensions as the system is used. The patient is positioned in various ways—supine, sitting, and bending. When the optimum site has been determined, the skin is tattooed with a 27-gauge sterile needle and India ink so that when the abdomen is opened and the anatomic relationships are distorted, the chosen site will not be mistaken. The stoma must be constructed so that it is visible to the patient (i.e., *not* located on the inferior surface of a pendulous abdomen) (Fig. 4-1). The stoma should be located away from the umbilicus, skin creases, scars, and bony prominences. Areas of skin damaged by irradiation or skin grafts also should be avoided.

In the immediate postoperative period, a pectin skin barrier is used for end stomas. A karaya washer is used for loop stomas because when the karaya reaches body temperature, it molds itself over the rod and creates a seal. A temporary ostomy pouch is used until the rod has been removed. When the rod is removed, the patient is fitted with an ostomy management system and given instructions on care of the stoma and the equipment. The patient must be competent and comfortable with care of the stoma before hospital discharge because deficiencies in care can have serious psychologic

A

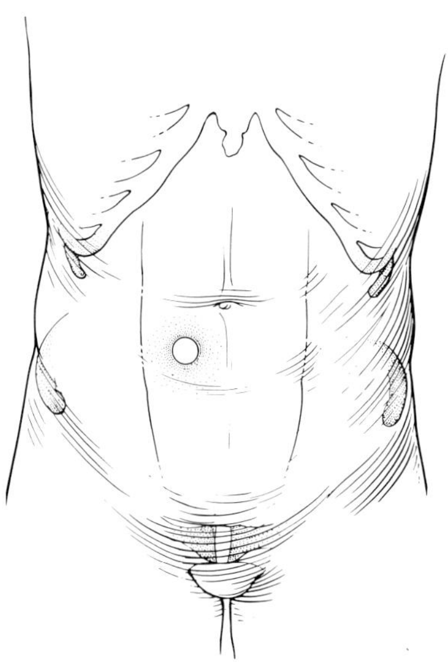

B

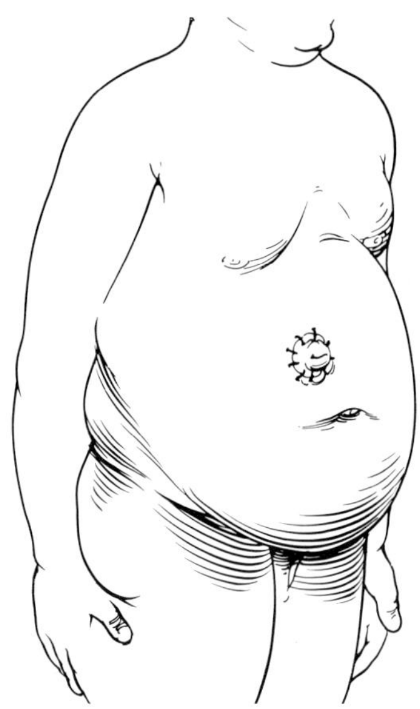

Fig. 4-1. A, The optimum site for an ileostomy is the apex of the subumbilical fat roll through the rectus muscle. **B,** In patients with a pendulous abdomen, the stoma needs to be located in the upper abdomen so that it can be seen by the patient. It also needs to be placed in an area of skin that is flat.

and physical consequences for the patient. Follow-up in the clinic usually takes place 1 month after discharge so that the situation can be assessed and the stoma can be remeasured as postoperative edema resolves. If necessary, self-care instruction can be continued by a home care ET nurse.

Since construction of a stoma creates an abnormal anatomic situation, complications may occur. However, such complications can be minimized through the surgeon's understanding of physiology and correct construction of the stoma.

GASTROINTESTINAL FUNCTION

Jejunostomy

Jejunostomy function usually begins within the first 48 hours after surgery. Initially the effluent is watery, clear, and dark green. Because the volume of output may approach 2400 ml in 24 hours, the patient should be monitored closely for signs of electrolyte imbalance. Absorption capacity depends on the length and functioning of the proximal bowel. The absorption of nutrients, fluids, and electrolytes may be deficient in the patient with a jejunostomy.

Ileostomy

An ileostomy generally begins to function within the first 48 to 72 hours after surgery. The initial effluent is viscous, green, and shiny. Such output does not necessarily indicate return of peristalsis; rather, it may represent the elimination of secretions that have collected in the distal small bowel. Once peristalsis has returned, the patient may enter a period of high-volume output known as the adaptation phase. Output during this period exceeds 1000 ml/day and frequently reaches 1500 to 1800 ml/day. The physiologic basis for this high-output phase is the loss of the colon's absorptive surface coupled with loss of the ileocecal valve. During this period the patient must be monitored closely for signs and symptoms of fluid and electrolyte imbalance. Replacement therapy, which is necessary at this time, can be managed via the intravenous route or with oral electrolyte replacement solutions, depending on the status of bowel function.

Over a period of days to weeks the proximal small bowel increases fluid absorption and the bowel adapts; gradually the volume of output decreases and the stool thickens to a toothpaste-like consistency and is light to medium brown. Initially the output from an ileostomy can vary from 500 to 1500 ml in a 24-hour period. After adaptation the average output decreases to between 500 and 800 ml daily.

Colostomy

The initial output from a colostomy varies, depending on the location of the stoma within the colon. Because the colon absorbs all but approximately 100 ml of the 1000 ml of contents that passes through the ileocecal valve daily, the output from distal colonic stomas has a thicker consistency and smaller volume than that of proximal colonic stomas.

Cecostomy

This stoma usually begins to function by postoperative day 3. The output may be projectile (because of the close proximity of the ileocecal valve) and initially is liquid. A cecostomy can be either skin-level or tubal. The location, output characteristics, and construction combine to make this a difficult stoma to manage. The tube cecostomy poses a particularly difficult management problem because stool tends to flow both through and around the tube. Tube cecostomies also are associated with a greater risk of intra-abdominal spillage.

Transverse Colostomy

A transverse colostomy usually begins to function on postoperative day 3 or 4. Output, which varies from pasty to soft, usually occurs after meals and at intervals throughout the day. In a loop transverse colostomy a support device (e.g., rod or bridge) placed during surgery is removed 5 to 7 days later. The alternative is to construct a fascial bridge at the time of surgery, which obviates the need for a stomal support device.

Descending or Sigmoid Colostomy

A descending or sigmoid colostomy takes the longest time to regain normal peristalsis and may not begin to function until postoperative day 5. Patients with active bowel sounds who have not passed flatus or stool by postoperative day 5 should be assessed for factors that would contribute to the delay in return of function (e.g., administration of narcotics). To stimulate function, a No. 20 Fr soft Foley catheter is well lubricated and then gently advanced into the stoma. A warmed solution of 500 ml of normal saline is instilled via gravity drainage and allowed to return. This procedure initiates a reflex contraction, provides relief of gaseous distention, and maintains peristalsis.

Once normal function has returned, the output from a descending or sigmoid colostomy usually is soft-formed stool. Elimination patterns generally are similar to those of the preoperative period.

The amount and consistency of stool from any gastrointestinal stoma is influenced by the amount of bowel resected, the length and condition of the proximal bowel, medications, and diet. Over a period of several months, the remaining bowel increases its absorptive capacity, and the effluent decreases in volume and becomes thicker.

POUCHING SYSTEM PROCEDURES

General issues that must be considered in establishing pouching system procedures include the following: organizational matters, timing of pouch change, frequency of pouch change, and sizing of the pouch or barrier opening.

Organization of Materials

It is helpful to organize all the products required for the pouch changing procedure in one area and to assemble all necessary supplies before the procedure is begun. Necessary supplies include a plastic trash bag (for disposing of soiled items), a wet washcloth or disposable wipes, the pouch itself, and any products for skin protection (e.g., skin barrier powder, sealants, or paste). When a cut-to-fit pouch is used, a measuring guide or pattern, pencil, and scissors also are needed. If hair is present in the peristomal area, an electric or disposable razor may be required. When a pouch is to be applied to a urinary stoma or a high-output fecal stoma, it is advisable to have an ample supply of absorbent materials, such as soft paper towels, nonsterile gauze, tampons, or dental wicks.

Timing of Pouch Change

Optimally the pouch is changed when the stoma is not highly active. A fecal stoma usually is most active within 2 hours of a meal. For a urinary stoma the best time for a pouch change usually is early in the morning before fluid consumption. Each patient learns his or her own best time for pouch changes.

Frequency of Pouch Change

There is no "correct" frequency for pouch changes. The goal is to establish a routine schedule that prevents leakage and provides the individual with control. The stoma that is appropriately sited and well constructed usually can be managed with a pouch change frequency of every 5 to 7 days. With more durable products some individuals can maintain secure seals for 10 days or even longer. In contrast, with a poorly sited or retracted stoma, a twice-weekly pouch change may be required to prevent leakage; occasionally daily or alternate-day changes may be required.

Establishment of the optimum frequency for pouch change requires individual adjustment and experimentation. In the immediate postoperative period the pouch is changed more frequently than usual to permit stoma assessment and to provide instruction in self-care procedures. After discharge the patient should be encouraged to gradually extend the interval between pouch changes until optimum frequency can be determined. This frequency then becomes the basis for routine pouch changes. The patient also is taught to recognize the signs of undermining and impending leakage (i.e., itching or burning of the peristomal skin, odor noted when the pouch is closed, or visible "meltdown" of the skin barrier) and to change the pouch promptly whenever any of these signs are present.

Sizing of Pouch or Barrier Opening

Most manufacturers of ostomy supplies include disposable stoma-measuring guides in each box of pouches. These guides are used to determine the size of a round stoma. An opening that clears the stoma and minimizes exposure of the peristomal skin should be selected. For irregularly shaped stomas it is necessary to make a pattern that can be used to size the barrier or pouch opening. One simple way to make a pattern is to use a transparent piece of plastic and a felt-tip marker to trace the contours of the stoma. The pattern is then cut out and altered as necessary until a good fit has been obtained. The pattern should be labeled with arrows indicating "head" and "foot" and "pouch side" and "skin side."

When a barrier is added to an adhesive pouch, the barrier is sized to fit closely around the stoma without impinging on the bowel mucosa; the pouch is sized to clear the stoma by at least one-eighth inch. This method prevents the rigid pouch opening from causing damage to the stoma; in addition, it prevents tunneling of the effluent between the barrier and the pouch (see box, p. 66).

Because edema decreases during the first 6 to 8 weeks after surgery, the size of the stoma decreases and the ostomy device opening needs to be resized at each pouch change during this period. Once shrinkage is complete, further resizing is not necessary unless the stoma changes. The condition of a patient who is not able to measure the stoma or who has an irregularly shaped stoma

APPLICATION OF ONE-PIECE FECAL POUCH*

1. Gather all supplies.
2. Gently remove soiled pouch by pushing down on skin while lifting up on pouch. Discard soiled pouch in odorproof plastic bag. *Save tail closure.*
3. Clean stoma and peristomal skin with water; pat dry. *If indicated,* shave or clip peristomal hair.
4. Use stoma-measuring guide or established pattern to determine size of stoma.
   Presized pouch. Check to be sure pouch opening is correct size. Order new supplies if indicated.
   Cut-to-fit pouch. Trace correctly sized pattern onto back of barrier or pouch surface, and cut stomal opening to match pattern.
   NOTE: Once stomal shrinkage is complete, this step may be omitted and preparation of clean pouch may be completed before soiled pouch is removed.
5. Apply skin barrier paste around stoma. (*Tip:* Wet finger to facilitate paste application.) An alternative approach is to apply skin barrier paste to aperture in prepared pouch or barrier. Allow paste to dry.
   Optional: Apply skin sealant to skin that will be covered by tape.
   Allow to dry.
6. Remove paper backing from pouch or barrier to expose adhesive surface; center pouch opening over stoma and press into place. Attach closure.
   Optional: Apply tape strips to "picture-frame" the pouch-skin junction.

NOTE: *Universal precautions* must be followed when this procedure is performed.
*From Erwin-Toth P, Doughty DB. Principles and procedures of stomal management. In Hampton BG, Bryant RA, eds. Ostomies and Continent Diversions. St. Louis: Mosby–Year Book, 1992, p 57.

must be followed closely during the first 6 to 8 weeks after surgery, either by a home care nurse or through follow-up at an outpatient clinic (Fig. 4-2).

Use of Pouch With Urinary Stoma

Issues that must be addressed in regard to applying a pouch to a urinary stoma include peristomal skin protection, pouching options, and modifications required for applying a pouch to a stoma with stents in place.

Peristomal Skin Protection

Urine contains no enzymes and is normally slightly acidic. Therefore skin damage from urine usually is caused by pooling of the urine on the peristo-

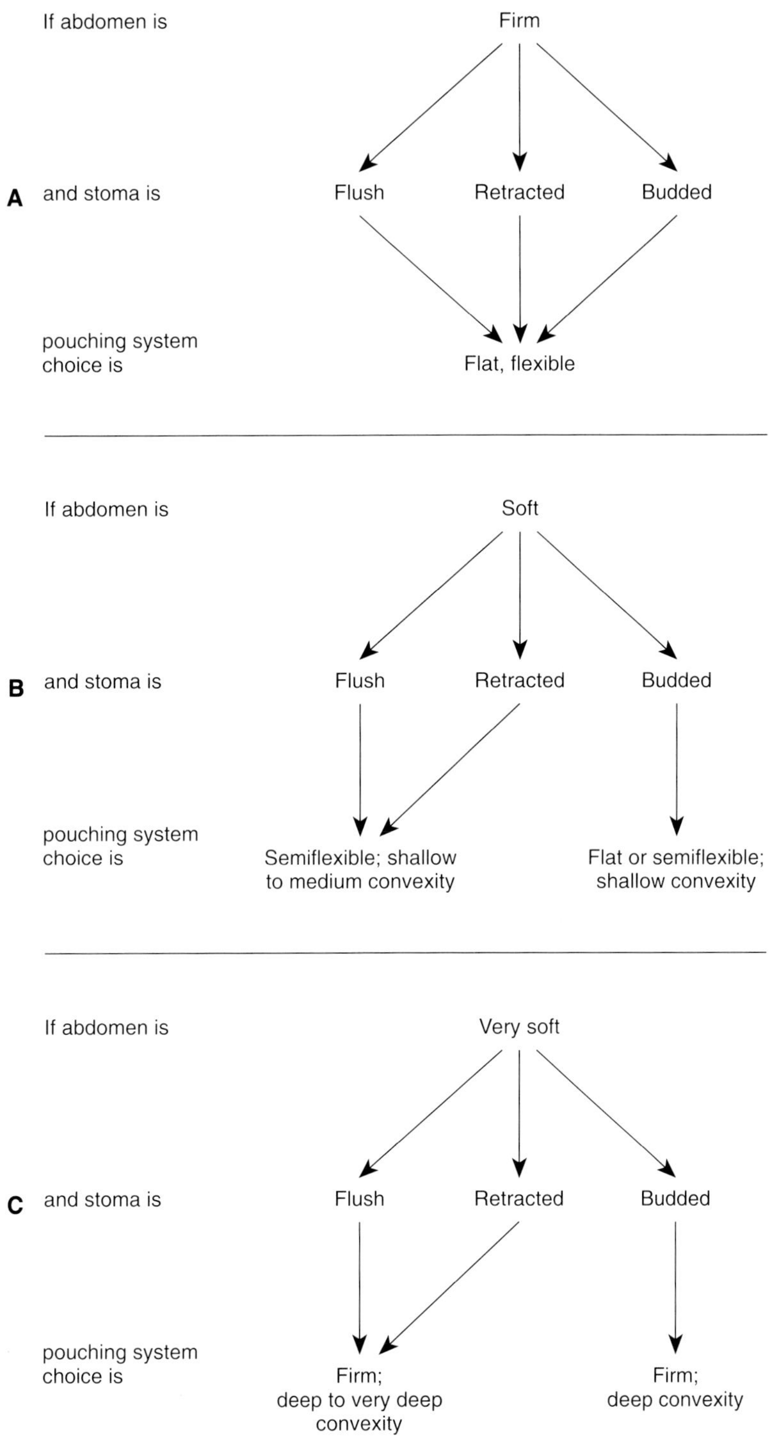

Fig. 4-2. When resizing of the barrier opening is necessary, the choice of a pouching system depends on the condition of the abdomen and the position of the stoma. This flowchart shows the possible choices when the abdomen is firm (**A**), soft (**B**), or very soft (**C**).

mal skin, which results in maceration. Alkaline urine can damage the skin and cause encrustations and crystal deposits. Therefore skin protection for the patient with a urinary diversion focuses on prevention of pooling and maintenance of acidic urine.

Pooling of urine is prevented by maintaining a tight seal between the skin and the pouch so that urine flows into the pouch and is not trapped under the pouch adhesive. Pouches with antireflux valves prevent or limit backflow of urine toward the peristomal skin. (Most disposable pouches and selected reusable pouches are constructed with antireflux valves.) Skin sealants also reduce the potential for maceration of the peristomal skin since they help to "waterproof" the skin.

Encrustations and crystal formation are prevented by maintaining an acidic and dilute urine.

Pouching System Options

In applying a pouch to a urinary stoma, two approaches can be taken: (1) a pouch with an attached skin barrier can be used (the skin barrier is sized to fit snugly around the stoma), or (2) an adhesive-only system with an antireflux valve can be used. In the latter approach the pouch opening is sized to adhere to a flat abdominal surface, even if cutting the pouch opening wide and leaving skin exposed are required. Both approaches are valid because the intent of each is to protect the skin from pooled urine. Skin barriers are not always required for urinary diversions, but their use may increase the wearing time of the pouching system.

Pouches with barriers are sized to fit closely around the stoma because the barriers are moldable and usually can adapt to peristomal contours. If the stoma is protruding (budded) and the pouch is equipped with an antireflux valve, any barrier that adheres well to the peristomal skin is appropriate. For example, karaya and pectin barriers are known to break down as a result of exposure to urine; however, they may be effective with a budded stoma if the pouch is equipped with an antireflux valve (because the urine projects into the pouch and backflow is limited by the antireflux valve). With a flush or skin-level stoma, however, it is important to select a barrier that is resistant to breakdown by urine. Urine from a flush stoma constantly washes over the barrier, and a barrier that is not resistant to urine quickly deteriorates. When a pouch with a barrier is being changed, the barrier and the peristomal skin are assessed to ascertain that the barrier is not absorbing the urine and causing peristomal maceration.

Some patients with urinary stomas obtain longer pouch seals and improved skin protection by using adhesive-only pouching systems. In the application of an adhesive-only pouch with an antireflux valve, the goal is to obtain

APPLICATION OF ONE-PIECE URINARY POUCH*

1. Gather all supplies.
2. Gently remove soiled pouch by pushing down on skin while lifting up on pouch. Discard soiled pouch.
3. Use stoma-measuring guide or established pattern to determine size of stoma.
   Presized pouch. Check to be sure pouch opening is correct size. Order new supplies if indicated.
   Cut-to-fit pouch. Trace correctly sized pattern onto back of pouch, and cut stomal opening to match pattern.
   NOTE: Once stomal shrinkage is complete, this step may be omitted. If a cut-to-fit pouch is used, pouch may be cut out before soiled pouch is removed.
4. Remove paper backing from pouch, and lay pouch to one side.
5. Clean stoma and peristomal skin with water; pat dry. *If indicated,* shave or clip peristomal hair.

Use wicks against stoma to absorb urine and to keep skin dry for steps 6 and 7.

6. *Optional:* Apply skin sealant to skin that will be covered by tape. Allow to dry.
7. Remove paper backing from pouch; center pouch opening over stoma and press pouch into place.
8. *Optional:* Apply tape strips to "picture-frame" the pouch-skin junction.

NOTE: *Universal precautions* must be followed when this procedure is performed.
*From Erwin-Toth P, Doughty DB. Principles and procedures of stomal management. In Hampton BG, Bryant RA, eds. Ostomies and Continent Diversions. St. Louis: Mosby–Year Book, 1992, p 59.

a good seal between the pouch and the peristomal skin in order to prevent pooling of urine. Adhesive surfaces cannot adapt to changing peristomal contours. If they are applied over irregular contours and deep creases, they may become partially detached and allow pooling. The pouch opening should be sized to permit adherence to a flat abdominal pouching surface. It must be emphasized that this approach requires the use of a pouch with an antireflux valve; backflow of urine must be prevented because the peristomal skin is exposed. The use of sealants or cements usually is recommended to further protect the skin from maceration (see box).

Control of Gas and Odor

The two major sources of intestinal gas are swallowed air and gas formed through bacterial action on undigested carbohydrates. Swallowed air is absorbed gradually during its transit throughout the intestinal tract. Therefore it is more likely to affect the patient with a small bowel stoma, especially one located in the proximal small bowel. Since swallowed air is increased by the use of straws, talking while eating, chewing gum, and smoking, the patient who swallows large amounts of air may benefit from reduction or elimination of these practices.

Gas formed by bacterial action on undigested carbohydrates is of greater significance to the patient with a large bowel stoma because most intestinal bacteria are located in the colon. Gas-forming foods (e.g., beans, cabbage, broccoli, brussels sprouts, and beer) are identified. The lag time between intake of gas-producing foods and actual flatulence is about 6 hours for the person with a colostomy (based on average transit time from mouth to colon). The individual can decide to omit these foods or to eat them only at times when flatulence will not cause embarrassment. Foods associated with reduced odor include yogurt, parsley, and orange juice. Measures for muffling flatus sounds include applying pressure to the stoma with the hand or elbow. Patients with large amounts of flatus but firm stool may benefit from pouches with deodorizing flatus filters. Such filters vent the gas through a charcoal filter, thus eliminating flatus odor while keeping the pouch relatively flat. Loose stool may seep into the filter and cause odor and leakage.

The most important odor-control measures are the use of odor-proof pouches and good hygiene (i.e., keeping the bottom of the pouch clean). The patient who is using an odor-proof pouch and keeps the pouch spout clean should have fecal odor only when the pouch is emptied or changed. Often it is helpful to remind the patient that fecal odor during elimination is normal. Additional options for odor control include pouch deodorants, room deodorants, and oral deodorizing agents. Agents used as pouch deodorants include commercial deodorants, commercial perineal cleansers, and mouthwashes, all of which contain antibacterial agents. Deodorizing agents for use in the pouch are added to the pouch after it has been emptied. Room deodorant sprays can be used when the pouch is being emptied or changed. They are particularly beneficial when the patient must empty the pouch in a public restroom, and they are available in purse or pocket size. Oral agents commonly used include bismuth subgallate (Devrom) and chlorophyllin copper complex. When taken consistently, these over-the-counter agents significantly reduce fecal odor. Again, it must be emphasized that the best odor-control measures are a secure, odor-proof pouch and good hygiene.

Management of Diarrhea

The person with a fecal diversion is just as susceptible to episodes of diarrhea as the individual whose bowel is intact. Diarrhea may occur as a result of a viral or bacterial gastroenteritis, antibiotic therapy, radiation therapy, chemotherapy, some medications (e.g., antacids containing magnesium), or food intolerance. Management of diarrhea depends on the location of the stoma within the gastrointestinal tract and the length and function of the proximal bowel. The principles of management are the same for all patients and can be summarized as follows:

1. Eliminate the cause of diarrhea, if possible; for example, the patient who is taking antibiotics may benefit from a lactobacillus preparation to restore normal bowel flora.
2. Maintain a bland, constipating diet. Recommended foods include rice, pasta, cheese, bananas, and applesauce.
3. Replace fluid and electrolytes. The patient is instructed to replace both fluid volume and fluid components (electrolytes). One approach is to drink a glass of replacement fluid each time the pouch is emptied. Suggested replacement fluids include sports drinks, fruit or vegetable juices, and broth.
4. Over-the-counter antidiarrheal medications usually are acceptable. One exception is for the patient receiving radiation therapy. Such patients should not take over-the-counter antidiarrheal agents because many of these preparations contain bismuth, which is a metallic agent.

Patients also should be instructed to notify their physician of signs and symptoms of fluid-electrolyte imbalance, such as weakness, lethargy, dry mouth and tongue, reduced urine output and increased urine concentration, abdominal cramps, and dizziness when standing. Notifying the physician is particularly important for patients with a small bowel or proximal large bowel stoma because these patients are at increased risk for fluid-electrolyte imbalance during episodes of increased fluid loss.

Recognition and Management of Food Blockage

Adherence to the guidelines for adding high-fiber foods to the diet usually prevents development of food blockage. The person with an ileostomy, however, should be taught the signs and symptoms of food blockage, appropriate home management, and indications for notifying the physician. Signs and symptoms of food blockage are the same as for any intestinal obstruction and vary depending on the degree of obstruction. A partial obstruction usually causes cramping abdominal pain, watery output with a foul odor, and possible abdominal distention and stoma swelling; nausea and vomiting also may occur. With complete obstruction, stoma output ceases; severe cramping pain, abdominal distention, stomal swelling, nausea, and vomiting usually occur. Patients are taught to notify their physician or ET nurse promptly if signs of complete obstruction do not respond to the use of mild analgesics and cessation of eating or drinking. These patients usually require ileal lavage, as outlined in the discussion of obstruction.

Prevention and Management of Fluid-Electrolyte Imbalance

Persons with an ileostomy have lost the absorptive functions provided by the colon. They lose approximately 500 to 750 ml of fluid daily through the stoma, compared with 100 to 200 ml lost by the average person with an intact colon. Thus individuals with an ileostomy are at much greater risk for fluid-electrolyte imbalance when increased loss occurs, for example, with gastroenteritis that causes diarrhea and vomiting. Self-care instruction for these patients should focus on the importance of vigorous replacement of fluid and electrolytes during periods of increased loss and the recognition and prompt response to signs and symptoms of fluid-electrolyte imbalance. The importance of notifying the physician promptly if fluids cannot be replaced during periods of increased loss also must be stressed.

FUNDAMENTALS OF PATIENT CARE

Special Considerations With Transverse Colostomy

Issues specific to patients with a transverse colostomy include dietary and fluid modifications and concealment of the stoma. Since transverse colostomies most commonly are performed for temporary diversions, an additional issue for many patients is incorporation of the colostomy into their own life-style on a temporary basis.

Dietary and fluid modification. Nutrients are digested and absorbed in the small intestine. Since the small intestine is not affected by a transverse colostomy, patients with a transverse colostomy have no absolute restrictions imposed by the colostomy. They do lose additional fluid through the stoma and should be instructed to increase fluid intake to 10 glasses of liquid per day.

Concealment of stoma. Patients with a transverse colostomy have a stoma located in the upper abdomen above the beltline. They frequently have concerns related to clothing and concealment of the stoma. Although suggestions must be individualized for the patient, general guidelines include wearing a layer of knit clothing next to the body to keep the pouch secure and smooth and adding a loose outer layer of clothing for concealment. Patients also may find vests, sweaters, scarves, and jackets to be helpful in concealing the stoma.

Prevention and management of constipation. The patient's previous bowel habits, including history of constipation, past management of constipation, and life-style factors (e.g., activity level and intake of fiber and fluid affecting bowel function), must be assessed. It should be explained to the patient that a colostomy does not prevent constipation, and specific recommendations must be made for maintenance of healthy bowel function and prevention of constipation. Routine preventive measures include daily exercise and an adequate intake of fluids and fiber. Individual recommendations are made based on usual fluid and fiber intake, past bowel patterns, and activity tolerance. For example, the sedentary patient with a history of constipation and the usual intake of fluid and fiber (limited to six glasses of fluid a day and one serving of fiber [<5 g]) may be instructed to begin a simple graduated walking program, add two glasses of fluid a day, and take a bulk laxative twice daily. An alternative suggestion would be to increase dietary intake of bulk or to add bran to the diet.

Colostomy irrigation. Education for the patient with a descending or sigmoid colostomy may include instruction in colostomy irrigation. The appropriateness of routine irrigation as a method of management is initially assessed, and the patient is then counseled regarding management options. The patient who is determined to be a candidate for routine irrigation and elects this management approach is instructed in the procedure.

Criteria for irrigation. Patients who meet the following criteria are good candidates for management with routine irrigation:

1. *Descending or sigmoid colostomy.* Routine irrigation is a management option only for patients with a descending or sigmoid colostomy. It is an inappropriate approach for patients with a more proximal stoma because such stomas produce a more fluid, higher volume output; since these patients are unable to regulate fecal output with irrigation, routine irrigation may induce fluid-electrolyte imbalance.
2. *Normal bowel function.* Routine irrigation is most appropriate for persons with a history of regular formed bowel movements. This method is least likely to be effective in individuals with frequent episodes of diarrhea or the irregular bowel pattern of irritable colon.
3. *Ability to learn and perform the procedure.* Patients must be capable of learning and performing the irrigation procedure. In addition, they must have access to adequate toilet facilities such as running water and indoor plumbing.
4. *Patient preference.* Irrigation is optional; it is not required to maintain normal bowel function. The decision to use this management approach should be made by the patient, not by the health care team.

Some conditions and situations that may be regarded as relative contraindications for routine irrigation include the following:

1. *Stoma prolapse or peristomal hernia.* Because of the potential for increased prolapse or bowel perforation, irrigation should be done only with appropriate equipment.
2. *Children and adolescents.* Routine irrigation may not be appropriate for younger patients because of the amount of time and the need to follow a regular schedule.
3. *Pelvic or abdominal radiation.* Irrigation is contraindicated in patients

who are receiving pelvic or abdominal radiation. It should not be initiated or resumed until the inflammation has resolved, as indicated by restoration of normal bowel function and healthy stomal mucosa.

4. *Temporary colostomy.* Routine irrigation usually is not recommended for patients with temporary colostomies because of the time required to master the procedure.
5. *Poor prognosis.* Routine irrigation usually is not recommended for patients who have a poor prognosis because of the time and energy required for the procedure. However, candidacy must be determined according to the individual's status and priorities.

Principles of Colostomy Irrigation

The goal of irrigation is to distend the bowel, making it contract and evacuate its contents. Routine irrigation causes the bowel to empty on a regular basis, which reduces the chance of fecal elimination between irrigations.

Scheduling of irrigation. Most individuals irrigate the colostomy daily or every other day, depending on their preoperative bowel pattern. The time of day is selected on the basis of their individual life-style and preference.

Type and volume of solution. Most patients use lukewarm tap water for irrigation. The alternative is saline, which can be made by adding 2 teaspoons of salt to 1 quart of water. The volume is titrated for the individual. The goal is to use enough irrigant to distend the colon but not enough to cause cramping pain. Most adults use between 600 and 1000 ml of water. The patient is instructed to instill the irrigant at a steady rate until a feeling of fullness has been achieved.

Equipment. A cone tip rather than a catheter is recommended. The cone tip prevents bowel perforation and also acts as a plug to prevent backflow of the irrigating solution around the device. An irrigation sleeve is snapped onto a two-piece wafer or belted into place around the stoma. Disposable adhesive irrigation sleeves also may be used. The end of the sleeve can be closed with a clip or placed in the toilet to direct the flow of return.

Time frame. The time frame required for the entire irrigation procedure is usually about 1 hour: approximately 10 minutes for setup and instillation of irrigant, 30 to 40 minutes for evacuation, and 10 minutes for cleanup. While waiting for evacuation, the individual is free to pursue other activities with the irrigation sleeve in place.

Teaching and Counseling for Self-Care

The initial focus in patient teaching is on self-care skills and daily management issues such as dietary alterations. Once these basic skills have been mastered, the focus shifts to how to incorporate the ostomy into the person's life-style. Common concerns include bathing and clothing; management of the ostomy at work, during exercise, in recreational activities and travel, and during sexual activity; and disclosure issues.

Bathing. Patients may take a tub bath or shower with the pouch left on or taken off. They are encouraged to bathe with the pouch on unless it is time to change the pouch (routine bathing with the pouch off may result in inadvertent removal of the skin barrier paste or washing of the skin barrier wafer or ring, which in turn contributes to premature disruption of the pouch seal). The patient may choose to "picture frame" the edges of the pouch with waterproof tape to increase the resistance; the alternative is to pat the taped edges dry or to dry them with a hair dryer.

Clothing. Snug undergarments over the pouch help conceal the presence of the stoma. Pouch covers protect the skin from the plastic of the pouch and also serve to conceal the pouch contents. For patients with a flush or slightly protruding stoma located in the lower abdominal quadrants, these measures usually are sufficient to conceal the stoma and allow preoperative clothing to be worn. Clothing modifications usually are minimal for these patients; for example, patients may wear slacks or skirts that have front pleats or are loose-fitting. Women are instructed that pantyhose and stretch panty girdles are permissible. Regular girdles also may be worn provided that the stays do not cross the stoma. Bathing suits are available that effectively conceal the stoma; women are advised to look for patterned suits with shirring or draping. Patients also should be made aware of specialty underclothing designed for the person with an ostomy.

Fecal diversions. When the distal bowel segment remains intact, as with a loop stoma, a double-barrel stoma, or an end stoma with Hartmann's pouch, the patient must be prepared for temporary output of stool per rectum once peristalsis returns. The distal bowel continues to produce mucus, and the patient periodically may feel rectal fullness and the need to evacuate the accumulated mucus. Patients who sense rectal distention but are unable to expel the mucus may benefit from a low-volume rectal enema to flush out the mucus.

The patient who has a double-barrel ostomy must be taught how to manage the nonfunctioning "mucous fistula" stoma. If the distal mucous fistula stoma is immediately adjacent to the proximal functioning stoma, it should be included in the pouch. If the nonfunctioning stoma is located at a distance from the proximal stoma, it can be managed with a light dressing, changed by the patient either daily or as needed, or with a stoma cap or cover.

Discharge Planning

Discharge planning is critical for the patient with an ostomy. As the length of stay after ostomy surgery has shortened, the time available for teaching and counseling also has decreased. The teaching focus during the postoperative phase must be survival skills, that is, pouch emptying and pouch changing procedures. Much additional teaching and counseling are required to support integration of the ostomy into the patient's life-style. All patients should have access to outpatient follow-up on a regular basis. In addition to such follow-up, many patients need home health care after discharge. The home care nurse can provide reinforcement and support for self-care and additional instruction regarding ostomy management and counseling regarding psychosocial issues. The ET nurse who provides instruction should evaluate the ostomy patient's potential need for home care follow-up and should initiate or contribute to the referral. Frequently it is beneficial to contact the home care nurse and provide that professional with additional information regarding the patient's care.

COMPLICATIONS

Metabolic Problems

The normal output from an ileostomy is approximately 800 ml/day. In the immediate postoperative period, the volume may be much higher because of partial obstruction caused by edema of the stoma. In the established stoma a bacterial or viral gastroenteritis commonly increases the output and may require intravenous fluid replacement until the volume of output diminishes. Chronic losses of electrolytes may alter the ratio of chemicals and predispose the patient to the precipitation of stones in the kidneys and gallbladder. If resection of an appreciable length of distal ileum has occurred, the possibility of a vitamin B_{12} deficiency needs to be considered.

Necrosis occurs because the terminal portion of the bowel has been deprived of an adequate blood supply. In the construction of an end ileostomy, the mesentery may be detached from the bowel for 5 cm without causing ischemia. The blood supply to the terminal ileum is transmitted through the submucosa (Fig. 4-3). In a patient with a thin abdominal wall, 5 cm is sufficient to construct a viable stoma and allow eversion of the bowel for nipple construction. Ischemia is readily recognized. In the postoperative period, if there is any doubt about whether a dusky color change is congestion or ischemia, a pinprick will clarify the issue. If ischemic, the stoma will need to be revised at laparotomy. If the level of ischemia is above the level of the fascia, the revision can be done at a convenient time. However, if there is no identifiable level of demarcation superficial to the fascia, laparotomy should be performed promptly.

In obese patients, even moderately obese ones, construction of an end ileostomy may result in compromising viability and/or having the nipple pro-

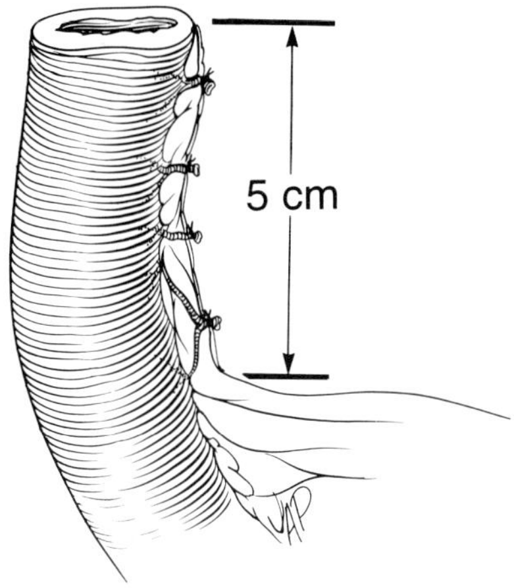

Fig. 4-3. The mesentery of the small bowel may be detached from the bowel for 5 cm without causing compromise of the blood supply to the terminal ileum.

trude above skin level. Construction of a loop end ileostomy as described by Turnbull and Weakley[1] allows the creation of a viable stoma with a nipple valve that looks and functions as an end ileostomy. In extremely obese individuals, fashioning even a loop end ileostomy may be very difficult. The small intestine needs to be mobilized and a generous incision (8-10 cm) must be made in the rectus muscle to allow the stoma to be delivered through the skin aperture. When the surgeon is satisfied with the length of the stoma supported by a rod, the defect in the muscle and fascia is closed cephalad and caudal to the bowel with interrupted nonabsorbable sutures. Closing the defect reduces or delays the development of a parastomal hernia.

Parastomal Abscess, Ulcer, and Fistula

In the early postoperative period, considering the local environment, parastomal abscesses are uncommon. When they do occur, they are related to revision or reconstruction of a stoma at the same site. An abscess, which is the result of an infected hematoma or a misplaced suture during maturation, requires surgical drainage. When an abscess develops at a mature stoma, it is usually the result of folliculitis or recurrent Crohn's disease in an ileostomy. At a colostomy, an abscess usually results from perforation of the intestine with an enema tip during attempted irrigation. A parastomal abscess needs to be drained if it has not done so spontaneously. An ileoscopy or stoma injection is performed to investigate the cause of the abscess and to determine if a fistula is present. If no fistula is present, the cause is invariably folliculitis. The abscess may be drained, but it will not heal unless the cavity is unroofed by excising the undermined skin. Reepithelialization then will occur. If the unroofed area is small (≤2 cm in diameter), the ulcer is managed with a small piece of nonadhesive dressing placed under the conventional ostomy management system and changed daily until it heals. If the ulcer is larger, healing is better if a Perry Model 51 ostomy management system (Perry Co., Minneapolis, Minn.) (or a modification of it) is used. The Perry system is kept in place with a belt rather than adhesive. This system allows changes of the nonadhesive dressing on the ulcer 3 to 4 times a day without damaging the skin, which would occur with such frequent removal of an adhesive type appliance. The dressing used is an absorbent paper pad (Micropad 3M; 3M Health Care, St. Paul, Minn.) moistened with Domeboro solution (aluminum acetate).

After an abscess has been drained, whether or not a fistula is present will become evident. Enteric content will be seen issuing from the drain site or under the ostomy management system and will create skin excoriation. A fistula in an ileostomy is invariably the result of prestomal Crohn's disease. Treatment requires resection of the prestomal disease and construction of a new stoma. It is preferable to relocate the stoma if a suitable site exists to avoid the infection present at the old site. This problem is the reason that a midline abdominal incision is advised in surgery for inflammatory bowel disease. A midline incision preserves all quadrants of the abdomen in the event that relocation of a stoma becomes necessary.

A parastomal abscess resulting from a perforated colon is a more serious and urgent problem since the perforation and abscess are usually within a parastomal hernia that precipitated the injury. This situation involves the potential for contamination of the peritoneal cavity. The abscess needs to be drained and laparotomy must be performed to resect the perforation. If possible, the stoma is relocated and the hernia is repaired. This procedure may be staged, depending on the toxicity of the patient.

Pyoderma gangrenosum around a stoma may mimic a parastomal ulcer. This condition is best managed locally with the Perry ostomy management system and conventional medical treatment of the pyoderma. Treatment consists of local applications of a 10% to 20% solution of benzyl peroxide, which kills bacteria and fungus. A high dose of tetracycline (100-200 g/day) is given orally. In some instances dapsone and colchicine are used. Since dapsone may produce anemia, the initial dose is 25 mg and this dose is increased to 100 mg over several months. In addition, patients should be given vitamin E, which has a beneficial effect on erythrocytes. Methotrexate or azathioprine and antibiotics can be used sparingly, and corticosteroids can be used systemically (Table 4-1).

Table 4-1. Common peristomal skin conditions

Condition	Cause	Solution
Allergic	Sensitivity to skin barriers, adhesives, tapes	Use patch test to determine what patient can tolerate
Bacterial	Folliculitis	Trim peristomal hair with scissors or electric razor Use adhesive remover to ease release of adhesives
Fungal	*Candida albicans*	Nystatin topical powder is applied with each pouch change Excess powder must be dusted off to allow appliance to seal
Chemical	Leakage of effluent under pouching system	Determine cause of leakage Check for peristomal fistula Refit into proper pouching system Dust skin with skin barrier powder prior to pouching Severe hyperplasia may require surgical debridement and use of nonadherent system until reepithelialization occurs
Mechanical	Skin stripping from adhesive removal	Gently pull skin away from adhesive with warm, moist gauze square or adhesive remover
	Laceration of stoma from pouching system due to shifting, improper sizing, or improper application	Remeasure stoma Observe pouching system while patient is sitting, supine, and standing Observe patient applying pouching system
Other peristomal abcess	Commonly caused by recurrent Crohn's disease	Unroof ulcer: If ulcer is <2 cm, cover with nonadherent gauze or hydrocolloid, apply pouch as usual, and change every 2 to 3 days If ulcer is >2 cm, apply nonadherent pouching system

Parastomal Hernia

Parastomal hernias are relatively uncommon with ileostomies; the reported incidence varies between 0.7% and 2.6%.[2-4] These hernias are more common with colostomies, with occurrence reported as between 3% and 10% of patients.[5,6] Predisposing conditions are obesity, a large abdominal wall aperture, placement of the stoma lateral to the rectus sheath, and weakness of the abdominal wall from age or multiple incisions. Parastomal hernias generally enlarge and may cause an unsightly bulge under clothing. If untreated, these hernias may enlarge and make it difficult to keep an ostomy management system attached. If a rigid faceplate is used, pressure necrosis may result from tightening the belt to keep the system attached. Less rigid ostomy management systems, such as those with a pectin base skin barrier, make this complication less likely. Smaller asymptomatic hernias can be managed by using a Velcro binder with an opening cut for the pouching system. The indications for surgery are difficulty with pouch application or with irrigation of the colostomy.

Surgery is most satisfactorily done by relocating the stoma, usually to the contralateral side. As a practical consideration, certain sites for relocating the stoma are less than optimal and local repair may be preferable. Local repair is done at laparotomy. The orifice through the abdominal wall is closed with interrupted nonabsorbable sutures. In a survey of patients at the Cleveland Clinic, the cumulative probability of recurrence was 46% after 6 years. Obesity was the only clinical factor investigated that significantly predisposed patients to recurrence of the hernia.

Stricture

It is still thought by some individuals that stomas need to be dilated after construction to prevent stricture formation. This idea originated when stomas were not matured primarily. When stomas are constructed correctly and matured primarily, there is *no* reason for "dilatation" of the stoma. Not only is this practice uncomfortable and unnecessary; it also can cause strictures from the scarring that develops as a result of the repeated trauma caused by the dilatation.

If a stricture develops as a result of ischemia or recurrent prestomal Crohn's disease, revision is necessary. Such revision may be done locally, but recurrent Crohn's disease usually requires laparotomy and resection of the terminal ileum.

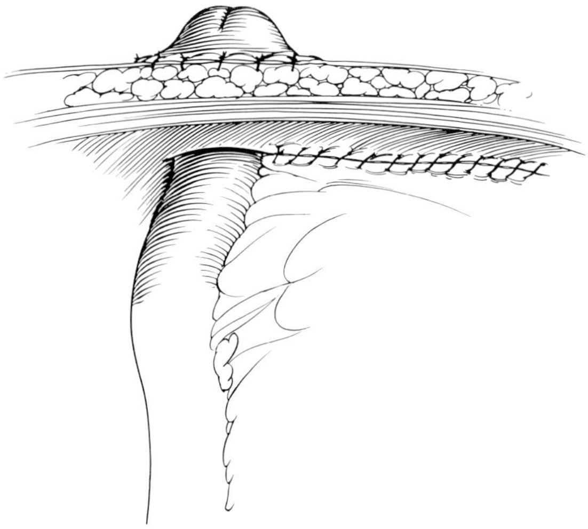

Fig. 4-4. Suturing the cut edge of the mesentery of the small bowel to the posterior rectus sheath obliterates the mesenteric defect through which the bowel may rotate.

Volvulus

Volvulus around an ileostomy is prevented by suturing the cut edge of the mesentery of the small bowel to the anterior abdominal wall (Fig. 4-4). This method closes the mesenteric defect, preventing the small bowel from rotating on the axis of the mesentery of the stoma. A volvulus may occur around a loop ileostomy where the mesentery is not divided; however, such an occurrence is uncommon, and it is not practical to attempt to close the mesenteric defect. We have seen three instances of volvulus around loop ileostomies during the latter half of pregnancy—possibly related to a change in the location of the small intestine.

Volvulus is manifest as an obstruction involving congestion of the stoma. Laparotomy is indicated to alleviate this condition.

Caput Medusae

Caput medusae is a circumferential burgundy halo around a stoma that blanches with pressure. It is the result of a portosystemic collateral circulation from portal hypertension. The underlying cause is cirrhosis caused by sclerosing cholangitis. Bleeding, the resulting complication, occurs at the mucocutaneous junction and may be profuse. Immediate control of the bleeding can be obtained by applying pressure precisely to the bleeding point. The bleeding will stop if there is no coagulopathy, as may occur with cirrhosis. Repeated episodes of bleeding should prompt surgical treatment. Such treatment involves interrupting the portosystemic circulation by separating the mucocutaneous junction.[7] The collateral circulation is located at this level. It is not necessary to mobilize the stoma completely down into the peritoneal cavity. Some of the vessels to be interrupted have a large caliber and require individual ligation. Blood loss may be more than expected if the portal pressure is high. Because of the pathophysiology of the caput medusae, recurrence is inevitable. Portosystemic shunting is not indicated. Sclerotherapy has been proposed as a treatment method, but those reported cases in which it was done required multiple injections and the effect was short-lived.

Obstruction

In the early postoperative period, obstruction is caused by edema at the level of the new stoma. The obstruction may result in some abdominal cramping and liquid output caused by excessive secretion of succus entericus. As the time from operation increases and the edema settles, so do the symptoms.

In a well-established ileostomy an adhesive bowel obstruction may occur (as after any abdominal operation). In specific relation to the stoma, obstruction caused by a food bolus needs to be considered. Direct questioning of the patient regarding recent ingestion of food with a high fiber content will give an indication of the degree of probability of such obstruction. If the patient has been indiscrete and has eaten a large volume of high-fiber foods, it is likely that a bolus of undigested food is the cause of the obstruction. The point of obstruction occurs at the fascia level of the abdominal wall. Management involves ileostomy lavage. The lavage is performed by inserting a No. 22 or No. 24 Fr Foley catheter into the distal bowel and irrigating it with several 100 ml aliquots of saline. A two-piece pouching system or irrigation sleeve can be applied to manage the flow. If the catheter can be inserted into the stoma for several inches and irrigation with several aliquots does not produce a return of fluid containing particulate matter of undigested food, the obstruction should be considered more proximal, probably an adhesive bowel obstruction. Further attempts to relieve the obstruction by irrigation should be stopped. If the irrigation produces a volume of undigested fibrous material, the procedure is continued until the bolus is broken up and there is some evidence of spontaneous evacuation. Treatment of a bolus obstruction by lavage usually does not require admission to the hospital.

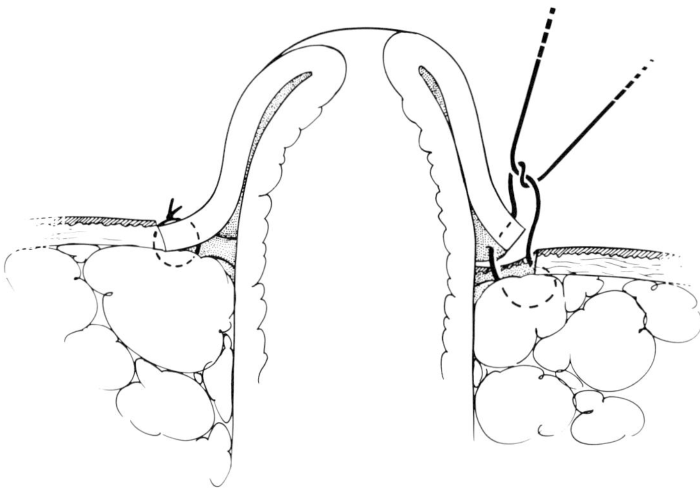

Fig. 4-5. During maturation of the stoma, sutures are placed through full thickness of the bowel and dermis of the skin.

Mucosal Implants

Mucosal implants are islands of mucosa that have lodged along suture tracts. They are avoided by the technique of stoma construction. During maturation of the stoma, the mucocutaneous sutures are placed through the dermal layers of the skin without entering the epidermis (Fig. 4-5). If mucosal implants create a problem, it is from the mucus that they secrete under the ostomy management system. The mucus reduces the adhesion of the pouch and causes leakage. It is not common for implants to cause a major problem, but if the implants are extensive, relocation of the stoma may be necessary. Precise destruction at skin level with a needle electrocautery will give temporary relief.

Trauma

Trauma to the stoma may occur in body contact sports, but this is uncommon because most patients with stomas are advised to avoid this type of activity. When the aperture in the pouching system is too small or misplaced, vigorous physical activity may result in a cut or circumferential ulcer and bleeding. If the cut is deeper, a fistula or complete transection of the stoma can occur. In less severe cases modification of the pouching system will allow healing of the ulcer.

At the Cleveland Clinic, McLeod et al.[8] conducted a survey of patients with conventional ileostomies to determine which factors affected the health and quality of life of these individuals. It was found that the only significant item that had any effect on the quality of life was the function of the ileostomy.

The most common reasons for stoma revision are technical errors and recurrent disease. Surgeons in concert with ET nurses must approach the construction of stomas with care and make every effort to minimize potential problems, both physical and psychosocial.

REFERENCES

1. Turnbull RB, Weakley FL. Atlas of Intestinal Stomas. St. Louis: CV Mosby, 1967, pp 32-39.
2. Carlstedt A, Tasth S, Hulten W, Nordgren S, Palselius I. Long-term ileostomy complications in patients with ulcerative colitis and Crohn's disease. Int J Colorectal Dis 2:22-25, 1987.
3. Goligher JC. Surgery of the anus, rectum and colon, 5th ed. London: Baillière Tindall, 1984, pp 703-704, 891-894.
4. Horgan K, Hughes LE. Para-ileostomy hernia: Failure of a local repair technique. Br J Surg 73:439-440, 1986.
5. Prian GW, Sawyer RB, Sawyer KC. Repair of peristomal colostomy hernias. Am J Surg 130:694-696, 1975.
6. Green EW. Colostomies and their complication. Surg Gynecol Obstet 1:1230-1232, 1966.
7. Beck DE, Fazio VW, Grundfest-Broniatowski S. Surgical management of bleeding stomal varices. Dis Colon Rectum 31:343-346, 1988.
8. McLeod RS, Lavery IC, Leatherman JR, Maryland PA, Fazio VW, Jagelman DG, Weakley FL. Factors affecting quality of life with conventional ileostomy. World J Surg 10:474-480, 1986.

SUGGESTED READING

Erwin-Toth P, Doughty DB. Principles and procedures of stomal management. In Hampton BG, Bryant RA, eds. Ostomies and Continent Diversions. St. Louis: Mosby–Year Book, 1992.

An excellent review of the practical aspects of nursing management of stomas.

5 QUALITY OF LIFE WITH A STOMA

Robin S. McLeod and Zane Cohen

Quality of life, which encompasses the physical, psychologic, and social well-being of an individual, is important in the assessment of the outcome of a procedure that will leave the patient with a permanent stoma. This issue is particularly important for patients who have several surgical alternatives, for example, those with ulcerative colitis. For most patients with an ileostomy, the quality of life is high, perhaps because of the excellent physical well-being they enjoy. Most patients with a colostomy also enjoy a good quality of life, although their concerns may be somewhat different because of age or indications for surgery.

Traditionally, the success or failure of a surgical procedure has been based on its associated operative morbidity and mortality. Earlier in this century this viewpoint was appropriate since patients often underwent surgery as a last resort, after all other treatment alternatives had failed. Operative mortality tended to be high and complications were frequent. Today, however, the diagnosis often is made at an earlier stage, and surgery is performed earlier in the course of the disease. In addition, improvements in anesthesia and preoperative and postoperative care have resulted in a low operative mortality, even with major operations. For these reasons operative mortality is less important in assessing outcome and in comparing operative procedures. Other outcome measures, such as the complication rate, duration of hospitalization, and postoperative quality of life, are of greater significance.

Assessment of quality of life is particularly important in patients who require surgery that will leave them with a permanent stoma. Not surprisingly, many patients faced with this possibility may be reluctant to undergo surgery for fear that they may be more disabled postoperatively than they were preoperatively. In deciding whether to agree to surgery and in choosing a specific operative procedure, the patient often considers quality of life to be a major determinant. This factor is especially important for patients with ulcerative colitis, who may choose from several surgical options, each with its advantages and disadvantages and varying complication rates. It also may be significant for selected patients with rectal cancer who have the option of local therapy or radiation therapy vs. radical surgery with a colostomy. Such patients may need to weigh quality of life against a higher risk of tumor recurrence when deciding on treatment.

ASSESSMENT OF QUALITY OF LIFE

Although all of us have a sense of what quality of life is, this factor is difficult to define and even more difficult to measure. The World Health Organization's definition of health as "a state of complete physical, mental and social well-being and not merely the absence of disease or infirmity" is often used to define quality of life. Shumaker et al.[1] define quality of life as "an individual's overall satisfaction with life, and one's general sense of personal well-being." In any consideration of quality of life, the major domains of physical well-being and functional status, psychologic function, and social interaction should be included.[2] Other domains such as somatic sensation and sexual function may be included, and some investigators even add a financial component. In addition, since quality of life is highly personal, it is often considered to be assessed best by the individual. A patient's assessment of his or her quality of life may vary according to the individual's cultural background, age, sex, previous life experiences, life-style, expectations, and work. What is acceptable to one person may be unacceptable to another.

Quality of life always has been important to the clinician, but it tended to be assessed in response to a question such as "How are you doing?" Although such an inquiry permits some assessment of the patient's status, the assessment is subjective—lacking accuracy, reliability, and validity. Unfortunately, most assessments of quality of life in stoma patients are still rather unsophisticated. Commonly, the components of quality of life are assessed by focusing mainly on physical well-being rather than functional status and psychologic well-being. Rarely are all domains considered and the results aggregated into one measure. Often assessments are made without validated instruments, and subjective responses are elicited. Since the quality of life is not measured quantitatively, comparisons before and after surgery and between different therapies or procedures cannot be made. Hopefully, in the future instruments that are sensitive, valid, and reliable will be developed so that the quality of life after surgery can be assessed quantitatively and comparisons can be made between different surgical procedures or therapies.

LIFE WITH AN ILEOSTOMY

Most patients who require a permanent ileostomy have ulcerative colitis; a smaller proportion of this group has Crohn's disease or familial adenomatous polyposis. Although this group has several surgical alternatives from which to choose, including the continent ileostomy (Kock pouch) or an ileal pouch–anal procedure, the conventional ileostomy is still considered by most surgeons to be the standard against which other procedures are compared.

Although patients may be reluctant preoperatively to accept a permanent ileostomy, most patients adapt well to it and achieve a very high quality of life. Of 273 ileostomy patients who underwent follow-up at the Cleveland Clinic, 72% considered that they led normal lives without restriction, 24% stated that they had minor restrictions or difficulties adjusting to an ileostomy, and only 4% said that they regretted having had the surgery.[3] Roy et al.[4] from the Mayo Clinic reported that 92% of their patients were satisfied with their postoperative status. The major reason for this appears to be that most patients regain their normal physical well-being following surgery. In a similar survey of patients with an ostomy at the Cleveland Clinic, 80% of patients considered their physical health to be good or excellent.[3] Similar results were reported by both Morowitz and Kirsner[5] and Roy et al.[4] Eighty-seven percent and 89% of patients, respectively, considered their postoperative physical well-being to be excellent.

Despite the good overall rating of quality of life, restrictions are encountered by individuals with an ileostomy (Table 5-1). Approximately 10% of patients who were surveyed experienced severe restrictions, and 40% to 50% had moderate restrictions postoperatively associated with diet, ability to participate in sports and hobbies, travel, and clothing selection.[6] However, often these patients had been restricted in their activities of daily living preoperatively and, with the exception of clothing selection, were generally less restricted postoperatively. In other surveys over 90% of patients stated that they were able to return to work and were unrestricted by the ileostomy.[7,8]

Table 5-1. Restrictions with conventional ileostomy in daily activities before and after surgery (%)*

	None		Moderate		Great	
	Before	After	Before	After	Before	After
Diet	24	39	45	48	30	12
Sports	37	42	31	44	27	10
Hobbies	35	51	43	39	19	8
Travel	34	57	39	34	24	8
Clothing selection	54	34	30	53	10	9

*From McLeod RS, Lavery IC, Leatherman JR, et al. Patient evaluation of the conventional ileostomy. Dis Colon Rectum 28:152, 1985. Copyright © American Society of Colon and Rectal Surgeons, Inc.

Problems encountered by patients with an ileostomy who were surveyed at the Cleveland Clinic included skin irritation (49%), offensive odor and noise (42%), and detection of the ostomy device by others (17%).[6] Twenty-nine percent stated that they had difficulties in maintenance of the ostomy management system. On the whole, however, all these problems were less troublesome than expected, and 90% of the patients stated that they devoted less than 1 hour per day to care of the ileostomy. Roy et al.[4] reported that 85% of patients felt that caring for the ileostomy was not difficult.

Despite concerns about the psychologic impact of a stoma, most patients do adjust well to the ileostomy. In a report from the Cleveland Clinic, approximately 80% noted that their emotional health was good or excellent and a similar proportion felt that they had a positive body image.[3] Only 10% experienced negative feelings from employers, friends, or family. Morowitz and Kirsner[5] also reported that 12% of patients with an ileostomy had some emotional problems related to the ileostomy. A survey by Burnham et al.[9] revealed that 12% of such patients believed that their marriages were adversely affected by the ileostomy. Rolstad et al.[10] reported that 30% to 40% of patients with an ileostomy felt that intercourse was more difficult physically or psychologically because of the ileostomy. Fifty to sixty percent of the same group felt less desirable sexually. Fortunately for this group of patients other surgical alternatives are available.

In predicting outcome, Morowitz and Kirsner[5] reported that the length of time patients had the disease before surgery was a significant variable. Ten of the 36 patients (28%) who felt that their health had deteriorated postoperatively had symptoms of ulcerative colitis for less than 1 year before they underwent surgery. In the Cleveland Clinic study the only significant variable was the function of the stoma.[3] Seventeen percent of patients with a poorly constructed stoma were dissatisfied with their quality of life, whereas only 2% of those with a well-constructed stoma were dissatisfied. This response emphasizes the need for a well-constructed and well-functioning stoma.

KOCK CONTINENT ILEOSTOMY

The continent ileostomy was developed by Professor Nils Kock in the late 1960s for those patients who were dissatisfied with the conventional ileostomy. A pouch that acts as a reservoir for stool and a nipple valve that maintains continence are constructed from the terminal ileum. Although the patient still has a stoma, it is flush with the skin and an ostomy management system is unnecessary. To empty the pouch, a catheter is inserted into the reservoir several times per day.

One of the major advantages of the continent ileostomy is that patients feel that they experience fewer restrictions. In a survey of 71 patients with continent ileostomies constructed at the Cleveland Clinic, only 10% noted having restrictions in activities related to work or leisure activities.[11] This response was markedly different from the responses of the 36 patients who had conventional ileostomies prior to conversion to continent ileostomies: 49% to 93% of these patients noted some restrictions in sports, work, hobbies, travel, or clothing selection. The most striking differences were with regard to clothing selection and sports activities. Only 15% of patients with continent ileostomies were limited in these areas, whereas approximately 90% of patients with conventional ileostomies complained of restrictions in these categories. The major restriction that individuals with a continent ileostomy did experience related to food intake. However, restrictions in diet were similar in frequency and severity to those experienced by patients with a conventional ileostomy.

For persons who have difficulty adapting to the conventional ileostomy for psychologic reasons, the continent ileostomy may be considered as a superior alternative. Nilsson et al.[12] reported that 98% of their patients had felt embarrassed or inhibited by the conventional ileostomy but only 24% had these feelings following conversion to a continent ileostomy. Eighty percent thought that their sexual lives were disturbed by the conventional ileostomy, but none of them felt inhibited by the continent ileostomy. Ojerskog et al.[13] reported that the most common reason for patients requesting a continent ileostomy was to achieve a better sex life. They also noted that 64% of patients felt that their overall sexual satisfaction was improved following construction of the continent ileostomy. Many of these patients also reported an improvement in body image and self-esteem. In our survey 80% of our patients noted that their body image was improved following conversion of their conventional ileostomy to a continent ileostomy.[11]

Despite the high surgical complication rate, most patients are extremely happy with what they perceive as a superior quality of life and are often willing to undergo multiple procedures in order to live without an ostomy management system. In fact, most would prefer to have revisional surgery rather than to have the continent ileostomy removed. In the Cleveland Clinic survey all patients stated that retrospectively they would have chosen to have a continent ileostomy.[11] Ninety-six percent found the result to be as good as or better than their preoperative expectations, and 97% stated that they would undergo revisional surgery rather than have removal of the continent ileostomy.

ILEOANAL POUCH PROCEDURE

As a result of the contributions of Sir Alan Parks and Professor J. Utsunomiya as well as others, patients requiring surgery now have another alternative: the ileoanal pouch procedure. In this procedure a reservoir is constructed from small bowel and is anastomosed to the preserved anal sphincter muscles. The major advantage of this operation is that patients do not have a permanent stoma and they evacuate via the normal route. Neither catheters nor ostomy management systems are necessary.

In a survey of our patients who have had this procedure, over 95% stated that their physical health was normal.[14] Eighty percent said that they had a good appetite and energy level. Approximately 50% of patients avoided some foods, particularly vegetables or gas-producing foods, or restricted the times at which they ate. However, only 15% stated that their bowel function interfered with their work or daily activities. Overall, 77% felt that they had an excellent result, 14% a good one, 5% a fair one, and only 4% a poor result.

Similarly, Pezim and Nicholls[15] surveyed 55 patients who had undergone the ileal pouch procedure at St. Mark's Hospital in London. All these patients had a temporary ileostomy constructed at the time of surgery. Eighty-seven percent of these patients preferred the reservoir to the ileostomy. A similar proportion felt more confident, had a better self-image, and felt that they were less restricted in their social and sports activities and work. Sixty-seven percent said that there was no significant disadvantage associated with the reservoir, whereas 20% saw the long convalescent period and 18% the requirement for catheterization as drawbacks to the procedure.

In evaluating the ileoanal pouch procedure, most reports have focused on the functional results. In order to assess domains other than physical status, we surveyed 50 patients who had an ileoanal pouch.[16] This group included patients who, in the opinions of the attending surgeons, had both good and poor results. Despite this fact, approximately 80% of the patients felt that they were not restricted in participating in sports, hobbies and leisure activities, traveling, and performing their jobs or attending school. Over 90% said that their confidence and self-esteem were good or excellent. Less than 10% of patients felt embarrassed by their bowel function. Eighty-five percent stated that they had normal sexual function.

This same group of patients was also asked to rate, on a scale of 0 to 10, the importance of 33 measures used to assess outcome.[16] Included in this list were factors in the physical domain (e.g., well-being, stool frequency, continence), the psychologic area (e.g., self-esteem, confidence, embarrassment), and the social domain (e.g., ability to perform activities of normal living, sports, work). Six of the 33 factors had mean ratings greater than 9: (1) the ability to perform normal activities, (2) the ability to pursue a career, (3) the ability to do leisure activities, (4) having a feeling of well-being, (5) having a good energy level, and (6) having normal sexual function. Stool frequency, which obviously affects the other factors, was, however, rated lower. Having fewer than 20 bowel movements per day was rated seventh, and having fewer than 5 bowel movements per day was rated as low as twenty-fourth. This survey confirmed our impression that continence (rated eighth) and absence of urgency (rated fourteenth) are important to the patient but stool frequency, as long as it is less than 10 bowel movements per day, is often less important. Indeed, a previous study had indicated that patients' recall of their stool frequency tended to be inaccurate.[17] The results of this survey also suggest that issues other than stool frequency may be more important in assessing the outcome of the procedure.

COMPARISON OF QUALITY OF LIFE

It is apparent that discrepancies arise in the assessment of the conventional ileostomy when the assessment is made by patients who have a conventional ileostomy or those who have a continent ileostomy or an ileoanal pouch. Patients who have had a conversion to a continent ileostomy complain of many more restrictions and inhibitions than those who keep a conventional ileostomy.[11] In part, this difference may be the result of a selection bias. Only those patients who are sufficiently dissatisfied with the conventional ileostomy actually choose to have a continent ileostomy. The difference also may be a result of the fact that the ileostomy is a temporary one, especially for patients undergoing the ileoanal pouch procedure. In this situation often the patient does not accept and adapt well to the ileostomy. In the case of a loop ileostomy, the ileostomy may not function optimally. However, patients differ in their life-styles and expectations, and the majority of patients with a conventional ileostomy adapt well to it. It is important to remember that all of the procedures have advantages and disadvantages and therefore one patient may be satisfied with one procedure whereas another may not. For this reason patients should be fully informed of all the surgical options and should be involved in the preoperative decision-making process.

Several studies have attempted to compare the quality of life of patients following the various procedures.[11-13,15,18-21] Unfortunately, these studies are not randomized controlled trials, which would not be ethical or feasible to perform, so there may be biases involved. Kohler et al.[18] surveyed patients who had undergone surgery for ulcerative colitis or familial adenomatous polyposis at the Mayo Clinic. The patients included 406 patients with a conventional ileostomy, 403 with a Kock continent ileostomy, and 300 with an ileoanal pouch. Patients who had an ileoanal pouch tended to be less restricted in their ability to participate in sports and sexual activity when compared to those with a conventional ileostomy. Patients with a Kock continent ileostomy were more restricted in food intake and ability to travel. Overall, however, over 90% of patients in all groups were satisfied with their current status.

In an attempt to quantitate quality of life following these procedures, our group used two techniques to measure quality of life—the time trade-off technique and the direct questioning of objectives.[19] These instruments are used for estimating the perceived worth or utility of a given health state. The utility scale ranges from zero for death to 1 for perfect health. Both instruments have been used to measure quality of life in other disease states and have been found to be both reliable and valid.[22,23] In our study three groups of patients were interviewed: those with a conventional ileostomy, those with a continent ileostomy, and those with an ileoanal pouch. Included in the samples were patients with a range of outcomes as judged by the attending surgeon. Some patients, in fact, were contemplating further surgery because of their desire for one of the other procedures or because of failure of the procedure at the time of the interview. When either technique was used, the mean utilities were similar for all three groups of patients, with utilities ranging from 0.86 to 0.97. The results of this study again confirmed that quality of life of patients following surgery is high, irrespective of the procedure. This study also demonstrated an improvement in quality of life postoperatively, with mean utilities changing from approximately 0.45 preoperatively to 0.9 postoperatively.

LIFE WITH A COLOSTOMY

There is even less written in the literature about the quality of life of patients with a colostomy than for those with an ileostomy. One can only speculate on the reason. Certainly cancer of the rectum, the most common indication for a permanent colostomy, is more common than inflammatory bowel disease and familial adenomatous polyposis. One reason for the lack of information may be that individuals with a colostomy are usually older than those with an ileostomy. A more likely reason, however, is that there is no other alternative for most patients and that survival is a primary concern. As a result, quality of life may be considered unimportant. Obviously, this attitude should not be the norm.

Wirsching et al.[24] reported on the psychosocial outcome of 114 patients who had an abdominoperineal resection for carcinoma of the rectum on average 10 years previously. Seventy-five percent of patients judged their present health status to be good. Many patients, however, complained of depression and loneliness. Devlin[25] reported that only 60% of patients with a colostomy claim to have an unrestricted social life. It is not clear, however, whether the difficulties experienced by these patients are related to the colostomy per se or to the underlying disease. Coe and Kluka[26] assessed 20 patients who underwent surgery for cancer, with 17 permanent colostomies and three ileal conduits resulting. The most common concerns of this small cohort of patients pertained to the cancer, whereas concerns related to the stoma, while present, were of lesser importance.

Von Smitten et al.[27] reported on 54 patients who had an end colostomy. Of these, 89% were able to care for their stomas. Only one patient experienced severe social restrictions as a result of the stoma, but another 13 (24%) reported some impairment. Surgical complications were frequent in these patients; they included paracolostomy hernias in 48%. In addition, stoma stenosis, retraction of the stoma, and peristomal irritation were experienced by a small number of patients.

SUMMARY

Quality of life is becoming increasingly important to the surgeon as well as to the patient. As patients become better informed, they demand more information about both the surgical procedure and their long-term outlook. It therefore behooves the surgeon to consider quality of life and to measure it objectively with instruments that are sensitive, reliable, accurate, and valid. The development of instruments to measure quality of life is also important so that modifications of techniques and new procedures can be evaluated adequately.

Despite the limitations of studies assessing quality of life, it appears that quality of life is good in most patients with an ileostomy or a colostomy. Although some restrictions may be encountered, most patients are able to lead a normal life.

REFERENCES

1. Shumaker SA, Anderson RT, Czajkowski SM. Psychological tests and scales. In Spilker B, ed. Quality of Life Assessments in Clinical Trials. New York: Raven Press, 1990, pp 95-114.
2. Schipper H, Clinch J, Powell V. Definitions and conceptual issues. In Spilker B, ed. Quality of Life Assessments in Clinical Trials. New York: Raven Press, 1990, pp 11-24.
3. McLeod RS, Lavery IC, Leatherman JR, Maryland PA, Fazio VW, Jagelman DG, Weakley FL. Factors affecting quality of life with a conventional ileostomy. World J Surg 10:474, 1986.
4. Roy PH, Sauer WG, Beahrs OH, Farrow GM. Experience with ileostomies. Evaluation of long-term rehabilitation in 497 patients. Am J Surg 119:77, 1970.
5. Morowitz DA, Kirsner JB. Ileostomy in ulcerative colitis. A questionnaire study of 1,803 patients. Am J Surg 141:370, 1981.
6. McLeod RS, Lavery IC, Leatherman JR, Maryland PA, Fazio VW, Jagelman DG, Weakley FL. Patient evaluation of the conventional ileostomy. Dis Colon Rectum 28:152, 1985.
7. Bone J, Sorensen FH. Live with a conventional ileostomy. Dis Colon Rectum 17:194, 1974.

8. Gruner OPN, Naas R, Fretheim B. Marital status and sexual adjustment after colectomy. Results in 178 patients operated on for ulcerative colitis. Scand J Gastroenterol 12:193, 1977.
9. Burnham WR, Lennard-Jones JE, Brooke BN. Sexual problems among married ileostomists. Survey conducted by the Ileostomy Association of Great Britain and Ireland. Gut 18:673, 1977.
10. Rolstad BS, Wilson G, Rothenberger DA. Sexual concerns in the patient with an ileostomy. Dis Colon Rectum 26:170, 1983.
11. McLeod RS, Fazio VW. Quality of life with the continent ileostomy. World J Surg 8:90, 1984.
12. Nilsson LP, Kock NG, Kylberg F, Myrvold HE, Palselius I. Sexual adjustment in ileostomy patients before and after conversion to continent ileostomy. Dis Colon Rectum 24:287, 1981.
13. Ojerskog B, Hallstrom T, Kock NG, Myrvold HE. Quality of life in ileostomy patients before and after conversion to the continent ileostomy. Int J Colorect Dis 3:166, 1988.
14. Fleshman J, Cohen Z, McLeod RS, Stern H. The ileal reservoir and ileoanal anastomosis procedure: Factors affecting outcome following the pelvic pouch procedure. Dis Colon Rectum 31:5, 1988.
15. Pezim ME, Nicholls RJ. Quality of life after restorative proctocolectomy with pelvic ileal reservoir. Br J Surg 72:33, 1986.
16. McLeod RS, Cohen Z. Unpublished data, 1990.
17. McHugh SM, Diamant NE, McLeod R, Cohen Z. S-pouches vs. J-pouches. A comparison of functional outcomes. Dis Colon Rectum 30:671, 1987.
18. Kohler LW, Pemberton JH, Zinsmeister AR, Kelly KA. Quality of life after proctocolectomy. A comparison of Brooke ileostomy, Kock pouch, and ileal pouch–anal anastomosis. Gastroenterology 101:679, 1991.
19. McLeod RS, Churchill DN, Lock AM, Vanderburgh S, Cohen Z. Quality of life of patients with ulcerative colitis preoperatively and postoperatively. Gastroenterology 101:1307, 1991.
20. Pemberton JH, Phillips SF, Ready RR, Zinsmeister AR, Beahrs OH. Quality of life after Brooke ileostomy and ileal pouch–anal anastomosis. Ann Surg 209:620, 1989.
21. Kock NG, Darle N, Kewenter J, Myrvold H, Philipson B. The quality of life after proctocolectomy and ileostomy. A study of patients with conventional ileostomies converted to continent ileostomies. Dis Colon Rectum 17:287, 1974.
22. Detsky AS, McLaughlin JR, Abrams HB, L'Abbe KA, Whitwell J, Bombardier C, Jeejeebhoy KN. Quality of life of patients on long-term total parenteral nutrition at home. J Gen Intern Med 1:26, 1986.
23. Torrance GW, Thomas WH, Sackett DL. A utility maximization model for evaluation of health care program. Health Serv Res 7:118, 1972.
24. Wirsching M, Druner HU, Herrmann G. Results of psychosocial adjustment to long-term colostomy. Psychother Psychosom 26:245, 1975.
25. Devlin HB. Colostomy: Past and present. Ann Coll Surg Phys 72:175, 1990.
26. Coe M, Kluka S. Comparison of concerns of clients and spouses regarding ostomy surgery for treatment of cancer: Phase II. J Enterostom Ther 17:106, 1990.
27. Von Smitten K, Husa A, Kyllonen L. Long-term results of sigmoidostomy in patients with anorectal malignancy. Acta Chir Scand 152:211, 1986.

PART TWO

OPERATIVE TECHNIQUES

6 END SIGMOID COLOSTOMY

David E. Beck

Creation of a colostomy is one of the oldest surgical operations. Due to advances in stapling techniques and procedures such as a coloanal pull-through, the frequency with which surgeons create end colostomies is decreasing. However, this ostomy remains one of the most common ones that a surgeon will perform. An ostomy is an anastomosis of the intestine to the skin, and, like any other anastomosis, it must be constructed with care. The principles of adequate blood supply, lack of tension, minimization of tissue trauma, and avoidance of contamination must be followed to achieve a good result.

INDICATIONS AND CONTRAINDICATIONS

The primary indications for an end sigmoid colostomy include (1) reconstruction after abdominoperineal resection for malignancy, (2) permanent diversion for radiation proctitis or rectal fistulas, and (3) temporary diversion for emergency surgery for peritonitis associated with diverticulitis, trauma, or bowel perforation.

Any patient undergoing intra-abdominal bowel surgery has some potential need for a stoma, and it is incumbent on the surgeon to consider this possibility in the preoperative period. Those patients with a high probability of requiring a stoma should be extensively educated by a stoma therapist and their surgeon. The site for the stoma should be selected according to the method described in Chapters 3 and 9. The sites commonly used for a sigmoid colostomy are depicted in Fig. 6-1. The left lower transrectus area is the primary choice because it can be conveniently reached by the patient and allows for the easy application of a pouch. If the patient's bodily characteristics make this site inappropriate or if available bowel length is a concern, an

☐ The opinions expressed in this chapter are those of the author and do not reflect the opinions of the United States Air Force or the Department of Defense.

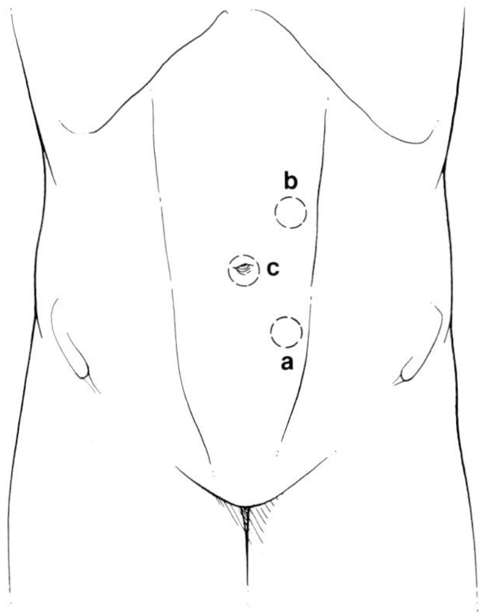

Fig. 6-1. Stoma placement options with sigmoid colostomy: *a,* left lower lateral rectus; *b,* left upper lateral rectus; *c,* umbilical area.

upper transrectus site may be used. Kodner and associates[1,2] have described excellent results with a midline site. I have used this site with good results in patients who do not have a transrectus site available, but I do not consider it as a primary choice.

If the creation of a permanent stoma can be avoided without harming the patient, the surgeon should do so. Although there are no absolute contraindications to creating a stoma, certain conditions are complicated if a stoma is required. Such conditions include ascites and portal hypertension. In addition, patients with physical disabilities such as arthritis or blindness may find it difficult to care for a stoma.

OPERATIVE TECHNIQUE

As with other resectional operations, the procedure performed should be determined by the patient's disease processes rather than whether the patient will need a stoma. Thus an adequate operation should be performed first, and consideration of the need for a stoma should be second. Since the end of the remaining proximal bowel will be brought through the abdominal wall to create a stoma, it is helpful to divide the proximal bowel with a linear cutting stapler. This method reduces the potential for contamination from bowel contents. After the bowel has been divided, the left colon must be adequately mobilized. The avascular peritoneal reflection is incised as shown in Fig. 6-2, *A.* The posterior surface of the left colon is mobilized by dissection in the

A

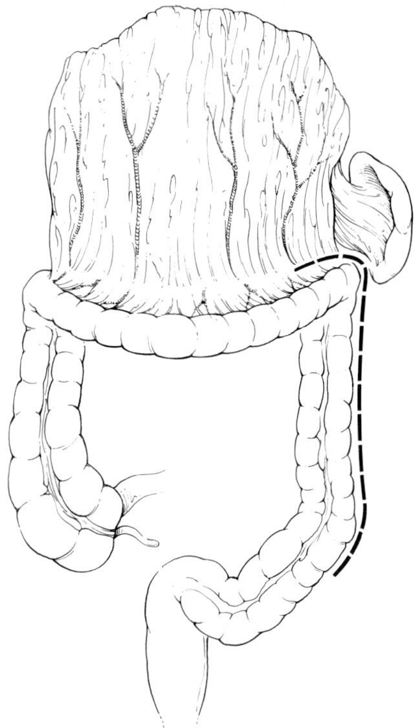

Fig. 6-2. **A**, Mobilization of left colon. **B**, Cross-section demonstrating line of incision for mobilization. **C**, Transection of mesentery, vessels, and colon: *a*, proximal inferior mesenteric artery; *b*, inferior mesenteric distal to left colic artery; *c*, left colic artery.

B

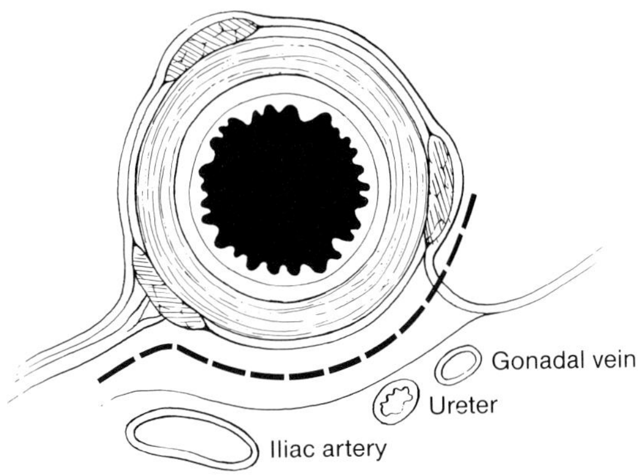

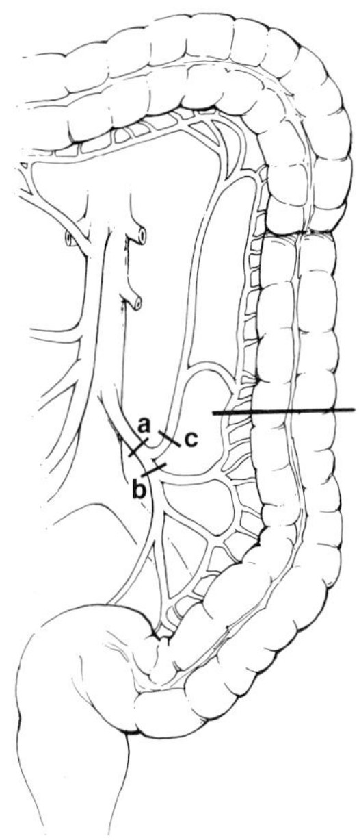

C

avascular plane between the posterior bowel wall and the retroperitoneum. Dissection in the correct plane leaves the gonadal vessels, ureter, and iliac vessels in their normal anatomic position and lessens the risk of injury (Fig. 6-2, *B*). An adequate length of well-vascularized bowel (enough to extend 3 to 4 cm above skin level) must be available. If a significant portion of the sigmoid or distal colon is resected, the splenic flexure often will need to be mobilized. In addition, it may be necessary to divide the inferior mesenteric artery at its takeoff from the aorta (Fig. 6-2, *C*).

To create the ostomy opening in the abdominal wall, the following techniques are used. First, clamps (e.g., Kocher clamps) are attached to the edges of Scarpa's fascia and the rectus sheath. The surgeon holds these clamps with equal traction to maintain the skin and the fascia in alignment.[3] A folded lap pad is placed under the stoma site. Using his left hand, the surgeon elevates the abdominal wall and retracts it to the anatomic midline. Next, a circular skin opening is made with a scalpel (Fig. 6-3, *A*). Proper technique allows a circular skin opening to be made. The practice of elevating the skin with a clamp and cutting a skin disk with scissors should be avoided because it often produces an oval skin opening, which results in pouching difficulties for the patient. After the dermis has been cut, the circular piece of skin is separated from the subcutaneous fat with electrocautery. An effort is made to leave as much fat as possible because retention of this tissue helps to support the stoma and reduces the potential for stomal hernias.

A vertical incision is then made in the subcutaneous fat with electrocautery. Retractors (e.g., Army-Navy retractors) are used to hold back the fat and expose the anterior rectus sheath (Fig. 6-3, *B*). This fascia is also incised in a vertical direction from the top to the bottom of the stoma site by making an incision approximately two to three fingerwidths in length. With the retractors kept in place, the ends of scissors (or a straight clamp) are inserted through the rectus muscle between its fibers to the posterior fascia. The instrument is rotated (perpendicular to the direction of the fibers) and opened so that it splits the muscle. With the instrument held open, the retractors are repositioned one at a time, engaging the rectus muscle and retracting each split edge laterally. Electrocautery is used to make a vertical incision in the posterior fascia two to three fingerwidths in length. The surgeon's left index finger and third finger are then passed through the stoma opening from inside to outside, and the retractors are removed. This maneuver tests the size of the stoma opening. For most patients the correctly sized opening should tightly admit two average-size fingers. Obese patients or those with dilated bowel or thick mesentery may require a larger stomal opening. A Babcock clamp is then passed from outside to inside through the stoma site by following the path of the surgeon's fingers. The tip of the clamp is then elevated, exposing the inner stoma opening for inspection. Any bleeding vessels can be identified easily, and the bleeding can be managed with ligatures or electrocautery.

Cutting the muscle or the fascia in a horizontal or cruciate direction should be avoided. Making vertical incisions and splitting the muscle parallel to its fibers allows the natural contraction forces of the muscle to work to-

A

B

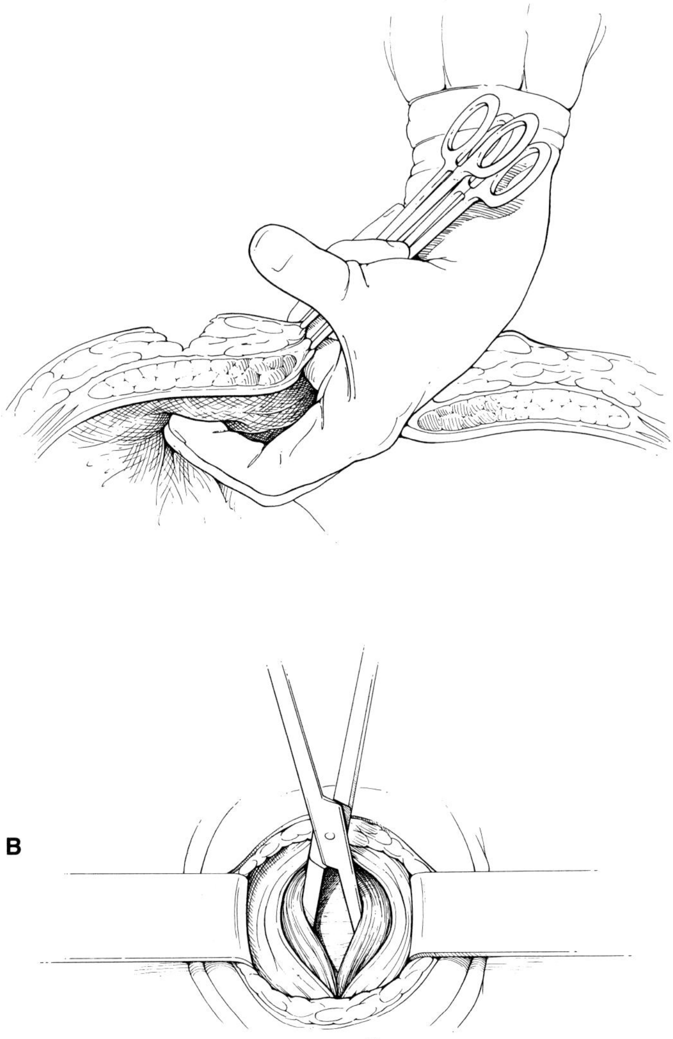

Fig. 6-3. Construction of end colostomy. **A,** Incision of abdominal wall at stoma site to create a circular skin opening. **B,** Rectus sheath has been incised in a vertical direction, and rectus muscle is split.

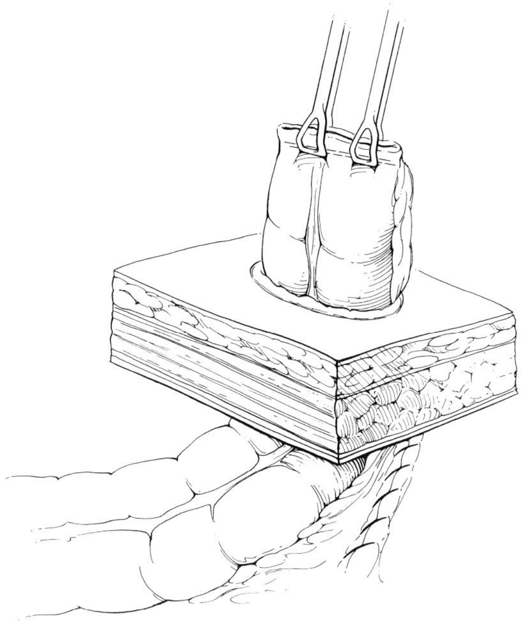

Fig. 6-4. Colon is delivered through stoma wound, and mesenteric defect is closed.

gether to support the stoma. Horizontal division of the muscle or the fascia results in distraction of the muscle ends and produces a tendency for the stomal opening to become larger. This situation increases the probability of stomal hernia.

The stapled end of the colon is then grasped with a Babcock clamp, and the bowel is maneuvered through the stomal opening in the abdominal wall (Fig. 6-4). The bowel should be pushed from the inside rather than being pulled with the clamp to prevent tearing of the bowel or its mesentery. The end of the bowel should be brought 3 to 4 cm above the skin level to allow adequate length for maturation. The surgeon should err by bringing out more rather than less bowel. The mesenteric defect may be closed or left completely open. Partial closure of this defect should be avoided because such closure creates a smaller opening, which increases the opportunity for a symptomatic internal hernia.

In patients with adequate length of bowel and in whom peristomal hernia or ascites may be a problem, an extraperitoneal stoma may be created. An extraperitoneal tunnel is created by incising the parietal peritoneum at the lateral abdominal wall. Blunt dissection with the surgeon's fingers or a clamp is done to create a tunnel from this lateral opening to the area posterior to the

A

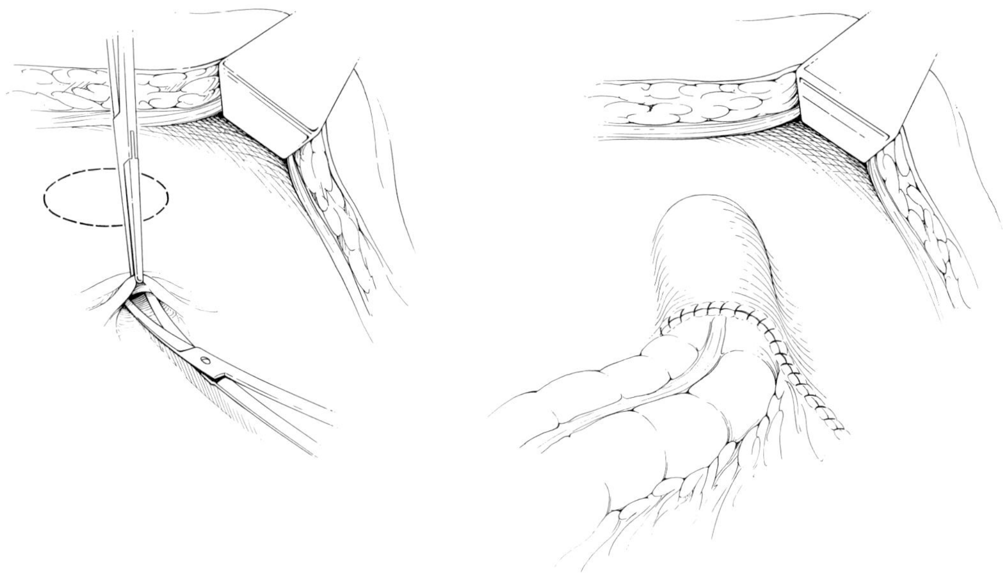

B

Fig. 6-5. Extraperitoneal colostomy. **A,** Peritoneum is opened, and an extraperitoneal tunnel is created with blunt dissection. **B,** Colon is brought through tunnel, and mesenteric defect is closed.

rectus stomal opening (Fig. 6-5, *A*). The bowel is brought through this tunnel and taken out of the ostomy opening (Fig. 6-5, *B*).

The midline abdominal wound is closed, and the skin is approximated in the usual manner. If the patient's condition dictates that the wound be left open, the skin adjacent to the stoma should be approximated and the subcutaneous tissue beneath it can be packed with gauze from the remainder of the open wound. A towel or lap sponge is placed over the closed incision, and the stoma is matured. Virtually no indication exists for delayed maturation in modern management of colostomies.[1] The staple line at the end of the bowel is excised with scissors or electrocautery, and a mucosal to deep dermal approximation is accomplished with interrupted 3-0 chromic sutures (Fig. 6-6). Eight properly placed sutures produce a circumferential mucocutaneous approximation. For obese patients or for those undergoing reconstruction of a stoma, additional sutures may be placed prior to maturation of the stoma. Three or four 3-0 chromic sutures placed from the serosa to Scarpa's fascia tend to pull in the subcutaneous tissue and "mound" the stoma. Stitching from the end of bowel to the bowel serosa to the deep dermis (three-point fixation) should be avoided because incorrect placement of such stitching can lead to a skin level fistula.

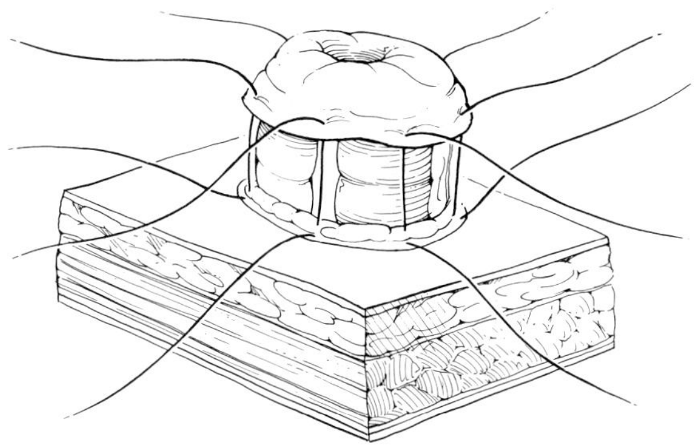

Fig. 6-6. Colostomy maturation. Sutures are placed from the bowel (full thickness) to the deep dermal layer of the skin.

COMPLICATIONS

Compared to other stomas, end colostomies are associated with fewer complications.[4] Potential complications are minimized when the procedures described in this chapter are followed. For ease of understanding, stomal complications have been divided into early and late complications.

The majority of early complications are technically related. Ischemia of the stoma results from inadequate arterial perfusion. Such ischemia occurs when the vascular arcade supplying the left colon is damaged or is inappropriately divided. Problems also can occur if the colonic vessels are placed under too much tension. Division of the inferior mesenteric artery at its origin (between the aorta and the takeoff of the left colic artery [see Fig. 6-2, *C*]) often will release excessive tension while maintaining adequate perfusion. If additional length is required, division of the inferior mesenteric vein at the inferior border of the pancreas may be necessary.

An ischemic stoma initially will appear edematous and then will progress to discoloration and finally necrosis. The depth of the ischemia can be assessed by a number of methods. Inspection of the stoma with the ostomy management system removed is helpful. An endoscope or a glass test tube with an external light can be inserted into the stoma to visualize the intrastomal mucosa. The stoma also can be punctured with a needle. Viable stomas will bleed at the puncture site, whereas nonviable ones will not.

If the ischemia is superficial, it should be observed closely. The ischemic mucosa will often sluff, but the remaining mucosa will grow to close the defect. Full-thickness necrosis above the fascia will result in stenosis after healing, but ischemia below the fascia requires urgent operative revision to prevent intra-abdominal contamination. Inadequate venous drainage usually results from injury of the venous arcade close to the bowel wall. Inadequate drainage causes stomal edema (associated with a bluish discoloration) but will rarely cause tissue loss. Division of the inferior mesenteric vein close to the splenic vein, as described above, does not cause this problem.

Mucocutaneous separation usually is caused by inadequate or improper approximation of the mucosa to the dermal layer or excessive bowel tension. If the separation is minor, observation is all that is required because wound contraction and healing will close the defect.[5] Complete separation usually requires revision.

Stomal retraction is caused by excessive tension on the bowel. Such tension usually results from failure to adequately mobilize the bowel. Significant retraction requires operative revision.

Hemorrhage can be caused by trauma to the stoma, or it may be a complication of the tissue loss resulting from ischemia. Bleeding from the divided end of the bowel can be controlled with digital pressure, cauterization, or suture ligation. Stomal lacerations or bleeding from denuded mucosa often will respond to topical pressure or application of an epinephrine-soaked sponge.

Infection, which is uncommon, is linked to contamination from the bowel. A peristomal or abdominal wall abscess requires immediate drainage. In performing such drainage, care must be taken to avoid injury to the bowel and to minimize wounds that would interfere with the stomal appliance. Cellulitis requires the administration of antibiotics. Significant or recurrent infections raise the possibility of an associated fistula.

Stomal fistulas result from trauma or disease processes. In colostomies such fistulas usually result from excessive fat clearing or inadvertent excision of a diverticulum. Almost all stomal fistulas require operative revision.

Late complications include stenosis, peristomal hernia (Chapter 15), prolapse (Chapter 16), skin problems (Chapter 19), varices (Chapter 20), and lymphoid hyperplasia. Stenosis results from ischemia or stomal retraction. An experienced, well-trained stomal therapist can help the patient cope with many of these problems. However, the patient with significant symptoms may require a local revision of the stoma.

Lymphoid hyperplasia is a benign condition that results from prolonged local trauma. It presents as a fungating nodule on the bowel that slowly increases in size. Occasionally, the lesion may bleed, and if it grows too large, it may make it difficult to place a stomal device. Small nodules can be removed by topical application of silver nitrate. For larger nodules a biopsy should be done to exclude the rare neoplasm of the bowel, which may have a similar gross appearance. Extensive lesions may necessitate a local revision of the stoma.

POSTOPERATIVE CONSIDERATIONS

A modern ostomy management system with a clear pouch should be placed after the stoma has been matured in the operating room. This method protects the stoma and the surrounding skin and facilitates nursing care. In addition, it allows health care providers to easily inspect the stoma.

Many patients can "train" their bowel and colostomy through dietary manipulations or irrigations, as discussed in Chapter 4.[6]

SUMMARY

Although fewer end sigmoid colostomies are being created, this type of colostomy remains an important procedure. Adherence to the principles described in this chapter will improve the chances for creating a well-functioning stoma.

REFERENCES

1. Kodner IJ. Colostomy: Indications, techniques for construction, and management of complications. Semin Colon Rectal Surg 2:73-85, 1991.
2. Kodner IJ, Dubrin PB, Fleshman JW. Comparison of midline and left lower quadrant transrectus colostomies. Presented at 88th Annual Convention of American Society of Colon and Rectal Surgeons, Toronto, Canada, 1989.
3. Kodner IJ. Colostomy and ileostomy. Ciba Found Symp 30:22, 1978.
4. Hawley PR, Ritchie JK. The colon. I. Complications of ileostomy and colostomy following excisional surgery. Clin Gastroenterol 8:403-415, 1979.
5. Thompson JPS. Caecostomy and colostomy. I. Surgical procedures and complications. Clin Gastroenterol 11:285-296, 1982.
6. MacLeod JH. Colostomy irrigation—A transatlantic controversy. Dis Colon Rectum 15:357-360, 1972.

BIBLIOGRAPHY

Beck DE, Welling DR. Patient Care in Colorectal Surgery. Boston: Little, Brown, 1991.
A concise, inexpensive handbook written for the medical student, junior resident, or nurse caring for colorectal patients. In addition to providing a summary of disease processes, it has an excellent chapter on stomas and stomal therapy.

Beck DE, Wexner SD. Fundamentals of Anorectal Surgery. New York: McGraw-Hill, 1992.
A comprehensive, up-to-date textbook of anorectal conditions that may require the creation of a stoma.

Kodner IJ. Colostomy and ileostomy. Ciba Found Symp 30(5):1-30, 1978.
The outstanding color illustrations in this article depict stoma construction and associated complications.

Turnbull RB, Weakley FL. Atlas of Intestinal Stomas. St. Louis: CV Mosby, 1967.
An outstanding atlas of stomas with beautiful illustrations. Currently out of print.

7 DIVERTING STOMAS

Russell K. Pearl and Herand Abcarian

The construction of diverting stomas is an integral part of many operations for colorectal tumors, trauma, and inflammatory bowel disease. These stomas are formed by exteriorizing and maturing a segment of small bowel or colon in which the continuity of the intestinal wall or mesentery is preserved, most often resulting in a loop or end-loop configuration. Traditionally they are used in clinical situations in which proximal fecal diversion must be performed expeditiously and usually on a temporary basis, such as to protect a low anastomosis, decompress obstructed bowel, or prevent fecal material from further contaminating an inflammatory mass. The advantages of diverting stomas include technical ease of construction and, more important, ease of closure (because a formal laparotomy is seldom required). For these reasons diverting stomas, particularly the loop variety, have become the most frequently used type of ostomy in surgical practice.

Several fundamental questions commonly arise during a discussion of diverting stomas. Perhaps the most common one is: Do diverting stomas completely defunctionalize the bowel? Another important and frequently overlooked issue is: How often are diverting stomas temporary? In addition, there has been considerable discussion about which type of diverting stoma—ileostomy or colostomy—is superior with respect to ease of construction, function, and complications. The aim of this chapter is to answer these questions and to review the indications, operative techniques, and complications associated with the construction of diverting stomas.

INDICATIONS

A loop or end-loop ileostomy is often created to protect an ileal pouch–anal anastomosis in a patient with chronic ulcerative colitis or familial adenomatous polyposis coli. Diverting ileostomy also has been used as a temporizing measure in patients with fulminant inflammatory bowel disease, although most surgeons would probably opt for a more definitive procedure if the patient's condition permits.

A diverting colostomy is used most frequently to provide proximal fecal diversion in patients with a large bowel obstruction or pelvic sepsis when a malignant tumor, diverticulitis, colorectal trauma, radiation injury, or a complication of inflammatory bowel disease is present. Recently, such a colostomy has been used to protect a coloanal anastomosis as part of a sphincter-saving procedure for midrectal cancer, radiation-induced stricture, or fistulas.

We would caution against performing a "blind" transverse loop colostomy in cases of large bowel obstruction without manually exploring the abdomen to ascertain the site and resectability of the obstructing lesion. This type of diverting stoma has no value in relieving an obstruction at the ileocecal region or an obstruction due to a sigmoid volvulus.

A tube cecostomy often has been recommended as a convenient and rapid method of decompressing obstructed large bowel. However, regardless of the diameter of the lumen of the tube, a tube cecostomy is relatively ineffective in diverting the fecal stream. It is also prone to leakage of liquid stool from around the tube, which may result in wound complications or intra-abdominal sepsis.

OPERATIVE PLANNING AND TECHNIQUE

Whenever possible, an enterostomal therapist should be involved in the preoperative planning of a stoma, both to provide information about stoma function and care and to offer support and reassurance to the patient and family. Proper selection and marking of the ostomy site is an important consideration in preoperative stoma planning because many complications of ostomies are related to improper siting of the stoma. For example, if an ostomy is brought out too close to a bony prominence, such as the costal margin or the iliac crest, or within skinfolds, scars, or drain sites, it is usually not possible to obtain an adequate skin seal around the stoma. This situation will invariably lead to leakage of liquid stool around the ill-fitting ostomy pouch, which often results in skin irritation.

The patient should be evaluated in the supine, sitting, and (when possible) standing positions to determine optimal ostomy placement. In emergency situations the stoma should be brought out through the rectus muscle in a location surrounded by 2 to 3 inches of flat skin to allow adequate adherence of a pouch. In obese individuals lower abdominal sites should be avoided because of numerous skinfolds created by the protruding abdomen. Many obese patients will be unable to manage or even see their stoma in these locations.

Diverting ileostomies usually are formed in the right lower quadrant, whereas diverting colostomies are brought out along the course of the transverse or sigmoid colon, depending on the site of injury or obstruction. In a survey of technical considerations in the construction of intestinal stomas, 28% of surgeons responded that they routinely bring a loop colostomy through the main laparotomy incision. We believe that this practice makes it difficult to obtain a leak-free seal around the stoma pouch and produces a generally unattractive result.

It is always preferable to mature a loop stoma in the operating room, even in cases of large bowel obstruction. In the past it was feared that this procedure would lead to an unacceptable incidence of sepsis because it was theorized that stool would reenter the peritoneal cavity around the stoma at the mucocutaneous junction. If the distended bowel is carefully decompressed with a needle attached to the suction tubing to minimize fecal spillage prior to opening the loop, this fear is unwarranted. The advantages of primary maturation of a loop stoma in the operating room setting far outweigh the risks of attempting to mature a stoma at the patient's bedside on postoperative day 2 or 3 with suboptimal lighting, equipment, and anesthesia.

Loop Ileostomy

Construction of a loop ileostomy is technically more demanding than construction of most other types of intestinal stomas. In contrast to colonic content, ileal effluent is liquid and rich in skin irritants, such as bile salts, and proteolytic enzymes. In order to avoid complications such as ileostomy dysfunction and skin irritation, the end of the ileum and its mesentery must be mobilized far enough to form a properly everted protruding ileostomy without compromising its blood supply.

A circular skin incision about 2 cm in diameter is made at the designated point and continued through the subcutaneous fat down to the anterior rectus sheath (Fig. 7-1). The space created by removing this cylinder of fat in continuity with the overlying skin provides room for the bowel mesentery in order to minimize vascular compromise. A cruciate incision is made in the anterior rectus fascia with each limb extending about 3 cm. A curved hemostat is used to spread the rectus muscle in the direction of its fibers to expose the posterior rectus sheath or transversalis fascia, and then a short transverse

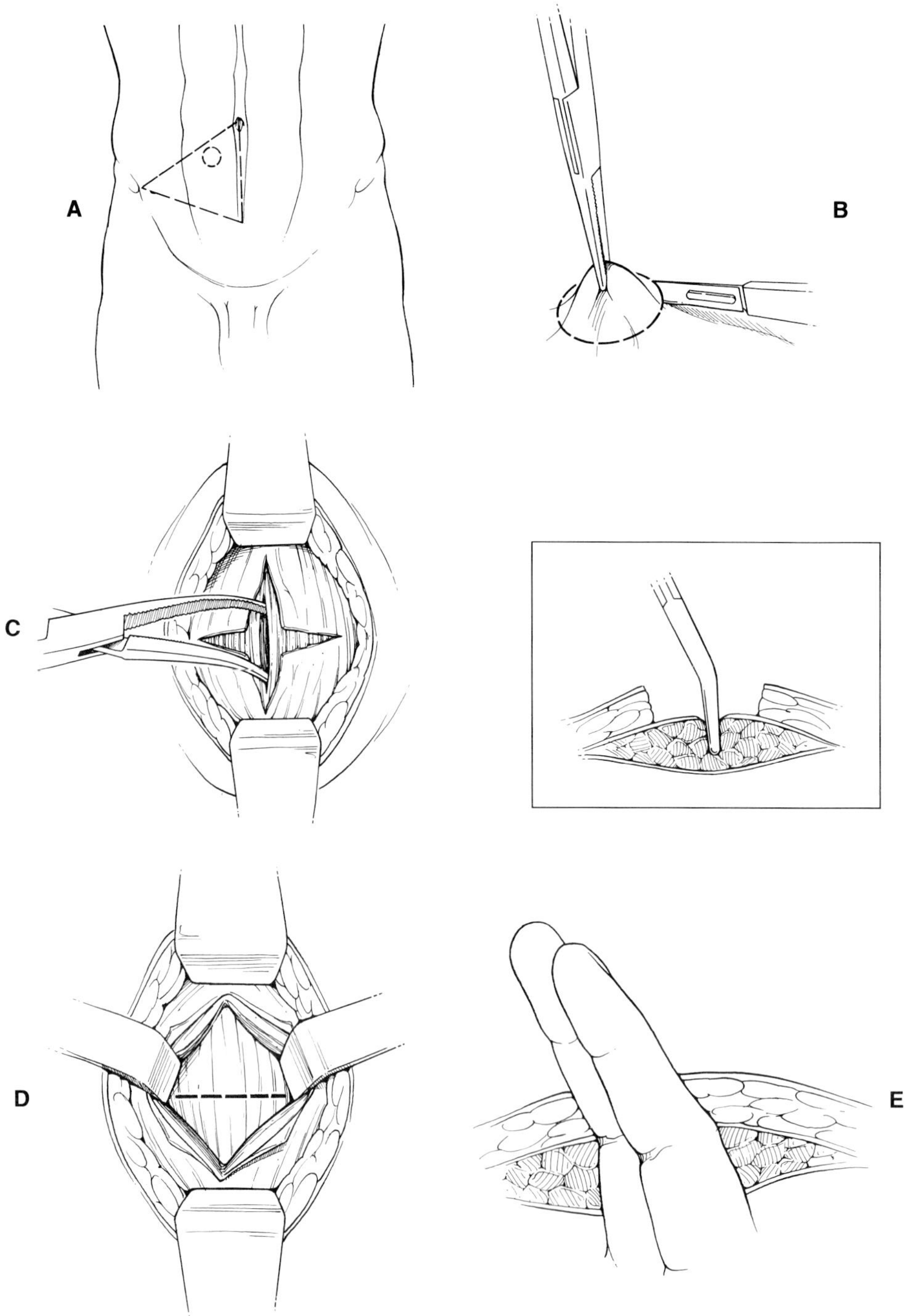

Fig. 7-1. Unplanned loop ileostomy. **A,** The incision should be placed within the triangle formed by the anterior superior iliac spine, the umbilicus, and the pubis overlying the rectus sheath. **B,** A circular skin incision approximately 2 cm in diameter is made. **C,** A cruciate incision is made in the anterior rectus sheath. A clamp is used to spread the rectus muscle in the direction of its fibers. **D,** A transverse incision is made in the posterior rectus sheath or the transversalis fascia. **E,** The opening in the abdominal wall should admit two average-size fingers. (After Pearl.)

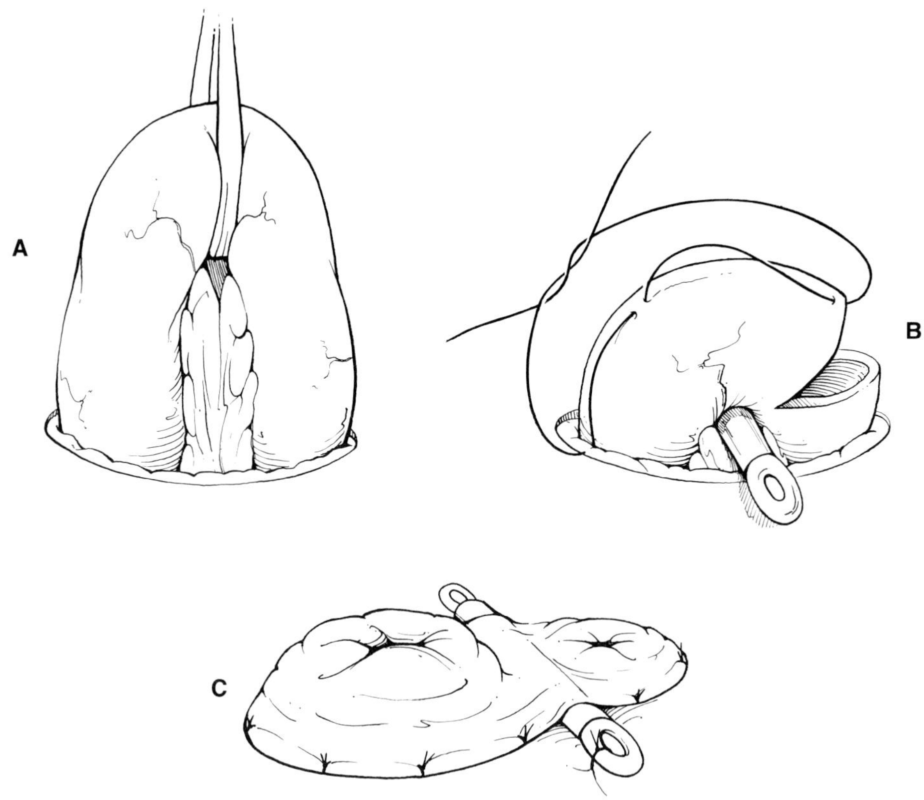

Fig. 7-2. Traditional loop ileostomy. **A,** A rubber drain is passed through a small hole in the mesentery of the segment of ileum to be exteriorized as a loop ileostomy. **B,** A plastic rod is placed through the mesenteric opening to support the loop on the skin and is sutured in place. The loop is opened transversely for about two thirds of its circumference toward the distal end. The longer proximal length of ileum is everted with interrupted absorbable sutures to form a protruding ileostomy. **C,** Completed loop ileostomy. Note the disparity in size and configuration between the proximal and distal lumens. (After Pearl.)

incision is made through this layer and the peritoneum. It is important to ensure that the opening in the rectus muscle is not oblique, and care should be taken to avoid injury to the inferior epigastric vessels. As a general rule, the opening in the abdominal wall should admit two fingers.

When fashioning a traditional loop ileostomy, the surgeon should mobilize the designated loop enough to reach the stoma site on the surface of the abdominal wall without creating undue tension (Fig. 7-2). A small opening is made in the mesentery of the loop adjacent to the ileal wall through which a small rubber drain or umbilical tape is passed. The ends of the drain are grasped with a hemostat, and the loop is gently drawn through the stomal aperture. A small rod or similar device is passed through the mesenteric opening of the loop in place of the drain; it is sutured in place to support the ileum on the abdominal wall. In contrast to the situation with a permanent end ileostomy, the mesentery does not need to be fixed intraperitoneally. It is useful to mark the distal portion of the loop with a silk suture at this point. After the abdominal incision has been closed, the loop is opened transversely for about two thirds of its circumference. This incision should be directed toward the distal end of the loop to ensure enough length to form a properly everted protruding ileostomy. The ileostomy and the defunctionalized ileal limb are sutured to the dermis with absorbable sutures to create a nipple and eversion of the functioning end. Skin protection, usually in the form of a properly fitted methylcellulose wafer (Stomahesive, ConvaTec [Bristol-Meyers Squibb], Princeton, N.J.), and an ostomy device are then applied before the patient leaves the operating room. The rod usually can be removed in 7 to 10 days.

Loop Colostomy

In many ways the construction of a loop colostomy and a loop ileostomy are similar (Fig. 7-3). However, because the colon is larger in diameter than the

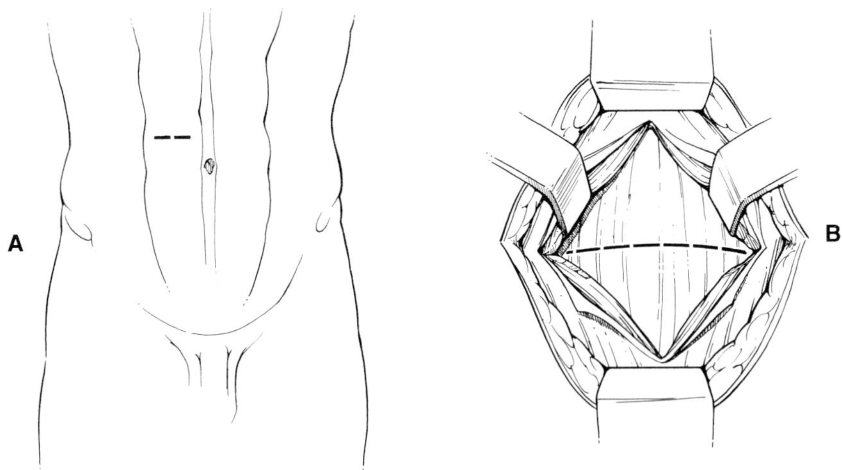

Fig. 7-3. Loop colostomy. **A,** A transverse incision is made in the right upper quadrant. **B,** The rectus muscle is often partially divided to allow for more complete eversion of the stoma. A transverse incision is made in the posterior rectus sheath.

small bowel, it is sometimes necessary to partially divide some of the rectus muscle at the ostomy site to allow for complete eversion of the stoma. The greater omentum should be dissected from the colon around the point of partial transection to facilitate maturation. As with a loop ileostomy, a rod is placed through the mesentery of the colon to support the loop on the surface of the abdomen; the rod is usually left in place for 7 to 10 days. Separate fascioseromuscular tacking sutures are not only unnecessary but may, in fact, interfere with the closure. The loop is opened in a transverse fashion for about two thirds of its circumference. The full thickness of the bowel wall of each limb is everted and sutured to the surrounding skin with interrupted absorbable sutures so that the bowel wall is nearly flush with the abdominal wall, and a colostomy management system is applied.

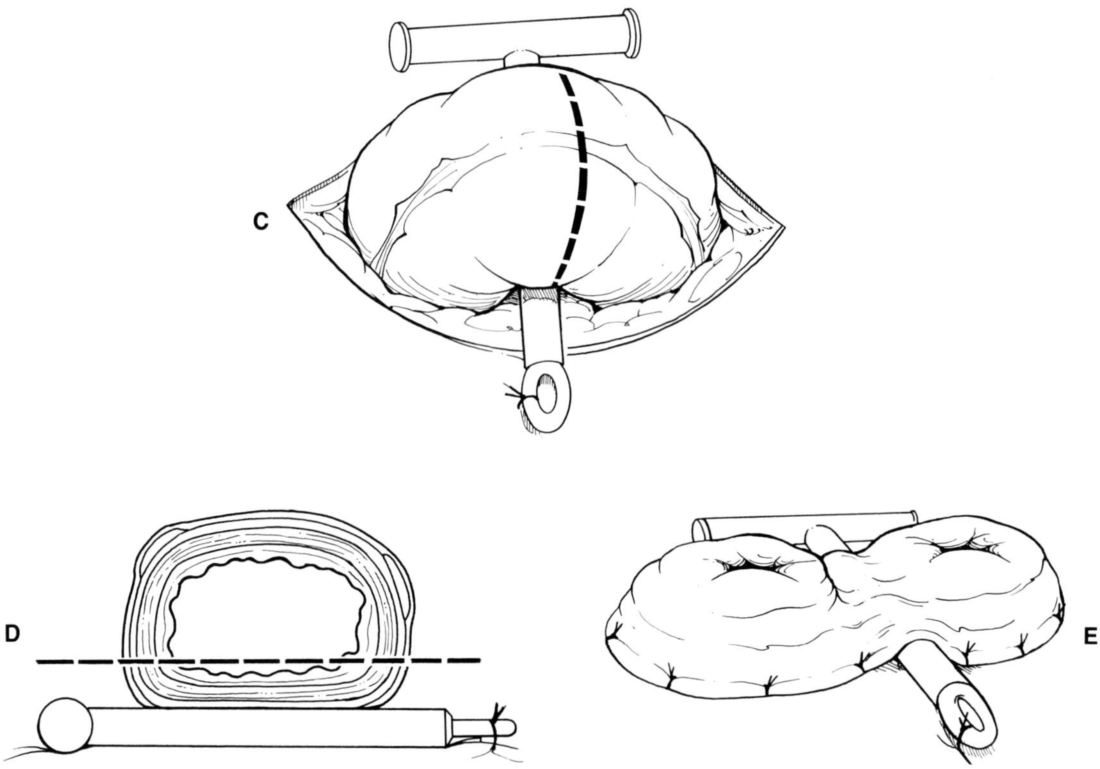

Fig. 7-3, cont'd. C, A supporting rod is placed and then sutured into position. **D,** The exteriorized loop of colon is opened transversely for about two thirds of its circumference. **E,** The loop colostomy is matured primarily with interrupted absorbable sutures. (After Pearl.)

End-Loop Stomas

The rodless end-loop stoma described by Prasad et al. (see Suggested Readings) is a simple modification of a loop stoma with several important advantages. First, it is technically easy to construct. Second, it does not require a supporting rod or a separate opening in the abdominal wall for a mucous fistula. These advantages facilitate stoma care because a single circular ostomy device readily covers the openings of both the proximal and distal limbs without the interference of a rod. End-loop stomas are also easy to close. A formal laparotomy is not required because of the proximity of the two limbs. This fact is a distinct advantage of the end-loop ileocolostomy over the more traditional approach of dealing with the divided ends of the ileum and the transverse colon in cases in which immediate ileocolic anastomosis is inadvisable after right hemicolectomy (e.g., right lower quadrant end ileostomy and left upper quadrant end transverse mucous fistula after penetrating trauma to the right colon). The technical details of the three variations of end-loop stomas are presented in Figs. 7-4 through 7-6.

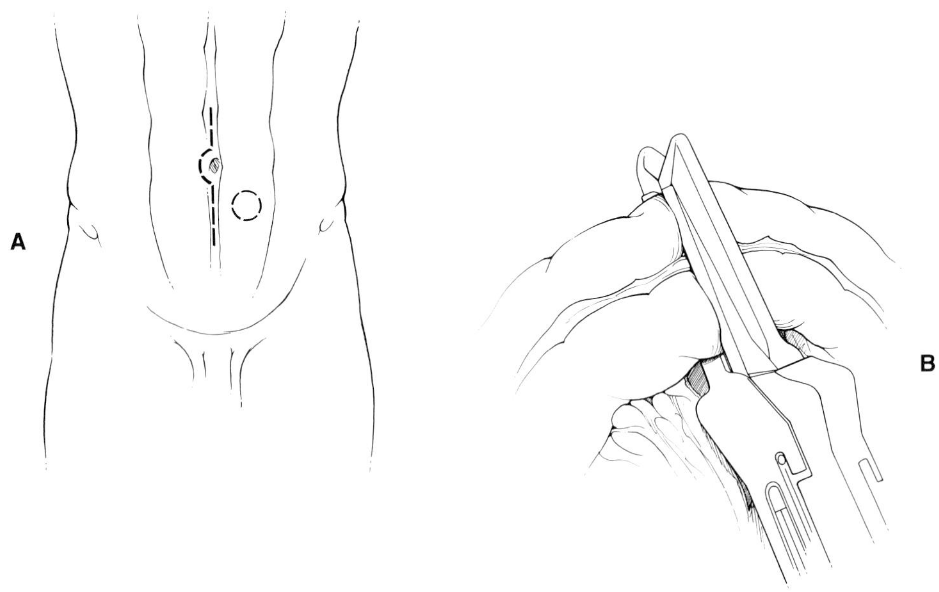

Fig. 7-4. End-loop colostomy. A, After abdominal exploration through a midline incision, a circle of skin is excised and an opening is made through the rectus muscle as for an end colostomy. B, The colon is divided with a linear-cutting stapler at a point where both the proximal and the distal limbs of the colon can be brought through the opening in the abdominal wall without tension.

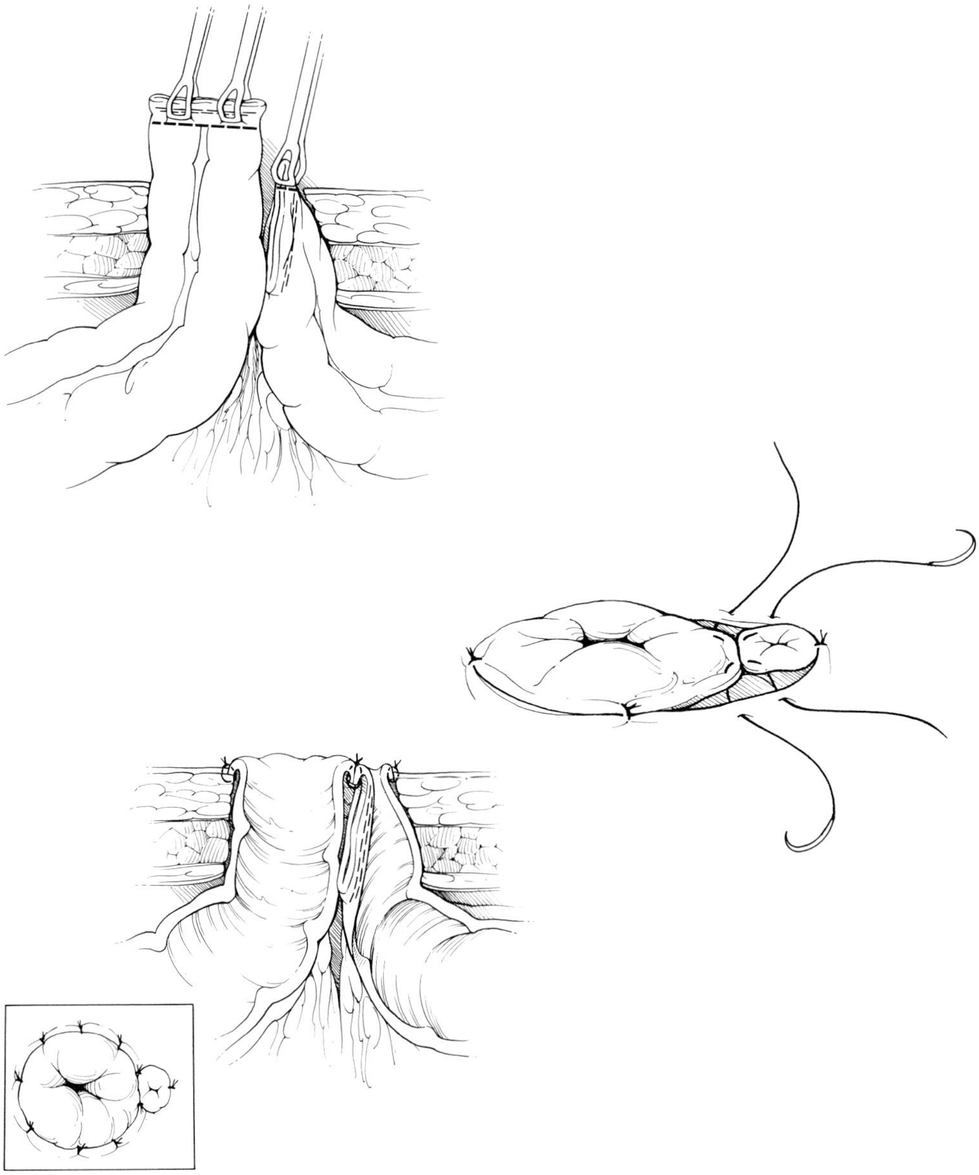

Fig. 7-4, cont'd. C, The entire divided edge of the proximal limb and the antimesenteric corner of the distal limb are gently drawn through the opening in the abdominal wall. After the abdomen has been closed, the staple line of the proximal limb is excised completely and only the antimesenteric corner of the distal staple line is removed. **D,** The proximal limb is matured flush with the skin by suturing full-thickness skin to full-thickness colon with absorbable sutures. Two transition sutures are placed to help mature the mucous fistula, which has the appearance of a "mini-stoma." **E,** Sagittal view of the completed end-loop colostomy. Note the position of the distal staple line in the subcutaneous tissue. (After Pearl.)

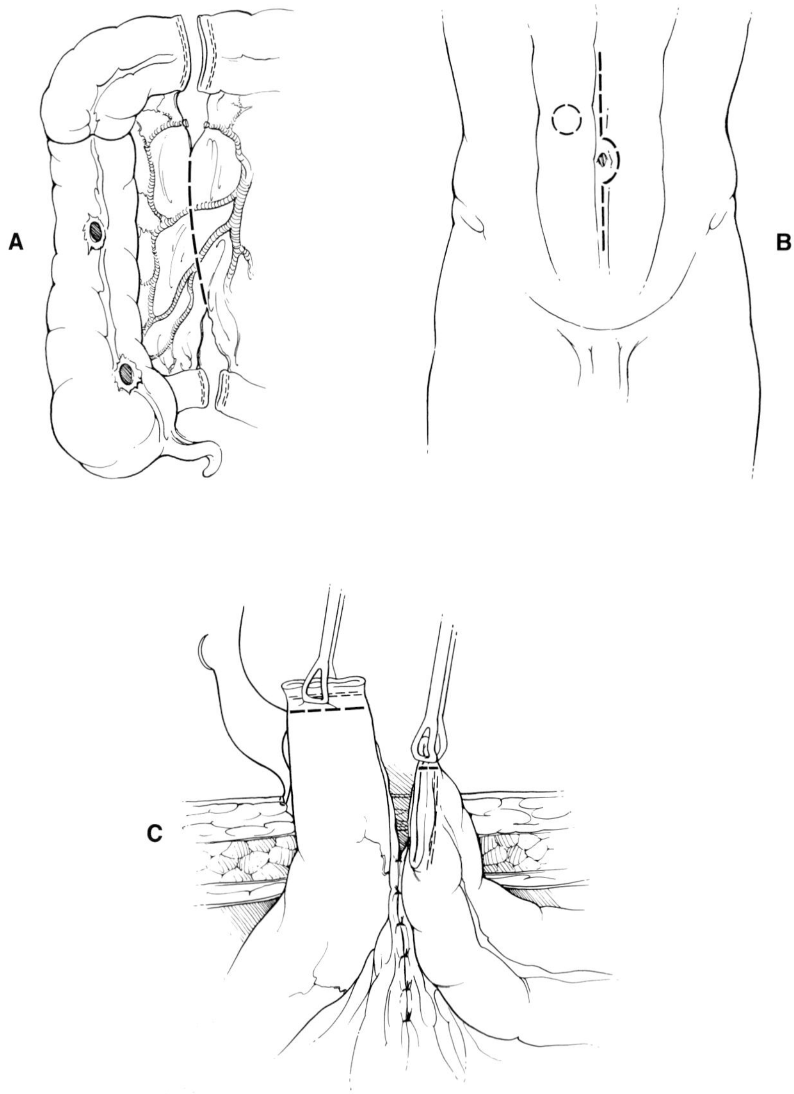

Fig. 7-5. End-loop ileocolostomy. **A,** Severe trauma to the right side of the colon, necessitating right hemicolectomy. The distal ileum and the right transverse colon have been divided with the linear-cutting stapler. **B,** Both limbs of the end-loop ileocolostomy are brought out through the rectus muscle in the right upper quadrant. **C,** The end of the distal ileum and the antimesenteric corner of the right transverse colon are gently drawn through the circular opening in the abdominal wall. The mesenteric defect created after removal of the right colon must be closed. The ileostomy is matured in the everted fashion.

D

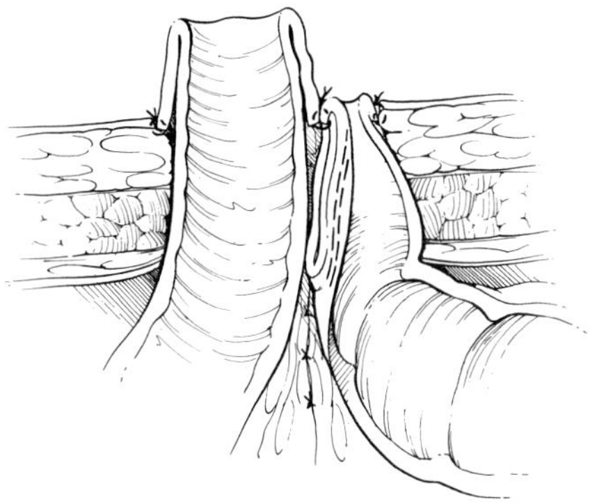

E

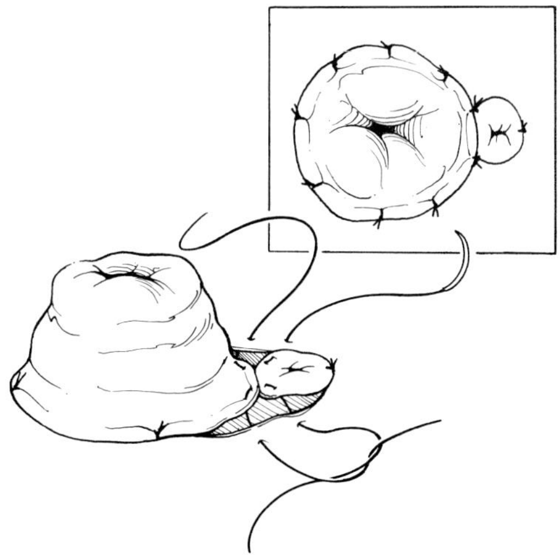

Fig. 7-5, cont'd. D, Sagittal view of the completed end-loop ileocolostomy. **E,** Two transition sutures are placed to help mature the mucous fistula. (After Pearl.)

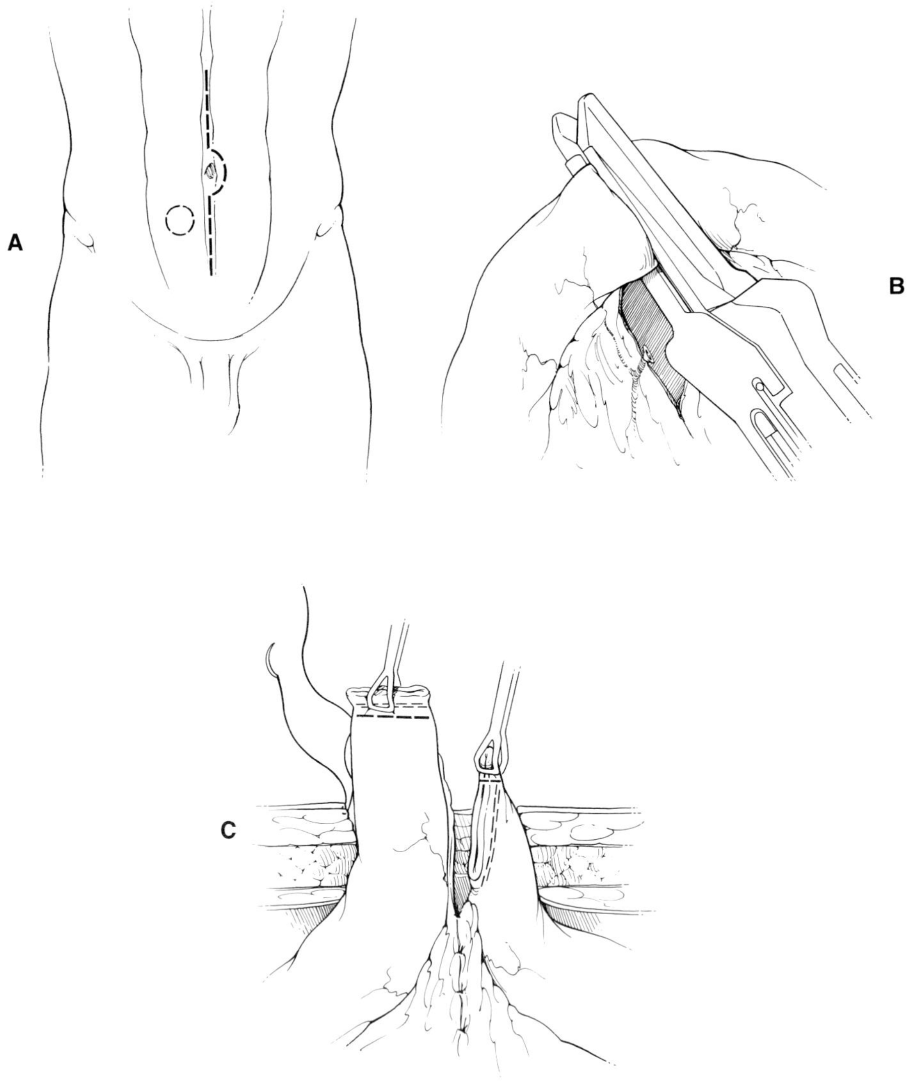

Fig. 7-6. End-loop ileostomy. **A,** The ileostomy incision is placed in the right lower quadrant overlying the rectus muscle. **B,** The ileum is divided with the linear-cutting stapler at a point where the proximal and distal limbs can be drawn through the abdominal wall without tension. **C,** The divided end of the proximal ileum and the antimesenteric corner of the distal ileum are gently drawn through the opening in the rectus muscle. The mesenteric defect is closed.

D

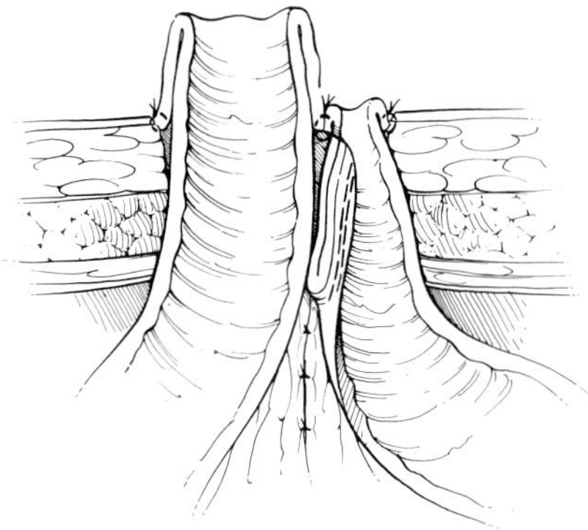

E

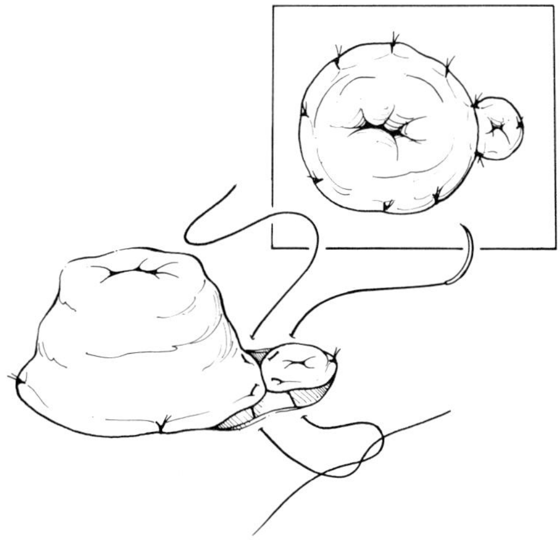

Fig. 7-6, cont'd. D, Sagittal view of the completed end-loop ileostomy. **E,** Two transition sutures are placed to help mature the distal "mini-stoma." (After Pearl.)

POSTOPERATIVE CARE AND CLOSURE

A sterile transparent ostomy pouch should be applied in the operating room so that the stoma can be inspected regularly in the postoperative period. If the margin of the stoma becomes dusky or edematous during the first 24 to 72 hours, it is usually not necessary to revise the stoma. However, a completely dark or black stoma needs to be evaluated for extension of the necrosis to beneath the fascia, in which case the stoma should be reconstructed on an emergency basis.

As a general guideline, closure of a diverting stoma should not be performed within 8 weeks of its formation. In addition, it is important to make sure that no distal obstruction or evidence of active inflammatory disease that might compromise the anastomosis is present. Endoscopic examination or a high-quality contrast study of the distal limb usually is performed to assess the integrity of the suture or staple line. A standard mechanical and antibiotic bowel preparation is used and may be supplemented with one to two perioperative doses of a cephalosporin administered parenterally.

An elliptical incision is made adjacent to the mucocutaneous junction of a loop or end-loop stoma and is continued downward along the serosal surfaces of both ends of the bowel until they are fully mobilized (Fig. 7-7). The skin and the fibrous tissue adherent to the edges of the bowel are excised, and a hand-sewn anastomosis is formed between the two ends. With many of the end-loop stomas, a side-to-side stapled anastomosis can be accomplished readily. The reconnected bowel is then returned into the peritoneal cavity, and the rectus sheath is closed. The skin may be left open to heal by secondary intention or, in selected cases, may be approximated loosely. The use of intraperitoneal drains is not recommended.

COMPLICATIONS

The formation and closure of diverting stomas is associated with an appreciable morbidity. The most important preventive measure is recognizing the magnitude of the potential problems that can develop and, with these in mind, paying strict attention to technical detail. When a complication does arise, it should be recognized promptly and dealt with in an appropriate manner.

Metabolic complications are more common with the formation of a loop ileostomy than with a loop colostomy. The volume of fluid lost from an established ileostomy averages 500 ml/day, including about 60 mEq of sodium. In cases of ileostomy dysfunction, significant sodium and water losses can occur and can lead to rapid dehydration. In one study, 23 of 117 patients with loop ileostomies (20%) required hospital admission because of dysfunction.[1] An-

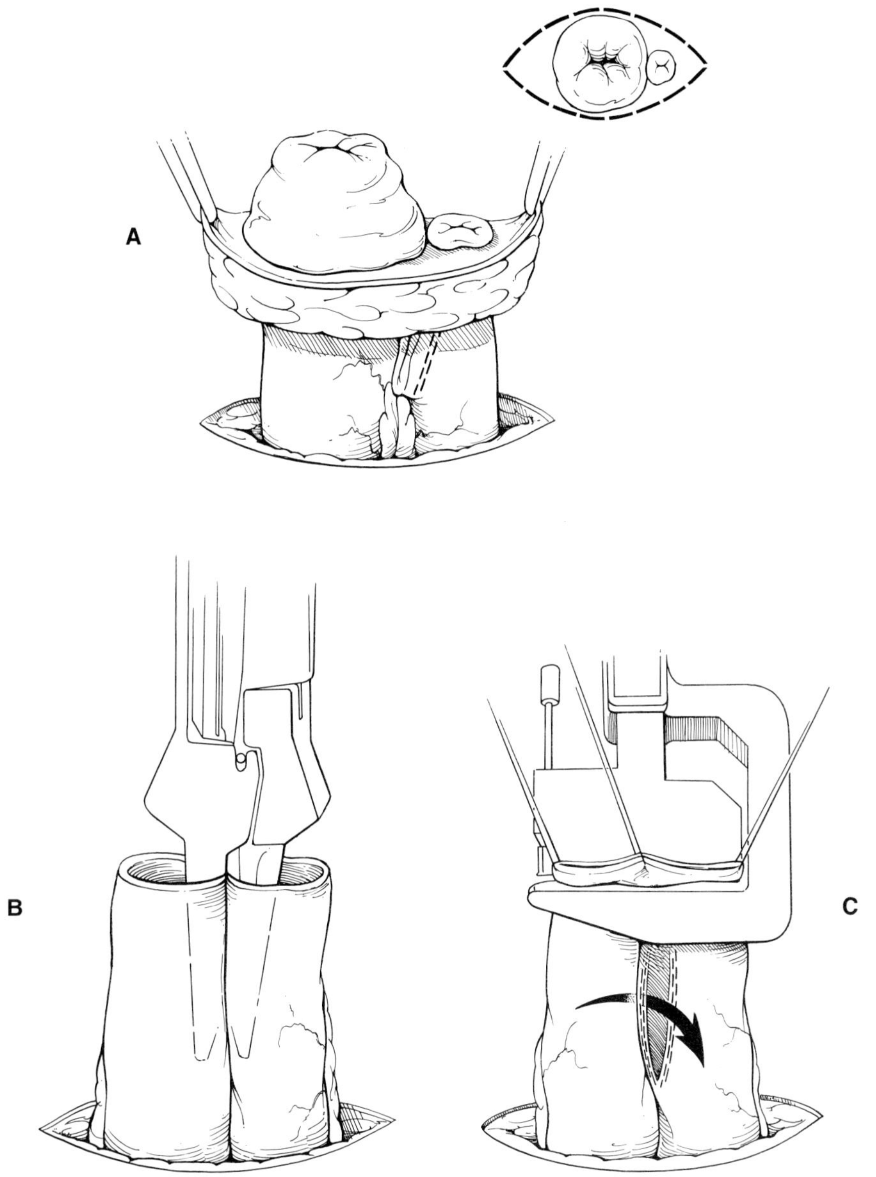

Fig. 7-7. Closure of a diverting stoma. **A,** An elliptical skin incision is made around both limbs of the ileum. **B,** After both limbs have been completely mobilized, the ends of the ileum and surrounding scar tissue are excised and a side-to-side stapled anastomosis is made. Care must be taken to avoid injury to the ileal mesentery. **C,** Closure of the loop is facilitated with a linear stapler. (After Pearl.)

other metabolic complication of ileostomy is the formation of urinary calculi. This complication occurs in 3% to 13% of patients and is related to chronic dehydration and sodium depletion. To avoid dehydration, patients with an ileostomy should be encouraged to drink several glasses of water daily.

Cholelithiasis occurs in up to 30% of patients with ileostomies. Gallstones form in these individuals because resection or inflammation of the terminal ileum interrupts the enterohepatic circulation, resulting in malabsorption or depletion of bile acids, conditions that favor the precipitation of cholesterol stones.

One of the most common problems associated with the formation of a loop ileostomy is local irritation and breakdown of peristomal skin, which occurs in about 15% of patients. This complication usually results from improper location of the stoma or other technical problems associated with stoma construction. In a prospective study comparing complications of loop ileostomy with those of loop transverse colostomy, the incidence of skin irritation was greater (30% vs. 13%) in those patients with loop colostomies.[2] The authors explain that, although the median daily effluent of the ileostomy group was nearly twice that of the colostomy group (438 ml vs. 265 ml), the spout of the ileostomy made collection of the effluent more efficient, thus minimizing leakage around the stoma.

Small bowel obstruction occurs in approximately 10% of patients with loop ileostomies yet is noted much less frequently with loop colostomies. This situation is probably so because the intact transverse or sigmoid mesocolon walls off the small bowel and prevents it from twisting. In contrast, a segment of small intestine can rotate around the base of a loop ileostomy at the point of fixation to the anterior abdominal wall, resulting in obstruction.

Retraction of loop stomas has been reported in 4% to 13% of patients. Such retraction usually results from inadequate mobilization of the mesentery of the bowel to be exteriorized. The special significance of retraction in loop stomas is that it has been considered as a cause of incomplete fecal diversion. The use of fascioseromuscular "tacking" sutures will not alleviate retraction of a loop stoma if the mesentery is under tension. In obese individuals it may be necessary to make one or more "relaxing" incisions in the peritoneum of the bowel mesentery in order to gain adequate length to properly exteriorize a loop stoma.

Prolapse of a loop stoma, another complication associated with incomplete fecal diversion, occurs in 5% to 10% of cases. Most frequently it involves the distal limb of a transverse loop colostomy, particularly when this procedure is performed on a patient with a distended colon. Treatment consists of closure of the stoma. In those patients in whom the loop stoma becomes permanent, local excision of the prolapsed segment can be performed and reconstruction of the functioning proximal component can be done.

In our experience with 229 patients with end-loop stomas, a total of 30 patients (13.1%) developed complications. Skin excoriation and retraction were most common, each having an incidence of 3.5%. Prolapse was observed in only one patient, probably because the tiny aperture of the mucous fistula prevents the distal bowel from prolapsing through it.

Loop stoma closure is associated with a morbidity reported to be between 10% and 50% and a mortality of 0% to 4%. Wound infections and anastomotic leaks are among the most common complications related to loop colostomy closure. In a large series of patients with loop ileostomies, 14% developed bowel obstructions within 30 days of closure, whereas anastomotic leaks and wound infections each developed in only 2.5% of patients.[1] One group of authors analyzed data from 93 consecutive colostomy closures in order to compare the morbidity and mortality of loop and end colostomies.[2] They concluded that loop colostomy closure is not associated with fewer complications than closure of end colostomy even though the latter takes longer and is more difficult.

Wound infections necessitate adequate drainage and aggressive local care. Small localized anastomotic leaks may be treated conservatively with parenteral nutrition or a low-residue diet that is high in protein and calories. If the patient begins to show signs of systemic sepsis or complete anastomotic disruption, proximal diversion and drainage or exteriorization of the anastomosis are indicated.

DISCUSSION

Perhaps the most compelling question regarding diverting stomas is: Do they completely divert the fecal stream? Several reports have addressed this issue (Table 7-1). The method of study involved either feeding the patients a barium meal or a radiolabeled tracer (chromium 51) and following the course of the

Table 7-1. Effectiveness of loop stomas in diverting fecal stream

Series	Year	Type	Method	No. of Patients With Complete Diversion (%)
Rombeau et al.[3]	1978	Colostomy	Barium	25/25 (100)
Schofield et al.[4]	1980	Colostomy	Chromium 51	10/10 (100)
Williams et al.[5]	1986	Ileostomy/colostomy	Chromium 51	10/10 (100)
Fontes et al.[6]	1988	Colostomy	Barium	53/62 (85)
Winslet et al.[7]	1991	Ileostomy	Chromium 51	22/26 (85)*

*When retracted stomas were revised, defunctioning efficiency approached 100%.

Table 7-2. Change of loop stoma from temporary to permanent state

Series	Year	Patients With Permanent Loop Stomas (%)
Winkler & Volpe[8]	1982	99/211 (47)
Boman-Sandelin & Fenyo[9]	1985	11/29 (38)
Rutegard & Dahlgren[10]	1987	35/56 (62)

marker through the intestinal tract with sequential abdominal radiographs or nuclear scans. As Table 7-1 shows, loop stomas diverted the fecal stream effectively in almost every instance, regardless of the consistency of the stool (liquid vs. solid) or a dependent location of the distal limb on the abdominal wall. The only significant factors that led to incomplete diversion were stomal retraction, revision of which reestablished effective diversion, and the presence of a loop stoma for longer than 3 months.

Another important but frequently overlooked question is: How often are diverting stomas actually temporary? Table 7-2 summarizes the results of studies concluding that nearly half of all diverting stomas that were intended to be temporary remain permanent. The usual causes for this change to permanency include patient preference and overall medical condition, nonresectability of the primary tumor, and limited life expectancy. These observations underscore the importance of careful preoperative planning and attention to technical detail when creating a "temporary" loop ostomy in order to minimize long-term morbidity.

Once the decision has been made to create a diverting stoma, the question arises about which type of loop stoma is best, colostomy or ileostomy. The most common method used to defunction the distal colon and rectum is the construction of a transverse loop colostomy. Although this type of stoma is relatively easy to fashion, it has several disadvantages. First, a traditional right upper quadrant transverse loop colostomy is often difficult to properly cover with an ostomy device because of its relative bulk and location. Second, the liquid consistency and corrosive nature of the effluent often lead to skin irritation in a relatively flush loop colostomy. Third, the offensive odor of colostomy output is a frequent patient complaint. Finally, closure of a transverse loop colostomy is associated with an overall complication rate of between 10% and 50%, with most complications secondary to wound infections and anastomotic leaks.

In contrast, a properly everted loop ileostomy may be a better choice for a diverting stoma because it circumvents most of the problems noted here. In a prospective controlled trial comparing loop ileostomy with loop transverse colostomy, ileostomy was associated with significantly less odor, a lower frequency of ostomy device changes, fewer complications of stoma management, and a lower wound infection rate following ostomy closure.[5]

In summary, the construction of a diverting stoma should be considered a major part of the overall operative procedure. If should be performed by a surgeon who is not only technically skilled but also understands the potential complications associated with an ileostomy or a colostomy. In the majority of cases loop stomas do seem to effectively divert the fecal stream. Almost half of all temporary loop stomas become permanent, a fact that underscores the importance of placing them in an optimal location on the abdominal wall and paying strict attention to technical details. Finally, loop ileostomy should be considered as a potentially superior alternative to transverse loop colostomy following various colorectal surgical procedures.

REFERENCES

1. Feinberg SM, McLeod RS, Cohen Z. Complications of loop ileostomy. Am J Surg 153:102-107, 1987.
2. Mileski WJ, Regs RV, Joehl RJ, et al. Rates of morbidity and mortality after closure of loop and end colostomy. Surg Gynecol Obstet 171:17-21, 1990.
3. Rombeau JL, Wilk PJ, Turnbull RB, et al. Total fecal diversion by the temporary skin-level loop transverse colostomy. Dis Colon Rectum 21:223-226, 1978.
4. Schofield PF, Cade D, Lambert M. Dependent proximal loop colostomy: Does it defunction the distal colon? Br J Surg 67:201-202, 1980.
5. Williams NS, Nasmyth DG, Jones D, et al. Defunctioning stomas: A postoperative controlled trial comparing loop ileostomy with loop transverse colostomy. Br J Surg 73:566-570, 1986.
6. Fontes B, Fontes W, Utiyama EM, et al. The efficacy of loop colostomy for complete fecal diversion. Dis Colon Rectum 31:298-302, 1988.
7. Winslet MC, Drolc Z, Allan A, Keighley MRB. Assessment of the defunctioning efficiency of the loop ileostomy. Dis Colon Rectum 34:699-703, 1991.
8. Winkler MJ, Volpe PA. Loop transverse colostomy—The case against. Dis Colon Rectum 25:321-326, 1982.
9. Boman-Sandelin K, Fenyo G. Construction and closure of transverse loop colostomy. Dis Colon Rectum 28:772-774, 1985.
10. Rutegard J, Dahlgren S. Transverse colostomy or loop ileostomy as diverting stoma in colorectal surgery. Acta Chir Scand 153:229-232, 1987.

SUGGESTED READINGS

Abcarian H, Pearl RK. Stomas. Surg Clin North Am 68:1295-1305, 1988.

Pearl RK. Complications of ileostomy. In Nelson RL, Nyhus LM, eds. Surgery of the Small Intestine. Norwalk, Conn.: Appleton & Lange, 1987, pp 499-509.

Pearl RK, Prasad ML, Orsay CP, et al. Early local complications from intestinal stomas. Arch Surg 120:1145-1147, 1985.

Pearl RK, Prasad ML, Orsay CP, et al. A survey of technical considerations in the construction of intestinal stomas. Am Surg 51:462-465, 1985.

Pearl RK, Prasad ML, Tan AB. Loop stomas: Indications, techniques for construction, take-down, and management. Semin Colon Rectal Surg 2:93-101, 1991.

Pearl RK, Tan AB. Stomas and stoma care. In Nyhus LM, Baker RJ, eds. Mastery of Surgery, 2nd ed. Boston: Little, Brown, 1992, pp 1218-1226.

Prasad ML, Pearl RK, Orsay CP. End-loop ileocolostomy for massive trauma to the right side of the colon. Arch Surg 119:975-976, 1984.

Unti JA, Abcarian H, Pearl RK, et al. Rodless end-loop stomas—A seven-year experience. Dis Colon Rectum 34:999-1004, 1991.

8 CECOSTOMY

Anthony Senagore

Pillore performed the first right inguinal cecostomy in 1776 to provide decompression for an obstructing rectal carcinoma.[1,2] This technique was not popularized until the 1950s, when cecostomy was advocated for several clinical conditions: (1) distal colonic obstruction, (2) proximal diversion to protect a distal anastomosis, (3) cecal volvulus, (4) decompression of toxic megacolon, and (5) intestinal pseudo-obstruction.[3,4] It should be recalled that cecostomy allowed for satisfactory colonic decompression with minimal anesthetic requirements at a time when large bowel obstruction carried a mortality of 12% to 56%.[5-8] Two other factors that increased the frequency with which this diversion procedure was performed were the reliance on three-stage resections for complicated diverticular disease and obstructing neoplasms and the perceived need to protect distal colonic anastomoses.

The use of cecostomy as an initial decompressive procedure for distal colonic obstruction has been very successful for decompression of the colon and subsequent preparation of the colon for definitive surgery.[9] However, in most series the mortality rate following decompressive cecostomy was alarmingly high (21.5%).[2,9] This situation is more a reflection on differences in perioperative care of the patient with large bowel obstruction rather than a specific disadvantage of cecostomy. At the time of cecostomy placement, as many as 10% of patients in these series had cecal perforations that would have been unnoticed if a blind transverse loop colostomy had been elected as the diversion procedure.[9] Conversely, complementary cecostomy performed to protect a difficult distal colonic anastomosis has been associated with few complications. However, it is disconcerting that leakage with subsequent mortality occurred as frequently (2%) at the cecostomy site as at the distal anastomosis. Such leakage is a factor that discourages wide application of this form of proximal diversion.[1] The treatment of nongangrenous cecal volvulus has included cecal resection, cecopexy, detorsion alone, and cecostomy with or without cecopexy.[10-14] A preference for nonresectional therapy with viable bowel has been noted, and the lowest recurrence rate appears to be associated with cecopexy and cecostomy tube placement.[10] In such cases cecostomy is most readily achieved through the appendicular stump unless the stump was previously resected. Overall, an approach involving cecostomy and cecopexy is highly successful and is associated with lower operative mobility and mortality than resectional therapy.[15]

The use of surgical cecostomy for intestinal pseudo-obstruction had been associated with operative mortality ranging from 25% to 44%, even with adequate decompression.[16-18] Mortality increases significantly with delay in diagnosis and associated full-thickness necrosis of the bowel wall, usually in the face of significant associated medical illnesses.[19] Successful decompression via colonoscopy has been achieved in 68% to 91% of such patients; however, recurrence rates have been as high as 22% and a significant risk of perforation remains with this approach.[20,21] However, the morbidity rates associated with endoscopic decompression are minimal compared to those of surgical cecostomy.

TUBE PLACEMENT

Throughout the years a number of techniques and tubes have been advocated for cecostomy. The two most frequently recommended techniques are exteriorization and blind tube cecostomy.[9,22-26] Typically the tube placement procedure is performed through a right lower quadrant incision, although Hughes[27] has advocated a formal laparotomy with placement of the cecostomy through a separate stab incision.

The procedure can be performed with the patient under local infiltrative anesthesia, although general anesthesia or a regional block method has been used, depending on the patient's medical condition. A transverse (McBurney) incision is made in the right lower quadrant to allow access to the peritoneal cavity (Fig. 8-1, *A*). On entry to the peritoneal cavity, the distended cecum should be readily identifiable. The cecum is carefully and gently inspected for perforations or serosal tears, which can occur in as many as 3% of patients with cecal distention greater than 10 cm.[2] If the surgeon encounters a collapsed cecum, bloody peritoneal fluid, or purulent exudate, the procedure should be terminated in favor of a formal laparotomy, which allows for clearer identification of the pathologic condition and definitive treatment. After the cecum has been identified, the cecotomy can be performed by exteriorization or the blind tube technique (Fig. 8-1, *B*). When exteriorization is used, the cecal pouch is allowed to protrude from the abdominal cavity to skin level. A row of seromuscular sutures is placed prior to opening the cecum to prevent spillage of cecal contents into the peritoneal cavity. A cecotomy is made, and the cecum is sewn to the skin circumferentially with seromuscular sutures (Fig. 8-1, *B-C*), completing the cecotomy.

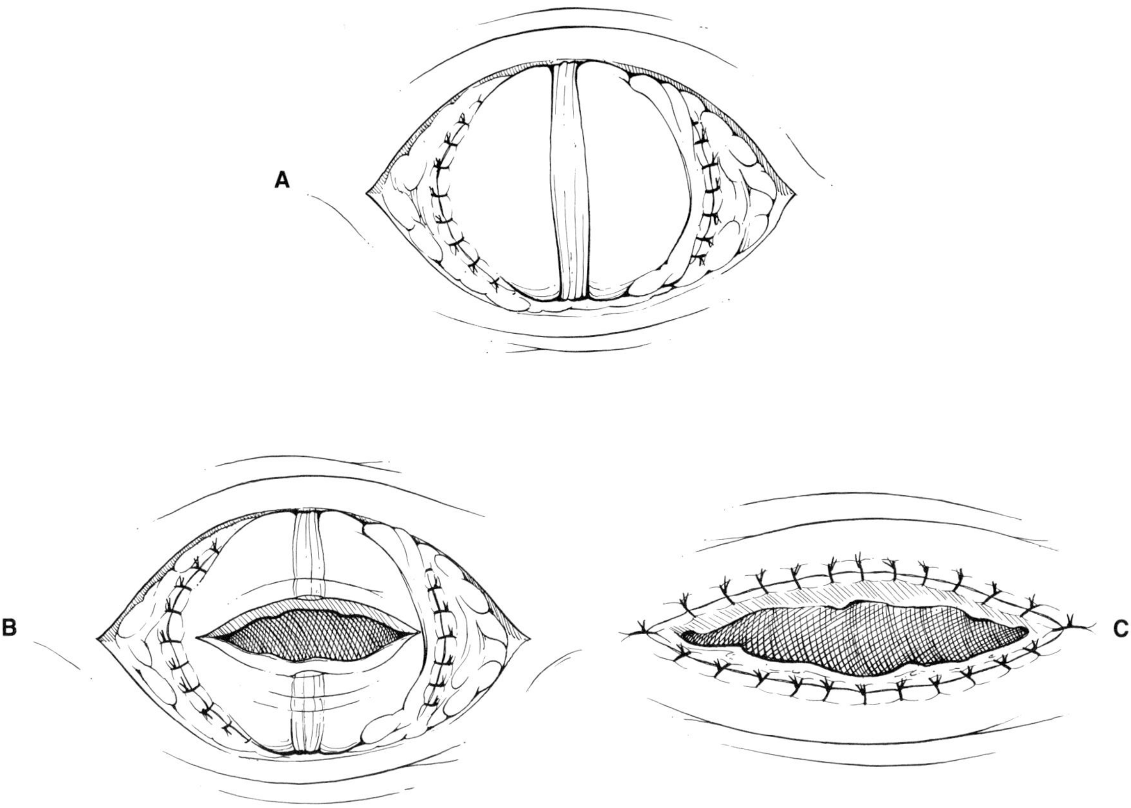

Fig. 8-1. A, A transverse (McBurney) incision is made in the right lower quadrant to expose the distended cecum, which is brought out to skin level through this incision. The peritoneal cavity is then closed circumferentially with seromuscular interrupted sutures. **B,** After the peritoneum has been approximated circumferentially, a cecotomy is performed. **C,** The cecotomy is matured by circumferential placement of full-thickness sutures through the cecum to the dermis.

When tube cecostomy is chosen, the cecum is initially sutured to the peritoneum circumferentially to prevent peritoneal soiling. Two concentric pursestring sutures of 2-0 silk are then placed in the cecum (Fig. 8-2, *A*). A small colotomy is made in the center of the inside pursestring, with suction readily available to aspirate the effluent. An important technical point is to place the suction tip at the opening of the colotomy rather than to insert it into the cecum because collapse of the cecum through suction may prevent adequate removal of the more distal contents. Once the effluent has been controlled, a 22 or 24 Fr soft rubber catheter is inserted through the cecotomy and both pursestrings are tied securely. A variety of catheters can be employed, including a de Pezzer catheter, Foley catheter, endotracheal tube, or even a soft rubber chest tube.[9,28] A water balloon catheter has the advantage of being more readily interchangeable, if a change should become necessary, compared to the de Pezzer catheter. In addition, the water balloon catheter offers a security advantage over a nonballoon-type catheter in that the balloon tends to retard accidental dislodgment. After the tube has been secured, the fascial skin layers are closed loosely around the catheter and a light dressing is applied (Fig. 8-2, *B*).

A

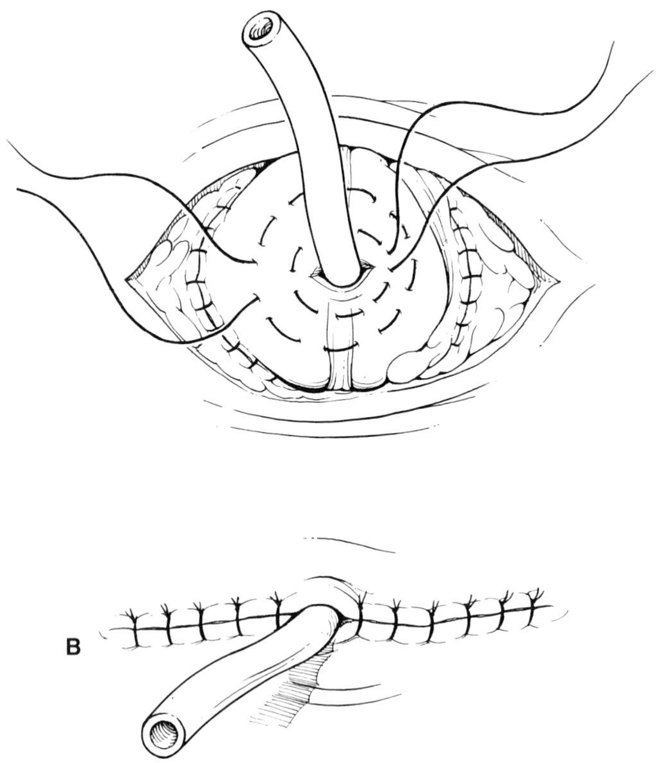

B

Fig. 8-2. A, The cecum is exteriorized through a right lower quadrant incision. The peritoneum may or may not be approximated to the seromuscular layer, according to the surgeon's preference. Prior to performance of a cecotomy, a double row of seromuscular pursestring sutures is placed around the proposed tube site for the cecostomy. A No. 24 Fr Foley catheter should be used as the cecostomy tube. First the inner pursestring sutures and then the outer ones are tied securely to hold the cecotomy around the tube and to keep it firmly in position. **B,** The skin is closed around the tube. The tube also should be secured at skin level with a separate stay suture.

In recent years CT-guided percutaneous cecostomy has been described.[29,30] For this technique the patient is rolled to the left lateral decubitus position. Only local infiltrative anesthesia is required at the site of tube insertion. A small incision is made, and under CT guidance a needle is placed through the retroperitoneum into the cecal lumen. The track then can be gently dilated via the Seldinger technique to allow catheter placement for decompression. Although most reports have involved a relatively small group of patients, the technique has resulted in successful rapid decompression of the cecum. Such decompression usually is achieved with the use of a 12 Fr catheter. In addition to the significant advantage of requiring only a local anesthetic, there have been no reported cases of major morbidity or procedure-related mortality with this approach.[29,31,32] Subsequently, Morrison et al.[33] have described a transperitoneal approach that excludes the need for CT guidance. This technique requires only fluoroscopy, thereby making the procedure readily available at most institutions. In addition, there are limitations associated with the retroperitoneal approach via CT guidance: (1) what appears to be an extraperitoneal cecum actually may be intraperitoneal because of a thin veil of peritoneal reflection that encircles the cecum, and (2) the posterior approach via CT guidance presents difficulties when the cecum is tremendously dilated or when it has twisted anteriomedially on its mesentery.[16,34] When the transperitoneal approach is used, the dilated cecum is located fluoroscopically and an area central to the cecum is identified. A 2-inch square of skin and abdominal wall is anesthetized with a local infiltrative anesthetic agent. A specially designed 18-gauge introducer needle loaded with a plastic T fastener is carefully inserted into the cecal lumen. The T fastener is launched from the introducer and is used to secure the cecum against the anterior abdominal wall. This step is repeated at each of the four corners of the selected site for tube insertion. After the cecum has been attached to the abdominal wall, the transcutaneous needle track to the cecal lumen is progressively dilated via the Seldinger technique to allow a 24 to 34 Fr tube to be placed at the initial setting. This technique has been advocated primarily for patients with cecal volvulus or those with distal colonic obstruction. In a small group of patients the technique has been very successful, with no procedure-related morbidity or mortality reported.[33]

For the first 12 to 24 hours after placement of a cecostomy tube, the tube should be gently irrigated with 30 ml of normal saline every 2 hours. Use of larger volumes may disrupt the seal between the cecum and the abdominal wall, increasing the chance for peritoneal contamination. During ensuing days the irrigation solution can be increased steadily to 500 to 1000 ml.[9] As the volume is increased, turning the patient in different positions can allow adequate preparation even as far distally as the descending colon. Between irrigation intervals, the tube must be carefully inspected to ensure that no obstruction has occurred as a result of accumulation of stool or kinking. If unrecognized obstruction occurs, the cecum may burst.[9]

TUBE MANAGEMENT

Tube management depends on the indication for placement of the tube. When the cecostomy is placed as protection for distal anastomosis, it should be left for 7 to 10 days. After this time adequate integrity of the colonic anastomosis should be ensured and the tube can be removed readily. In most cases the cecal cutaneous fissure will close spontaneously. Westdahl and Russell[2] have advocated the use of a pressure dressing with a rubber sponge placed over the stoma site to speed closure of the defect. If the cecostomy was placed for initial decompression, it obviously is used for the entire time the decompression is required and should be maintained as a protective measure for the ensuing distal anastomosis. If adequate anastomotic integrity has been ensured, the tube can be removed as previously described.

The incidence of management complications associated with cecostomy is generally related to the indications for performance of the procedure, with the highest rates occurring with acute colon obstruction. Specific complications directly related to cecostomy include wound contamination, leakage around the tube, and failure of spontaneous closure.[9] Local wound inflammation occurs in virtually all patients after tube cecostomy; however, major subcutaneous infections occur in only 3.3% to 7.5% of cases.[2,9] In most instances wound inflammation is secondary to reflux of cecal contents around the tube. Such reflux tends to be more severe when the cecostomy has been placed for decompression rather than for simple protection of a distal anastomosis.[2] If leakage occurs around the tube, the tube should be replaced with one of a smaller caliber. Inserting a larger tube simply increases the size of the defect and worsens the situation. In several days the stoma should retract around the smaller tube, allowing replacement of the original tube and control of the fistula.[9] The most troublesome complication following cecostomy is failure of closure of the cecal cutaneous fistula, which occurs in 15% to 33% of cases.[2,9] In most instances this complication occurred when the tube initially inserted was larger than a 30 Fr catheter or when formal exteriorization and maturation of the cecostomy with skin sutures were involved.[1,2,9] Operative closure of the cecostomy is required, and a laparotomy is recommended so that the cecum can be mobilized adequately and closed without producing undue tension or injury to the cecum.[2]

SUMMARY

Cecostomy was originally employed as a means of colonic decompression for distal obstruction requiring minimal surgical insult. In most cases the procedure can be performed with the patient under local anesthesia to achieve prompt decompression of the colon. In fact, the fluoroscope-guided percutaneous technique may be the most efficient, least morbid approach to achieving cecostomy tube placement. Although the need for cecostomy as a diverting procedure has decreased significantly in recent years, as perioperative medical management has improved and reliance on staged procedures has diminished, it is still useful for the surgeon to be familiar with the technique.

REFERENCES

1. Jackson PJ, Baird RM. Cecostomy: An analysis of 102 cases. Am J Surg 114:297-301, 1967.
2. Westdahl PR, Russell T. In support of blind tube cecostomy in acute obstruction of the descending colon. Analysis of ninety-three emergency cecostomies. Am J Surg 118:577-581, 1969.
3. Becker WF. Acute obstruction of the colon. An analysis of 205 cases. Surg Gynecol Obstet 96:677, 1953.
4. Klein SH, et al. Emergency cecostomy in ulcerative colitis with acute toxic dilatation. Surgery 47:399, 1960.
5. Westdahl PR. A comparison of cecostomy and colostomy in the management of acute obstruction of the left colon. Am J Surg 96:324, 1958.
6. Gerber A, Thompson RJ Jr. Use of tube cecostomy to lower the mortality in acute large intestinal obstruction due to carcinoma. Am J Surg 110:893, 1965.
7. Albers JH, Smith LL. Comparison of cecostomy and transverse colostomy in complete colon obstruction. Surg Gynecol Obstet 95:410, 1952.
8. Rack FJ, Clement CW. Cecostomy and colostomy in acute colon obstructions. JAMA 154:4, 1954.
9. King RD, Edelman S, Kirschner PA, et al. An evaluation of catheter cecostomy. Surg Gynecol Obstet 123:779-786, 1966.
10. Anderson JR, Welch GH. Acute volvulus of the right colon: An analysis of 69 patients. World J Surg 10:336-342, 1986.
11. Todd GJ, Forde KA. Volvulus of the cecum: Choice of operation. Am J Surg 138:632-634, 1979.
12. O'Mara C, Wilson TH Jr, Stonesifer GL, Cameron JL. Cecal volvulus: Analysis of 50 patients with long-term follow-up. Ann Surg 189:724-731, 1979.
13. Burke JB, Ballantyne GH. Cecal volvulus. Low mortality at a city hospital. Dis Colon Rectum 27:737-740, 1984.
14. Smith WR, Goodwin JN. Cecal volvulus. Am J Surg 126:215-222, 1973.
15. Andersson A, Bergdahl L, Van Der Linden W. Volvulus of the cecum. Ann Surg 181:876-880, 1975.

16. Vanek VW, Al-Salti M. Acute pseudo-obstruction of the colon (Ogilvie's syndrome): An analysis of 400 cases. Dis Colon Rectum 29:203-210, 1986.
17. Wojtalik RS, Lindenauer SM, Kahn SS. Perforation of the colon associated with adynamic ileus. Am J Surg 125:601-606, 1973.
18. Nanni G, Garbini A, Luchetti P, et al. Ogilvie's syndrome (acute colonic pseudo-obstruction): Review of the literature and a report of four additional cases. Dis Colon Rectum 25:157-166, 1982.
19. Johnson CD, Rice RP, Kelvin FM, et al. The radiologic evaluation of gross cecal distention: Emphasis on cecal ileus. AJR 145:1211-1217, 1985.
20. Strodel WE, Nostrant TT, Eckhauser FE, et al. Therapeutic and diagnostic colonoscopy in nonobstructive colonic dilatation. Ann Surg 194:416-421, 1983.
21. Nivatvongs S, Vermeulen JD, Fang DT. Colonoscopic decompression of acute pseudo-obstruction of the colon. Ann Surg 196:598-600, 1982.
22. Maynard A de L, Turell R. Acute left colon obstruction with special reference to cecostomy versus transversostomy. Surg Gynecol Obstet 100:667, 1955.
23. Hunt CJ. Surface cecostomy versus right colon colostomy as the procedure of choice in decompressing the acutely obstructed colon due to extensive cancer. West J Surg 67:101, 1959.
24. Gerber A, Thompson RJ Jr. Use of a tube cecostomy to lower the mortality in acute large intestinal obstruction due to carcinoma. Am J Surg 110:893, 1965.
25. Stainback WC, Christiansen KH. The value of Foley catheter cecostomy in conjunction with resection of the left colon and rectosigmoid. Surg Clin North Am 42:1475, 1962.
26. Florer RE. Cecostomy: Indications and technic. Am J Surg 93:865, 1957.
27. Hughes ESR. Cecostomy: A part of an efficient method of decompressing the colon obstructed by cancer. Dis Colon Rectum 6:454, 1963.
28. Ingoldby CJH, Dawson A, Addison NV. A new technique of cecostomy using endotracheal tubes. Ann R Coll Surg Engl 71:211-212, 1989.
29. Haaga JR, Bick RJ, Zollinger RM. CT-guided percutaneous catheter cecostomy. Gastrointest Radiol 12:166-168, 1987.
30. Crass JR, Simmons RL, Frick MP, et al. Percutaneous decompression of the colon using CT guidance in Ogilvie syndrome. AJR 144:475-476, 1985.
31. Casola G, Withers C, van Sonnenberg E, et al. Percutaneous cecostomy for decompression of the massively distended cecum. Radiology 158:793-794, 1986.
32. Quinn SF, Jones EN, Maroney T. Percutaneous cecostomy in the management of cecal volvulus: Report of a case. J Intervent Radiol 2:137-139, 1987.
33. Morrison MC, Lee MJ, Stafford SA, et al. Percutaneous cecostomy: Controlled transperitoneal approach. Radiology 176:574-576, 1990.
34. Rubenstein WA, Auh YH, Zirinsky K, et al. Posterior peritoneal recesses: Assessment using CT. Radiology 156:461-468, 1985.

9 END ILEOSTOMY

John R. Oakley

INDICATIONS

Inflammatory bowel disease remains the most common indication for end ileostomy despite the development of the ileal pouch–anal anastomosis, which allows many patients with ulcerative colitis to avoid having a permanent stoma. Nevertheless, for many patients with ulcerative colitis end ileostomy is the preferred option after proctocolectomy, and it remains the only alternative if proctocolectomy is required for Crohn's disease. An end ileostomy is also created after total abdominal colectomy performed for inflammatory bowel disease, particularly when the surgery is performed on an emergency basis for acute or toxic colitis. In such circumstances the stoma may not be permanent if the patient's condition is considered to be suitable for a subsequent ileorectal anastomosis or ileal pouch–anal anastomosis.

Proctocolectomy and ileostomy also may be performed in the treatment of familial adenomatous polyposis when ileorectal anastomosis is contraindicated (due to carpeting polyps in the rectum or the presence of carcinoma) or in the patient who is not considered suitable for, or declines, restorative ileal pouch–anal anastomosis.

On rare occasions an end ileostomy may be required when multiple synchronous carcinomas are present in the large bowel. Occasionally an end ileostomy is performed without colectomy, for example, after small bowel resection for massive mesenteric ischemia or in severe inflammatory bowel disease to allow the patient's general condition to improve before subsequent colectomy.

A "temporary" end ileostomy also may be indicated after resection of the terminal ileum or the right colon when the surgeon thinks that immediate anastomosis would be unwise. This situation may exist under any of these circumstances: (1) after resection for perforating Crohn's disease; (2) in the presence of generalized peritonitis; (3) when a residual inflammatory nest remains after drainage of an intra-abdominal abscess; (4) after complex fistula surgery; (5) after right colon resection for volvulus or an obstructing colonic carcinoma; (6) after ileocecal trauma; or (7) when the patient's nutritional status or general condition mitigates against safe anastomosis. With most of these circumstances a delayed takedown of the ileostomy and bowel reanastomosis is possible, although these procedures should be delayed for about 3 to 6 months.

No real contraindications to end ileostomy exist, although individual clinical situations sometimes may favor the use of a loop (or diverting) ileostomy. In the obese patient a thick abdominal wall may make it difficult to prepare sufficient length of bowel with adequate blood supply to reach the skin, and a loop-end ileostomy may be preferred. In a patient who has previously had a diverting loop ileostomy and requires colectomy, it is preferable to convert the loop ileostomy into a loop-end stoma (by dividing the efferent limb just inside the peritoneal cavity) rather than to create a new end ileostomy.

OPERATIVE TECHNIQUE

Preoperative Preparation

The surgeon should discuss with the patient and family the implications of life with an ileostomy. Preoperative education is greatly enhanced by a meeting with the enterostomal therapist and sometimes by a visit from a trained lay person who has a stoma. In addition, books and brochures, available from national and local stoma associations or from the surgeon's institution, are invaluable in the preoperative preparation of the patient.

Selection of Site

Accurate preoperative selection of the stoma site is essential. The site should be selected with the patient in the sitting position, which will make any skin creases or folds become more apparent. The site is then checked with the patient in a supine position.

The following basic principles should be followed in the marking of a stoma site:

1. The stoma should pass through the middle of, or within the surface marking of, the rectus abdominus muscle (upper illustration).
2. When possible, the stoma should be placed at the apex of the infraumbilical fat mound. In obese patients, however, it may be necessary to place the site above the umbilicus to enable the patient to see the stoma.
3. The mark for the site should be made at least 4 cm from the planned incision.
4. The stoma should be placed far enough from the umbilicus and from any bony prominence, scar or incision site, or skin crease or prominence to allow proper application of the stoma management system. The use of a commercially available standard-size faceplate template will greatly aid in correct placement (lower illustration).
5. Areas of skin that have been previously damaged from radiation, burns, or skin grafting should be avoided for the site.

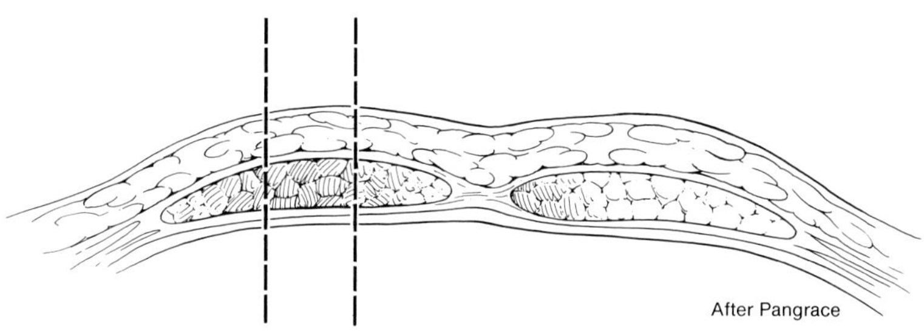

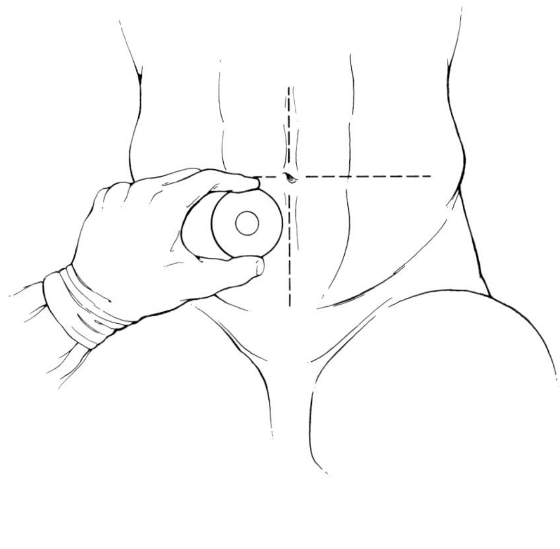

Marking of Site

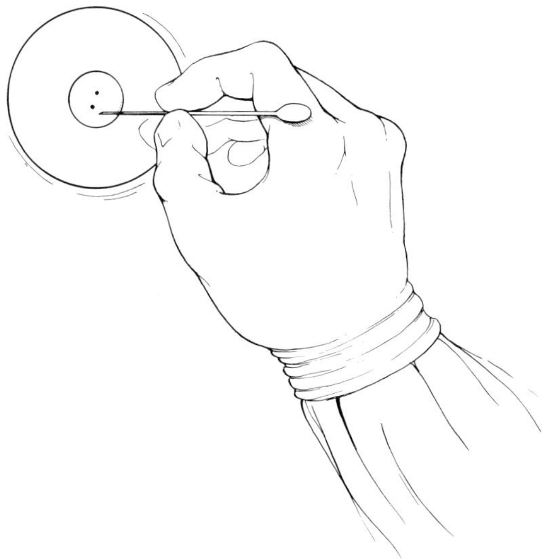

Once the optimal position of the faceplate has been determined with the patient in the sitting position, the patient is asked to lie down while the faceplate is held in position. An indelible mark is then tattooed at the center of the stoma site by placing a drop of India ink or methylene blue at this point and pricking the skin two or three times with a narrow-gauge needle. The resultant mark will not wash off during preoperative bathing or sterile skin preparation in the operating room.

The Incision

The exact site and size of the incision are determined by the extent of the surgery and the primary pathologic condition requiring ileostomy. However, whenever possible, a midline incision that closely passes the umbilicus on the left should be employed. A paramedian incision should be avoided because it destroys potential future stoma sites, especially in patients with Crohn's disease, who often require later ileostomy revision or relocation.

Preparation of Terminal Ileum

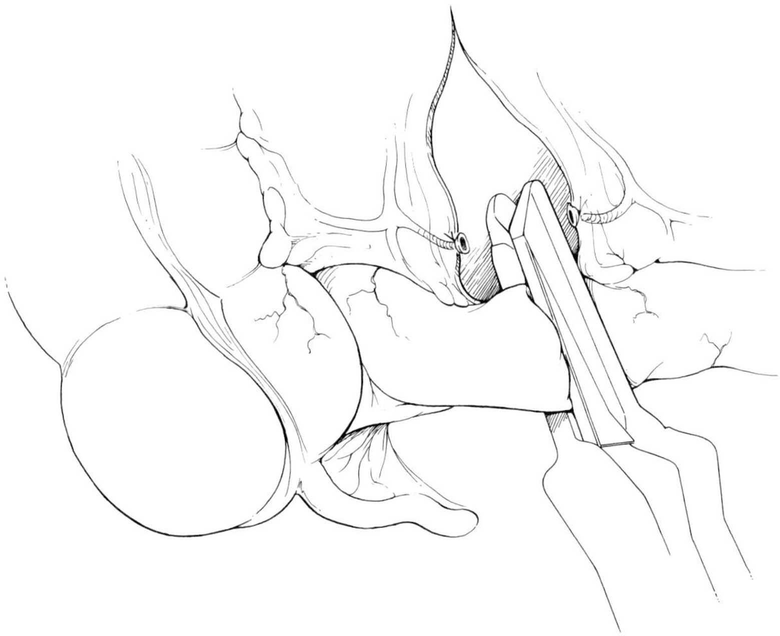

The terminal ileum usually is transected 7 to 10 cm from the ileocecal valve. However, for patients with right-sided colonic cancer or terminal ileal Crohn's disease more ileum may need to be resected. If a subsequent ileal pouch–anal anastomosis is contemplated, the division should be made within 1 to 2 cm of the ileocecal valve. The use of a linear-cutting stapler reduces contamination and will facilitate drawing the divided end of bowel through the abdominal wall aperture later.

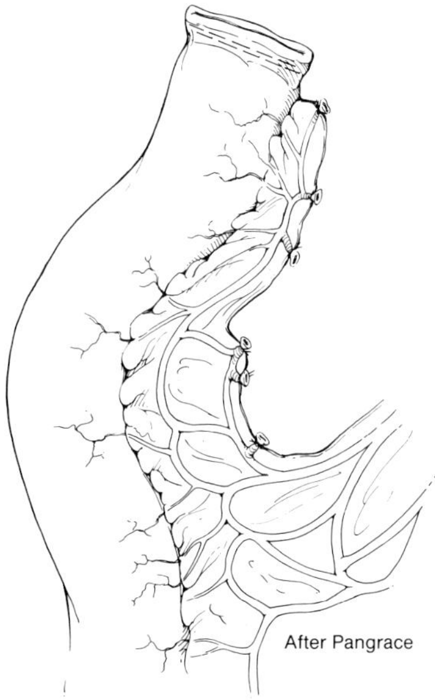

The mesentery of the terminal ileum is divided 0.5 to 1 cm from the bowel wall to preserve a vascular arcade close to the bowel. The bulk of the mesentery should be reduced as much as possible without compromising blood supply. Such reduction usually requires a stepwise division of the vascular arcades. Sufficient length of bowel should be prepared to allow the bowel end to protrude 5 to 6 cm beyond the skin level. Suture ligation of the vessels will help to prevent the ligatures from being dislodged as the bowel is brought through the stoma aperture. If arterial bleeding is not present at the distal end of the bowel or if a dusky coloration becomes apparent, the bowel should be trimmed further until adequate vascularization has been obtained.

Ileostomy Aperture

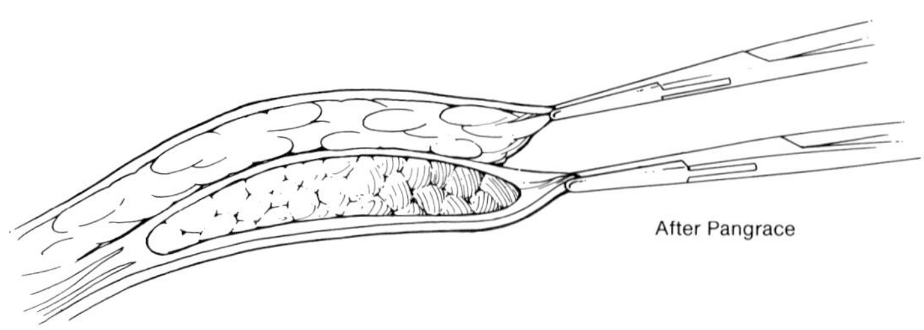

To provide even medial traction on the abdominal wall, the wound edge adjacent to the ileostomy site is grasped with Kocher clamps (or similar clamps) applied to the linea alba and the dermis.

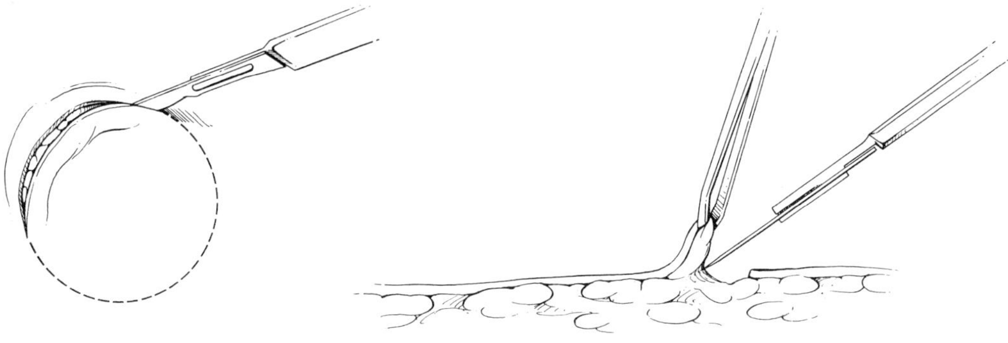

A circumferential skin incision approximately 2 cm in diameter is made around the tattoo mark, and the disk of skin is excised. The underlying fat is preserved to avoid a dead space and to provide support for the bowel as it passes through the subcutaneous tissue. Bleeding from the fatty tissue can be treated with cautery, but bleeding at the skin edge should be left to stop spontaneously because cautery in this area can damage the skin and lead to mucocutaneous separation.

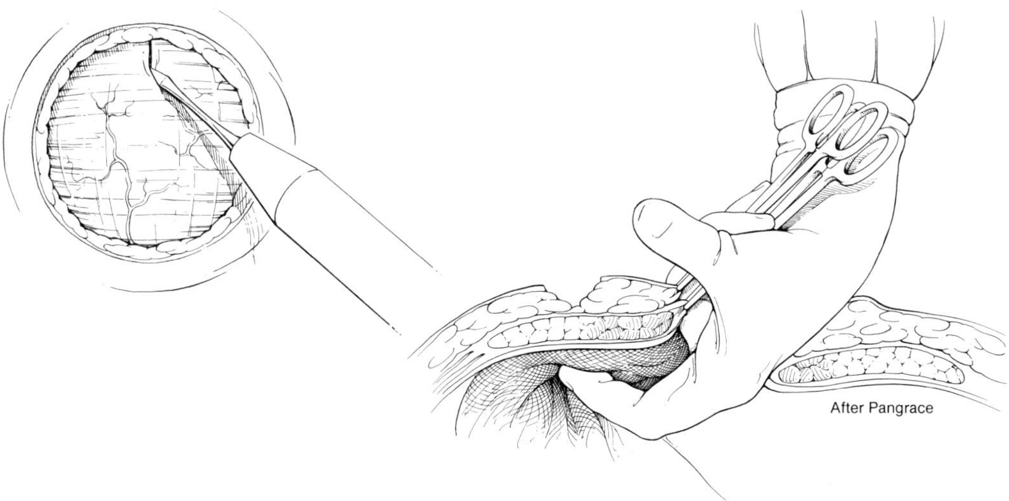

With the cutting cautery a vertical incision is made through the subcutaneous tissue to the level of the anterior rectus sheath. A small folded laparotomy pad is placed beneath the abdominal wall, and upward pressure is applied with the index and middle fingers while medial traction on the Kocher clamp is maintained with the same hand.

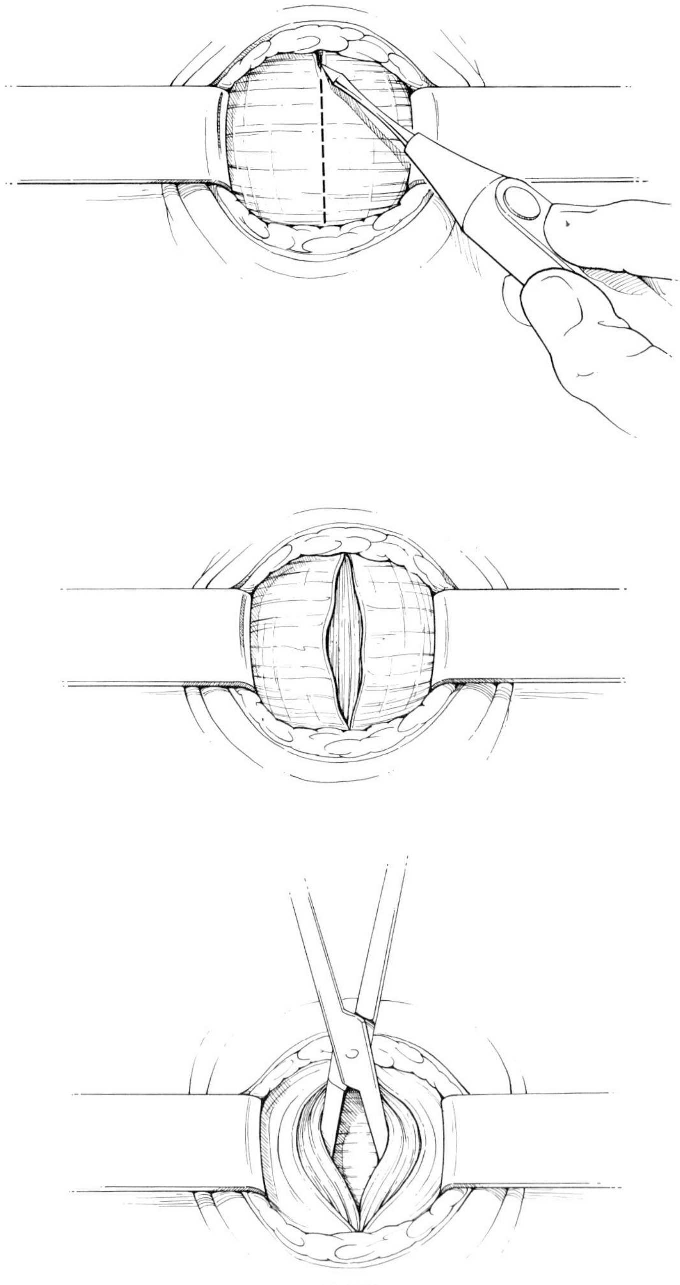

Two small right-angle retractors are used to allow access to the anterior sheath. The sheath is divided vertically to expose the fibers of the rectus muscle. The rectus muscle is separated with a blunt artery forceps.

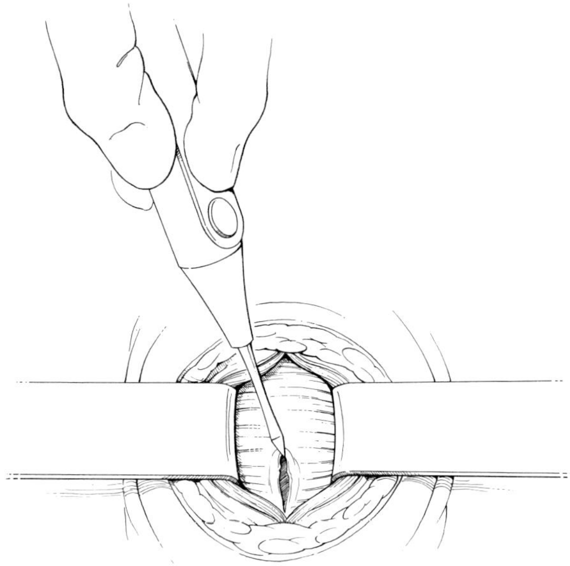

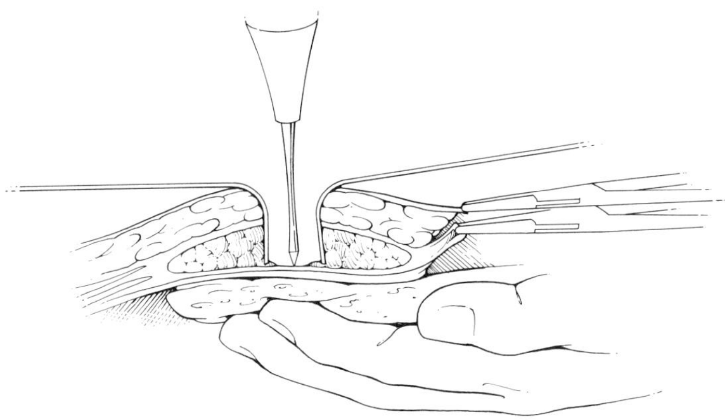

After Pangrace

The right-angle retractors are repositioned individually to expose the posterior rectus sheath. The cautery is used to cut vertically onto the underlying abdominal pack.

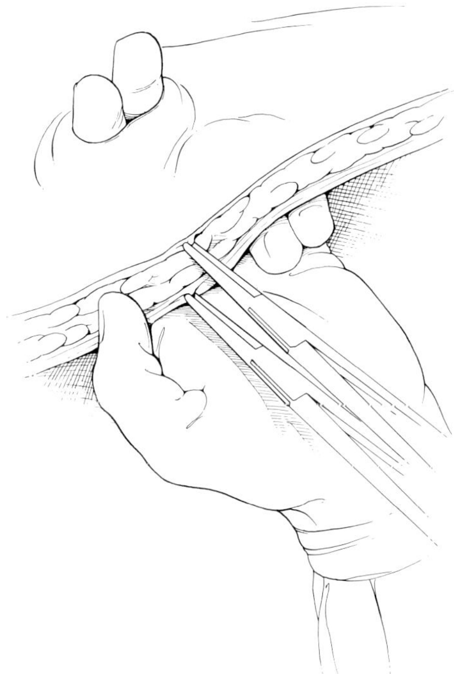

The vertical incisions in the rectus sheaths should be approximately 3 to 3.5 cm in length to produce a snug two-finger aperture so that the distal interphalangeal joint of the middle finger and the pulp of the index finger can be seen. An aperture of this size reduces the chance of hernia or prolapse (too large an aperture) or obstructive symptoms (too small an aperture). When the mesentery of the ileum is bulky, a slightly larger incision may be needed in the posterior sheath. Lateral cruciate incisions are not necessary. A vertical muscle split, rather than a transverse cutting procedure, is used to minimize the risk of postoperative hernia or prolapse of the ileostomy.

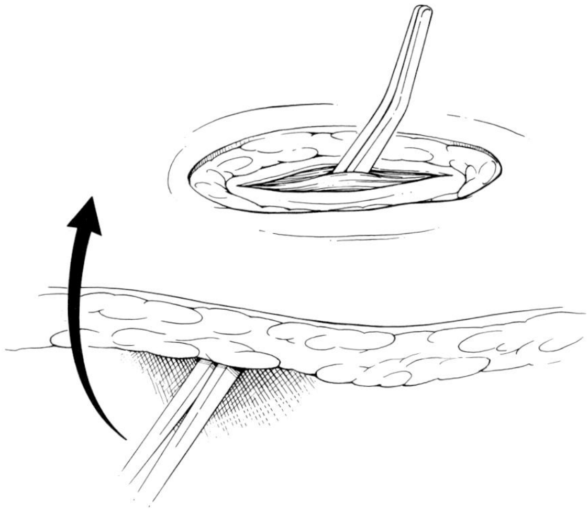

Blunt separation of the rectus muscle fibers helps to prevent damage to the inferior epigastric vessels. If bleeding does occur, a useful maneuver for gaining exposure is to pass a large artery clamp through the aperture and to use it as a retractor.

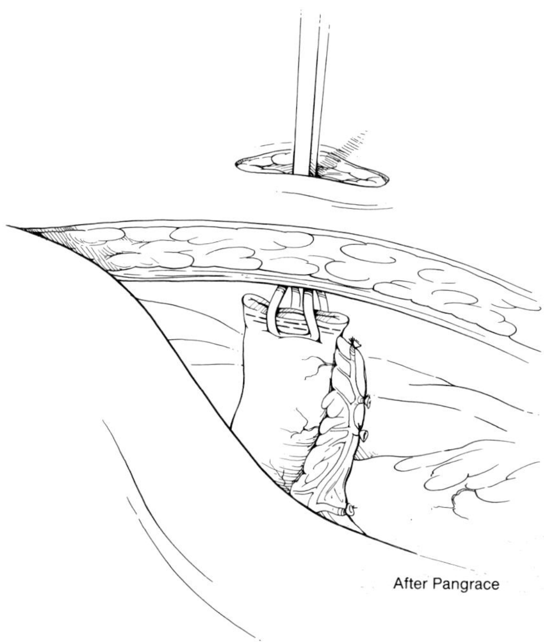

A Babcock clamp is passed through the stoma aperture to grasp the prepared ileum and draw it through the abdominal wall so that the ileal mesentery is not twisted. The mesentery is placed so that it lies cephalad in order to facilitate later closure of the mesenteric defect.

Fixation of Mesentery

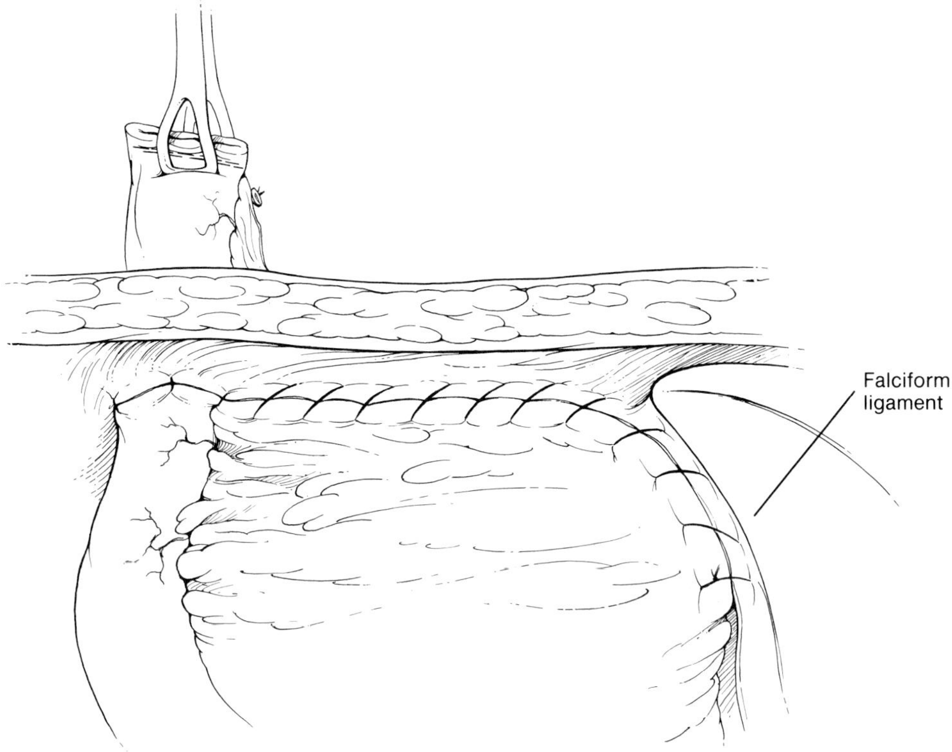

The free edge of the small bowel mesentery is sewn to the back of the anterior abdominal wall with interrupted or continuous sutures. The suturing is started adjacent to the stoma aperture, and at least a 2.5 cm gap is left between the suture line and the edge of the abdominal wound. The cephalad edge of the suture line is continued onto the free lower edge of the falciform ligament. Care must be taken to avoid damage to the vessels in the edge of the mesentery.

Several stabilizing sutures of 3-0 absorbable material usually are placed between the seromuscular layer of the ileum and the peritoneum around the internal aperture. This step provides another protection against ileostomy prolapse and recession, but in patients with Crohn's disease such suturing should be omitted or the sutures should be inserted more superficially into the bowel wall to minimize the chance of subsequent fistula formation.

Maturation of Stoma

The maturation of the stoma is normally completed after the abdominal incision has been closed, and the stoma is isolated with drapes to minimize contamination. The staple line closing the distal ileum is excised.

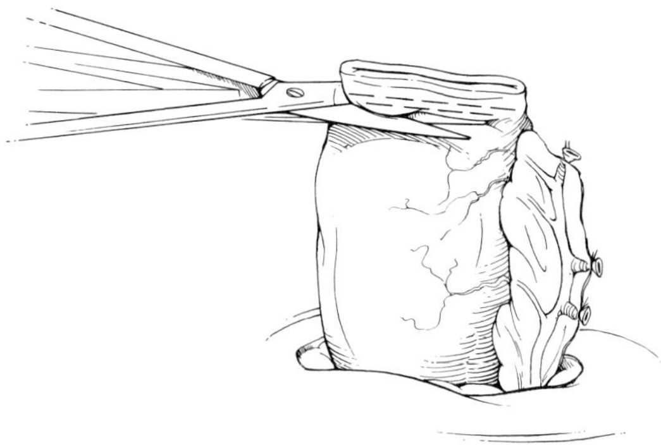

After Pangrace

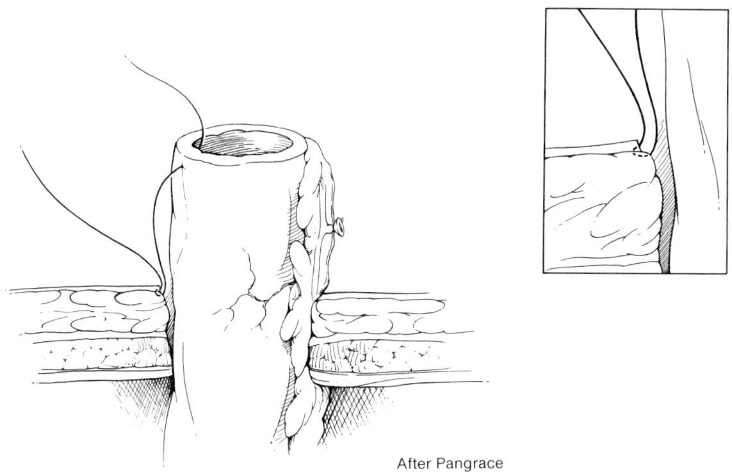

After Pangrace

Sutures of 3-0 chromic catgut are placed at the four compass points of the ileostomy through the full thickness of the bowel and the subcuticular layer of the skin (see inset).

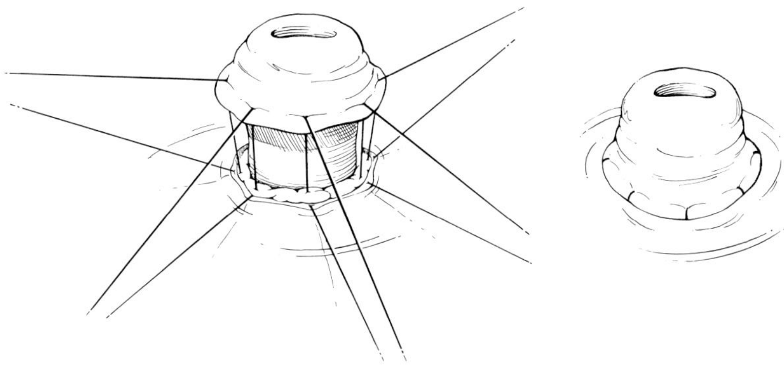

Another four sutures are placed midway between the initial four sutures. All sutures are placed vertically, rather than horizontally, through the subcuticular skin to avoid small areas of ischemia, which may cause mucocutaneous separation. Placing the sutures through the external skin should be avoided because of the risk of ileal mucosal implantation in the skin, which can lead to mucous secretion under the stoma device. After all sutures have been placed, they are tied down to produce eversion of the stoma.

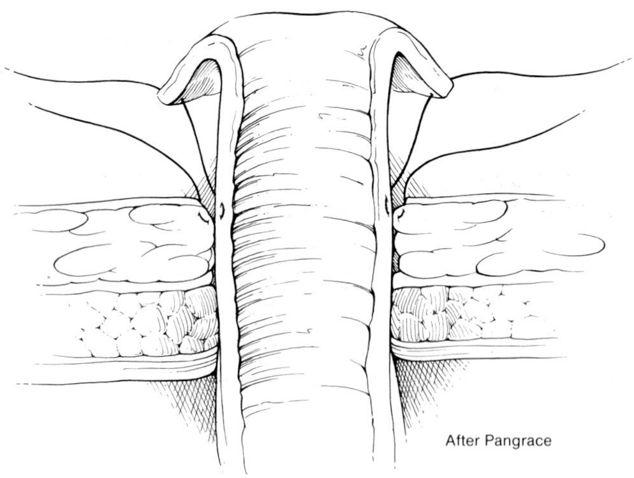

Two alternative methods of suture placement are sometimes valuable. A 3-0 suture inserted through full-thickness bowel and the seromuscular layer of the bowel wall at skin level, before being passed through the subcuticular layer of the skin, helps to maintain eversion of the ileostomy. This method is particularly useful in patients with flabby subcutaneous tissue, which provides little support for the stoma, but it should be avoided in patients with Crohn's disease because of the risk of producing a skin level fistula.

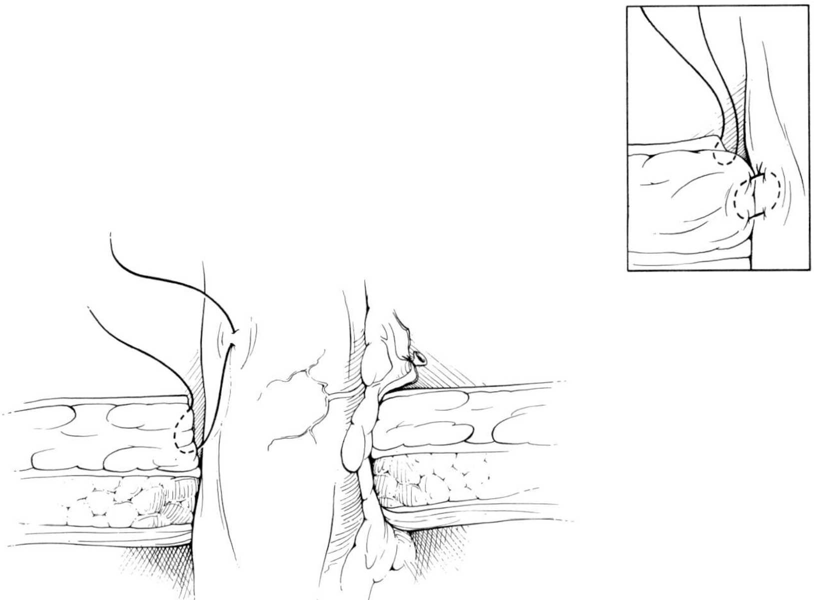

After Pangrace

The second alternative method of suture placement helps to prevent the formation of a gully or "moat" at the mucocutaneous junction. Such a formation can occur in obese patients without firm supporting subcutaneous tissue or in patients who gain weight after having ileostomy surgery. To help avoid this problem, the skin edge can be everted slightly more by placing radial sutures of 3-0 catgut between the bowel wall and the subcutaneous fat. If the seromuscular suture is placed approximately 1 cm above the skin level and through the superficial level of the fat, a slight concertina effect is produced as it is tied, reducing any tendency toward formation of a parastomal gully. The standard mucocutaneous sutures are then placed as a second layer (see inset).

Application of Postoperative Pouch

On completion of ileostomy construction, the perianal skin is cleansed and dried and a postoperative pouch is applied. The most suitable skin barrier for the pouch is a large karaya disk to which is attached an open-ended transparent postoperative pouch with adhesive backing. Hypoallergenic paper tape is used to secure the periphery of the pouch to the skin. The clear pouch allows easy inspection of the stoma during the postoperative period, when special attention must be given to stoma color, swelling, and mucocutaneous separation.

COMPLICATIONS

By strictly adhering to the principles and techniques described here, the number of postoperative ileostomy complications can be reduced but not eliminated. The most common early complications are ischemia (with possible mucocutaneous separation), high ileostomy output, and bowel obstruction. Problems that may develop later include stoma stenosis and retraction, stoma recession and prolapse, and parastomal herniation. Parastomal abscess, ulceration, and fistula, although sometimes the result of poor surgical technique, are often caused by recurrent disease, particularly Crohn's disease.

Ischemia

If bright-red or "nuisance" bleeding from the cut end of the ileostomy has been observed during maturation of the stoma, postoperative ischemia is unlikely to occur. Most instances of ileostomy ischemia result from excessive trimming of the mesentery (more than 5 or 6 cm). When such trimming has been done, the stoma usually appears dusky at the time of maturation. Excessive tension or delayed thrombosis in the mesenteric vessels adjacent to the ileostomy may be a contributing factor in some patients.

Ischemia usually is apparent within 24 hours and may vary considerably in severity. In the extreme situation the stoma appears dark purple or black and the mucosa loses its normal shiny appearance. Failure to produce any bleeding after a needlestick indicates that the ischemia involves both bowel wall and mucosa. In this situation it is important to assess the proximal extent of the ischemia through inspection of the lumen of the stoma by using gentle retraction with a cotton-tipped swab or a pediatric anoscope or proctoscope. A small well-lubricated test tube carefully inserted into the stoma also may be helpful in assessing the level of ischemia. If the ischemia extends deep to the fascia and involves intraperitoneal ileum, immediate revision is required to prevent later perforation and peritonitis. In addition, when extensive superficial ischemia is present, even if confined above the fascia, early revision is advisable because full-thickness ischemia that extends more than 1 or 2 cm is likely to produce stricture and require later revision.

With lesser degrees of ischemia, especially if only the mucosa appears to be involved, observation alone is indicated. Subsequently, sloughing of part of the mucosa, or mucocutaneous separation, may occur, resulting in delayed stoma healing. If the mucocutaneous separation is circumferential, late fibrosis and scarring (Bishop's collar deformity) may occur. However, as a rule, early revision for ischemia is not indicated except when the stoma is obviously necrotic or wide circumferential separation occurs at the mucocutaneous junction.

High Ileostomy Output

In the early postoperative period the ileostomy output may be a watery green effluent, sometimes of high volume, that contains clumps or strands of gray-white mucus. This type of output should not be regarded as a sign of return of normal bowel function, and oral intake should be withheld until a thicker brown effluent is noted. If the volume continues to be high after normal eating and drinking has been resumed, it can be reduced with Imodium, Lomotil, codeine, or tincture of laudanum, alone or in combination. Psyllium seed derivatives also may be helpful in thickening the stool.

Bowel Obstruction

Small bowel obstruction can be noted at any time after construction of an ileostomy. However, its incidence appears to be higher after surgery for inflammatory bowel disease than for cancer or other conditions. The reason for this difference is unclear.

Extrinsic mechanical bowel obstruction is most commonly caused by adhesions. Often these adhesions are related to the ligature site of the right, middle, or left colic vessels; the sigmoid or inferior mesenteric vessels; or the retained greater omentum (after subtotal colectomy or proctocolectomy). Although adhesions do occur in the pelvis after proctocolectomy, closure of the pelvic peritoneum does not reduce the incidence of small bowel obstruction and actually may increase it. Volvulus and internal herniation, which also can produce mechanical obstruction, are more likely to occur if the free edge of the small bowel mesentery is not firmly attached to the anterior abdominal wall at the time of ileostomy construction.

Obstruction caused by a food bolus also may occur after ileostomy construction, especially within 3 months of surgery. The obstruction usually is located at or near the fascia level; however, it also can occur at a point of low-grade angulation or narrowing caused by adhesions or as a result of recurrent Crohn's disease elsewhere in the bowel. Ingestion of poorly digestible food, such as corn, coconut, popcorn, stringy vegetables, nuts, or fruit skins, usually is responsible for the obstruction. The obstruction is often sudden in onset and usually complete, with total cessation of ileostomy output occurring at about the same time as the onset of abdominal pain. The diagnosis usually can be confirmed, and the problem can be treated conservatively through gentle irrigation of the stoma with 50 to 100 ml of saline introduced through a small soft catheter passed into the terminal ileum. The irrigation breaks up the bolus, which is washed out through the stoma. Lavage should be continued until the food particles are removed and an adequate return is obtained.

In the early postoperative period, making a distinction between a prolonged ileus and a mechanical obstruction can be difficult. If gentle stoma irrigation excludes (or relieves) a bolus obstruction, the initial management should be expectant and supportive, based on the generally accepted principles of fluid and electrolyte replacement and nasogastric suction. Operative intervention should be reserved for the patient who develops increasing pain or signs of peritonitis or if failure to resolve suggests a continuing mechanical obstruction.

Stoma Stenosis and Retraction

Stoma stenosis may occur as a late sequela of ischemia and mucosal sloughing. Recurrence of Crohn's disease is another common cause of stenosis. In either situation the underlying process also can produce scarring and retraction of the stoma, sometimes resulting in a flush stoma, which leads to pouching difficulties, leakage, and skin irritation.

Dilatation of a stenotic stoma is contraindicated because it usually aggravates the problem. If stoma stenosis is severe enough to produce symptoms, revision of the stoma is generally advisable. Minor degrees of retraction sometimes can be managed by a change in pouching technique, often by incorporation of a convex insert into the faceplate. More severe degrees of retraction, especially with associated stenosis, require revision. When the segment of diseased or involved bowel is short, the revision can be performed locally through a circumferential incision made exactly at the mucocutaneous junction. The ileostomy and adjacent small bowel are mobilized completely from the abdominal wall aperture, the diseased segment is resected, and sufficient healthy bowel is drawn through to produce eversion of the stoma. When the diseased segment is extensive or when sufficient mobilization of the bowel cannot be achieved, revision at laparotomy is indicated.

Ileostomy Recession and Prolapse

Intermittent recession, or telescoping of the stoma (which should be distinguished from progressive or fixed retraction), results from inadequate fixation of the bowel wall and the free edge of the small bowel mesentery to the abdominal wall. This complication usually can be prevented by avoiding too large an aperture and by the fixation techniques already described. When recession of the stoma into the abdomen results in pouch leakage and skin irritation, revision is indicated. Revision often can be done locally through reduction in the size of the fascia defect and refixation of the bowel to the abdominal wall, but occasionally laparotomy is needed to anchor the bowel and the mesentery more securely.

Ileostomy recession is often associated with ileostomy prolapse and para-ileostomy hernia, with inadequate bowel fixation and large abdominal wall apertures playing a major part in the etiology. Parastomal herniation and prolapse are discussed in more detail in Chapters 15 and 16, respectively.

Skin Problems

Multiple skin problems can follow ileostomy surgery. These problems may result from poor surgical technique, unsatisfactory pouching arrangements, recurrent disease in the stoma, allergies, and a host of primary skin and other conditions. The management of these problems is discussed in Chapter 19.

LONG-TERM FOLLOW-UP

The initial follow-up visit takes place approximately 6 weeks after discharge from the hospital. At this time it is usually necessary to remeasure the diameter of the stoma because shrinkage commonly occurs. This visit offers an opportunity to detect any problems with the pouching system and to assess the adequacy of skin care.

After the initial postoperative visit patients usually are encouraged to return to the surgeon or the enterostomal therapist if they notice any new problems with the stoma. In the absence of any particular problems, an annual review is recommended. Such a review gives an opportunity to detect any unrecognized problems or complications, including recurrent disease, and allows the patient to keep abreast of any new developments in stoma equipment and management.

SELECTED READINGS

Fazio VW. Complications of intestinal stoma. In Ferrari BT, Ray JE, Gathright JB, eds. Complications of Colon and Rectal Surgery—Prevention and Management. Philadelphia: WB Saunders, 1985.

Kodner IJ. Colostomy and ileostomy. Clin Symp 30:2-36, 1978.

Oakley JR, Fazio VW. Ileostomy. In Carter DC, Russell RCG, eds. Rob and Smith's Operative Surgery, 5th ed. London: Butterworth-Heinemann, 1993.

Turnbull R, Weakley F. Atlas of Intestinal Stomas. St. Louis: CV Mosby, 1967.

Woods RT, Fazio VW. Brooke ileostomy. In Bayless TM, ed. Current Management of Inflammatory Bowel Disease. Philadelphia: BC Decker, 1989.

10 CONTINENT STOMAS

Stephen R. Gorfine, Joel J. Bauer, and Irwin M. Gelernt

The achievement of continence, the ability to control the time and place of evacuation of intestinal waste, is one of the earliest developmental milestones in nearly all human societies. Until relatively recently, surgical creation of any kind of intestinal stoma was almost certain to result in the loss of this most basic function. Over the past 25 years considerable effort has been devoted to the development of means by which continence can be reestablished for the individual with an enterostomy.

CONTINENT ILEOSTOMY

Early work in the field of stoma continence was performed in the 1960s by Professor Nils G. Kock at Sahlgren's Hospital in Göteborg, Sweden.[1] In working with experimental models, Kock found that a double-folded ileal pouch provided a low-pressure reservoir capable of "storing" the intestinal effluent.[2] Early clinical results with the use of this technique were encouraging, but not all patients achieved satisfactory continence. Reliable stoma continence was realized in 1972, when a "nipple valve" formed by intussusception of the intestinal segment distal to the reservoir was added.[3]

Kock's continent ileostomy was enthusiastically embraced by patients who would have otherwise required a permanent Brooke ileostomy. Most candidates for the procedure were young adults suffering from chronic mucosal ulcerative colitis. The majority of them felt that the reservoir ileostomy had improved the quality of their lives. Many were quite willing to undergo multiple procedures rather than return to using an external ostomy device.

Despite widespread initial enthusiasm, it soon became obvious that Kock's intussuscepted valve was both the heart and the Achilles' heel of the procedure. Incontinence resulting from slippage or desusception of the valve was reported in nearly 50% of early cases.[4-7]

By the early 1980s a wealth of experimental and clinical evidence had been gathered that conclusively demonstrated that intermittent ileal occlusion with or without an ileal reservoir was safe, feasible, and without significant metabolic consequences.[8-11] Growing patient demand for a reliable continent stoma stimulated the pursuit of a method of improving long-term results and decreasing associated morbidity.

The search for better results yielded novel experimental and clinical techniques. For example, continence was achieved with nonreservoir ileostomies through intestinal intussusception[12] and indwelling catheter occlusion.[13] Neither approach gained widespread acceptance. Most investigators concentrated on improving the valve mechanism of the Kock ileostomy. Many believed that the intussuscepted nipple valve was basically a sound concept and that improved long-term stability could be achieved by modification of construction techniques. Others reasoned that the intestinal valve was intrinsically flawed and that its replacement by a prosthetic occlusive device would be a better option. The middle ground was taken by those who thought that supporting the intussuscepted nipple with a prosthetic or natural girdle would offer a better solution.

Steps to improve the reliability of the original Kock nipple valve were undertaken early in the evolution of the procedure. Stripping the serosa from the intussuscepted segment, staple fixation of the valve, and application of a special "rotational suture" proved to be useful and effective adjuncts.[1] Prolonged postoperative pouch intubation also helped to reduce valve complications.[14]

Concurrently, complete replacement of the valve by various prosthetic mechanisms was under investigation. The Mayo Clinic group found that a cuffed Silastic catheter, similar to an endotracheal tube, restored continence in "failed" Kock ileostomies[15] (Fig. 10-1). Fendel and Fazio[16] replaced the nipple valve by a porcine aortic valve in an experimental model. A mucosal "flap" valve was created in another experimental setting.[17] Magnetic closing caps were implanted successfully in two patients.[18] Although the devices subjected to clinical trials were able to maintain continence, various complications and limited patient acceptance prevented widespread adoption of their use.

A different approach was taken by Fazio, Cohen, Barnett, and others. They found that the intussuscepted nipple valve was more stable when it was mechanically supported at its junction with the pouch and the outflow tract. A strip of fascia,[19] Marlex or Prolene,[20] and, later, an ileal limb[21] were used to buttress the valve. Short-term results were promising. A dramatic decrease in the rate of valve desusception was reported. However, an equally dramatic rise in the rate of late fistula formation was associated with use of the various plastic materials.[22,23]

Even as evolutionary improvements in the reservoir ileostomy were being made, revolutionary change was beginning. In 1977 Martin et al.[24] reported successful preservation of continence after total colectomy by mucosal proc-

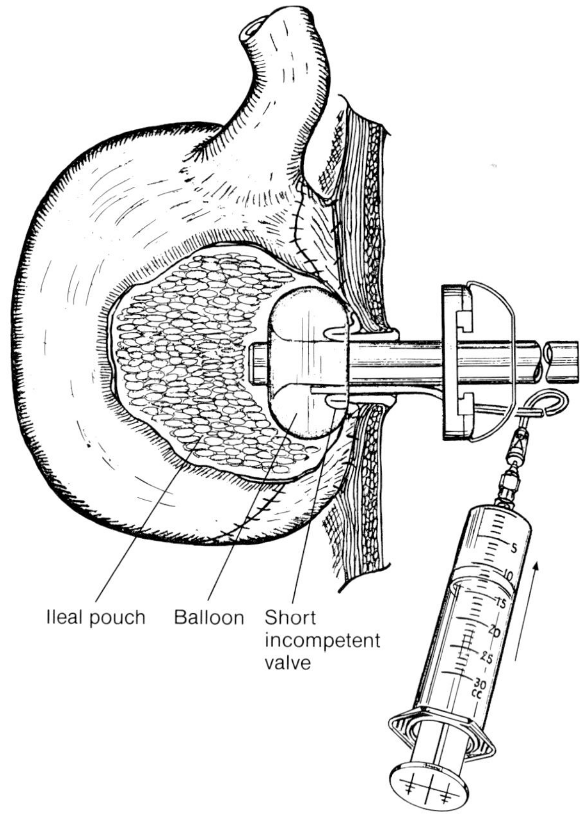

Fig. 10-1. Inflatable cuffed Silastic occlusion catheter in place in "failed" continent (Kock) ileostomy. (Courtesy Gauthier, Rochester, Minn.)

tectomy and ileoanal anastomosis. In 1980 Sir Alan Parks combined abdominal colectomy and mucosal proctectomy with an ileal pouch and pouch-anal anastomosis.[25] This new procedure completely eliminated the need for a permanent abdominal stoma. Use of the anal sphincter as the pouch closing mechanism effectively solved the valve problem. Although the new procedure had its own complications, enthusiasm for restorative proctocolectomy by ileal pouch–anal anastomosis grew quickly among patients and surgeons. By the mid 1980s, demand for the continent ileostomy had virtually vanished.[26]

Indications and Patient Selection

Continent ileostomy remains a therapeutic option open to selected patients who would otherwise require a permanent end ileostomy. Most candidates for this procedure will have the diagnosis of chronic mucosal ulcerative colitis or familial adenomatous polyposis. Some patients will choose the continent stoma as a primary or secondary procedure because of personal life-style considerations. For others, reservoir ileostomy may be the only continence-preserving alternative when the anal sphincter is unsuitable because of weakness, disease, surgical extirpation, or failure of a previous ileoanal procedure.

Selection of appropriate candidates for reservoir ileostomy is of the utmost importance. The risk of complication is significantly greater in certain patient populations. Long-term management of the stoma requires both cognitive and manual skills. All candidates must demonstrate the physical and emotional maturity needed to cope with ordinary, and occasionally extraordinary, stoma maintenance.

Patient education is equal in importance to patient selection. The mechanics of the reservoir ileostomy and its potential risks and benefits must be clearly, completely, and honestly explained to all suitable candidates. Candidates must become familiar with the concept of the reservoir and the valve. They must accept the possibility that the procedure may be abandoned intraoperatively because of unexpected findings or circumstances. The risk that repeated revisional surgery may become necessary must be clearly understood. We find it helpful to have a candidate for surgery speak to a patient who has undergone the procedure.

Continent ileostomy is not recommended in patients with Crohn's disease, suboptimal nutritional or immunologic status, or short bowel syndrome.[26-28] These conditions raise the risk of complications to an unacceptably high level. Emergency surgery, extremes of youth or age, obesity, and inability to intubate the pouch because of mental or physical impairment also are considered contraindications to a reservoir ileostomy.[26-28]

Operative Technique

Preoperative preparation includes standard mechanical and antibiotic bowel preparation and enterostomal counseling. With the patient under general anesthesia, the abdomen is entered through a midline incision. When indicated, proctocolectomy, proctectomy, or takedown of a standard ileostomy is performed in the standard fashion. In all cases every effort is made to preserve the ileal blood supply and conserve maximal ileal length.

The complete continent ileostomy is constructed from the terminal 45 cm of ileum. The nipple valve, outflow segment, and stoma are created from the most distal 15 cm. The reservoir is made from the proximally adjacent 30 cm of intestine.

The antimesenteric border of the ileum is grasped with a Babcock clamp

30 cm from the cut end. This distance should be measured accurately with a marked scalpel handle or a sterile ruler. The bowel is then folded upon itself with the 30 cm point resting at the apex of the loop.

The antimesenteric borders of the ileal loop are approximated with running 3-0 long-term absorbable sutures. The suture line runs for a distance of 15 cm from the loop's apex (Fig. 10-2). The approximated ileal limbs are opened with electrocautery parallel to the suture line. The incision in the afferent limb is continued proximally 2 to 3 cm beyond the distal termination of the incision in the efferent limb. This method will allow the afferent and efferent limbs to be separated when the pouch is closed. Both enterotomies are continued to the tip of the loop where they meet. A second layer of running 3-0 long-term absorbable sutures joins the two cut edges, leaving a U-shaped pouch of small bowel open toward the inflow and outflow tracts (Fig. 10-3).

The nipple valve is constructed from the 10 cm of distal ileum adjacent to the reservoir. The intussuscepted valve will be about 5 cm long. Multiple techniques are employed to promote permanent fixation of the valve in the intussuscepted position. These include thinning of the valve mesentery, scarification of the intestinal surface, and placement of sutures and staples. Barnett[29] recommends encirclement of the outflow tract with an ileal "collar." However, we do not routinely employ this technique.

Preparation of the ileal segment for valve intussusception begins by reducing its mesenteric bulk. This reduction is accomplished by excising the fat between the blood vessels (Fig. 10-4). Exceptional care must be exercised during this maneuver so that injury to the segment's blood supply is avoided. The serosa is then abraded with a fine rasp and scored with electrocautery. Scattered subserosal injections of a concentrated tetracycline solution are also helpful in promoting adhesion between the opposing surfaces.

Three 3-0 silk seromuscular sutures are placed on both sides of the mesenteric border, equidistant from the point of intussusception (Fig. 10-5). When tied, these sutures will help to maintain the intussusception. We think that rotation of the valve is not necessary. A Babcock clamp is passed from the pouch into the distal ileal segment, and the wall is grasped 5 cm from its junction with the reservoir. Gentle traction applied in the direction of the pouch lumen will cause intussusception of the segment. The previously placed silk seromuscular sutures are sequentially tied as the segment is intussuscepted (Fig. 10-6).

The valve is further stabilized by three rows of staples, one placed on either side of the mesentery and the third on the antimesenteric border (Fig. 10-7). These staples are most easily placed with a *bladeless* linear-cutter sta-

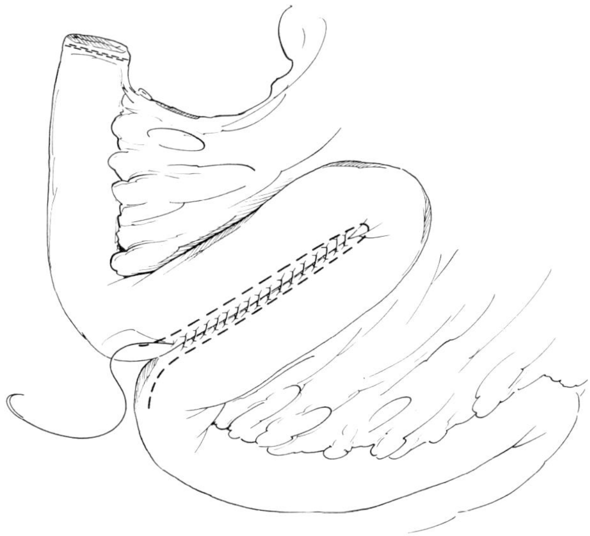

Fig. 10-2. Construction of continent ileostomy from distal 45 cm of ileum. Most distal 15 cm is used to form the valve and the outflow tract. Adjacent 30 cm of small bowel is folded on itself to form the pouch. Running 3-0 absorbable sutures approximate the antimesenteric borders. Both limbs are then opened parallel to the suture line (dashed line). Note that incision in proximal limb extends 2 to 3 cm beyond the end of the suture line.

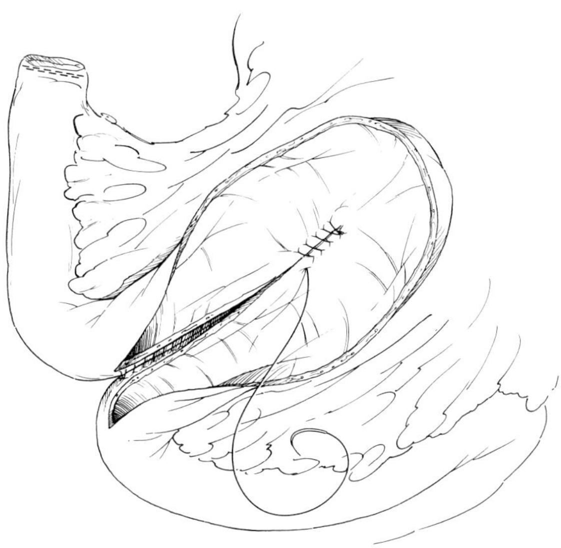

Fig. 10-3. Continent ileostomy with cut edges joined, leaving U-shaped pouch of small bowel. A second layer of running sutures is placed.

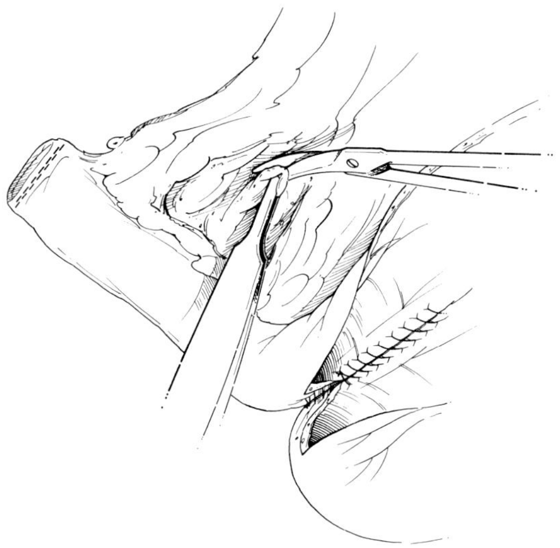

Fig. 10-4. Mesenteric fat between blood vessels is excised in preparation for valve intussusception.

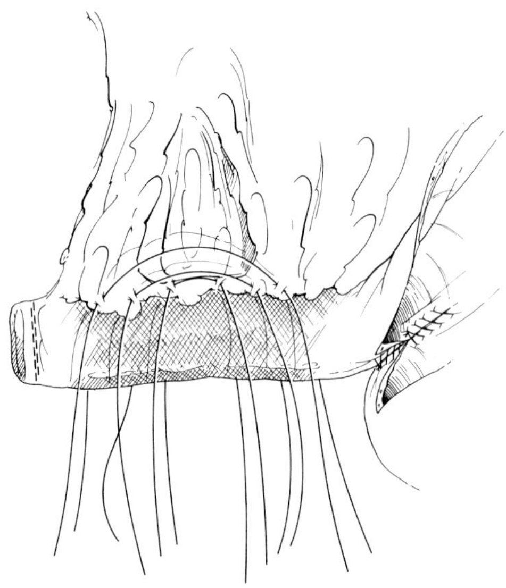

Fig. 10-5. Serosal surface of the valve segment is abraded. Silk seromuscular sutures are placed on both sides of the mesentery.

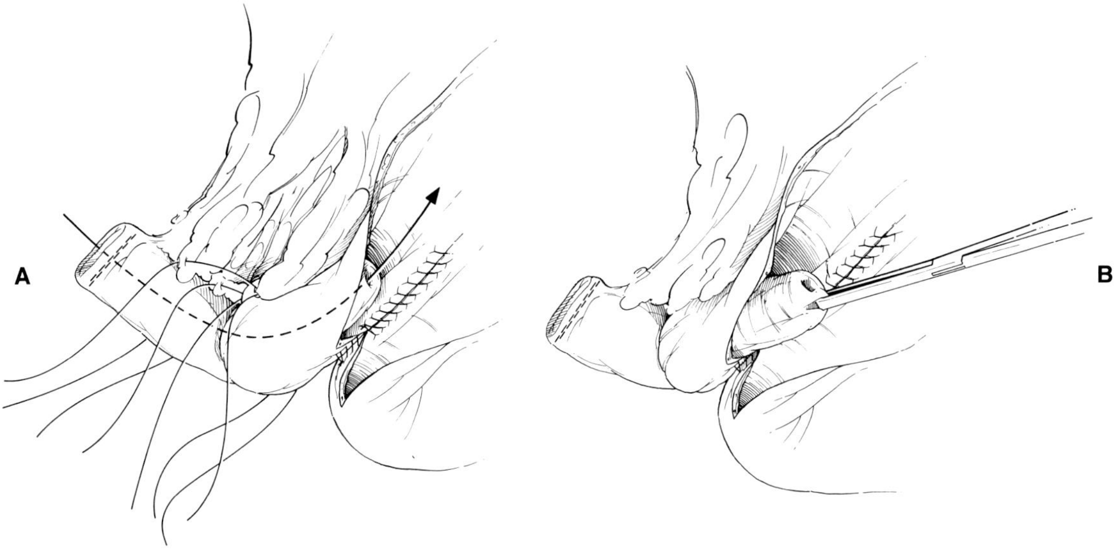

Fig. 10-6. A, Valve is intussuscepted and seromuscular sutures are tied. **B,** Intussuscepted valve.

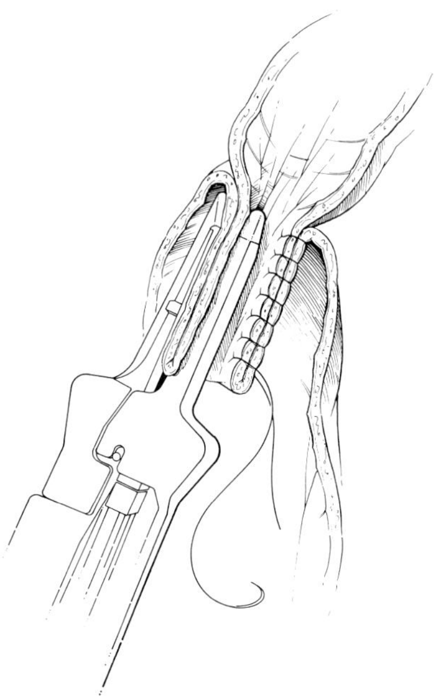

Fig. 10-7. Valve is secured with three rows of staples or silk sutures. Staples are placed with a bladeless instrument.

pler. In addition, six to eight 3-0 silk sutures are passed through all layers of the valve. To minimize the risk of nipple fistula, these sutures should enclose only a small bridge of tissue and should not be tied so tightly as to strangulate the encircled bowel. Last, a row of interrupted 3-0 silk sutures is used to fix the base of the valve to the surrounding pouch wall at its point of exit (Fig. 10-8).

The pouch is closed by bringing the apex of the U to the base of the valve (Fig. 10-9, *A*). A double layer of running 3-0 long-term absorbable sutures is used to close the enterotomy (Fig. 10-9, *B*). When the reservoir is complete, competence of the valve is tested. The inflow tract is occluded with an intestinal clamp. A bullet-nosed catheter is passed into the pouch through the outflow tract and valve. Air is insufflated and the catheter removed. The pouch should remain distended.

The position of the stoma is determined after the reservoir has been placed in the pelvis. The outflow tract should traverse the midportion of the right rectus muscle without angulation or redundancy. In most cases the stoma will lie just above the pubic hairline. The stoma defect in the anterior abdominal wall is created by excising a 2 cm disk of skin. The subcutaneous fat is retracted, and the fascia is opened by a cruciate incision. The fibers of the rectus muscle are split, and the peritoneum is incised. The defect should easily admit two fingers.

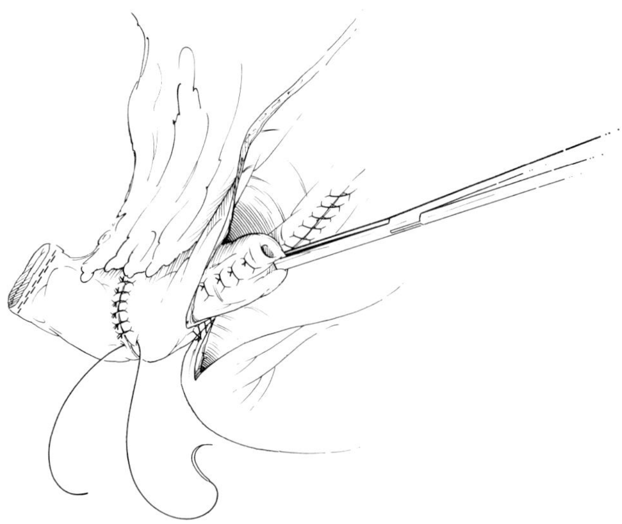

Fig. 10-8. Interrupted silk sutures are used to secure the base of the valve to the outflow tract.

A

B

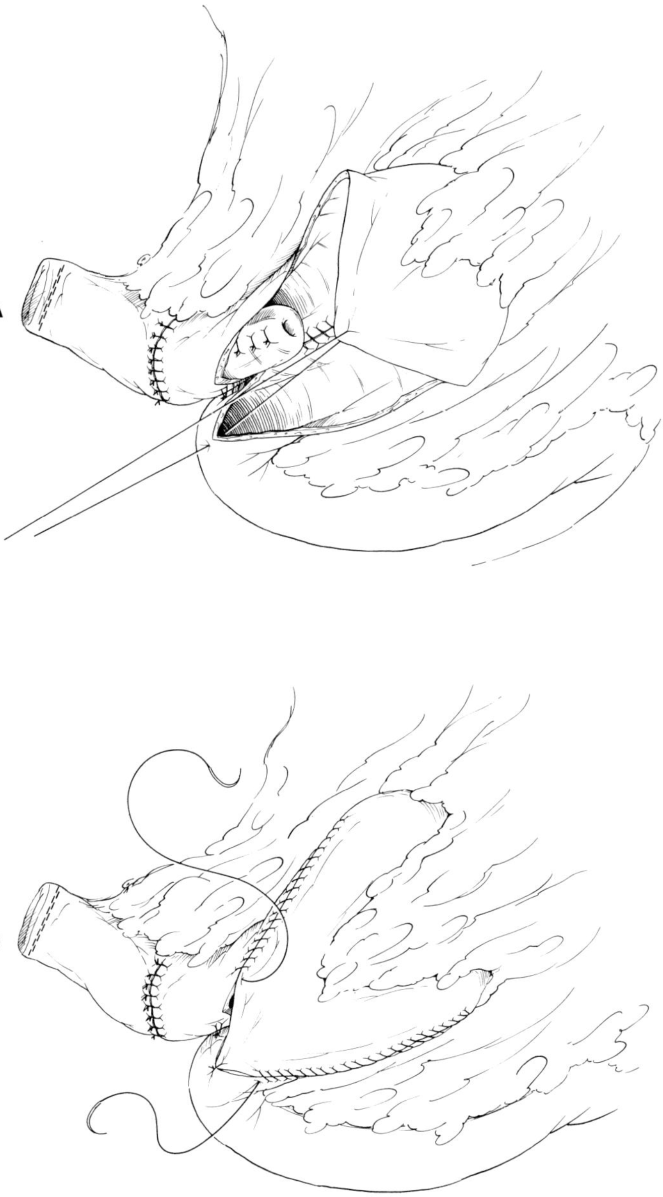

Fig. 10-9. **A,** Pouch is closed by folding the apex of the U to the base of the valve. **B,** Pouch is completed by placing running absorbable sutures from the corners to the apex.

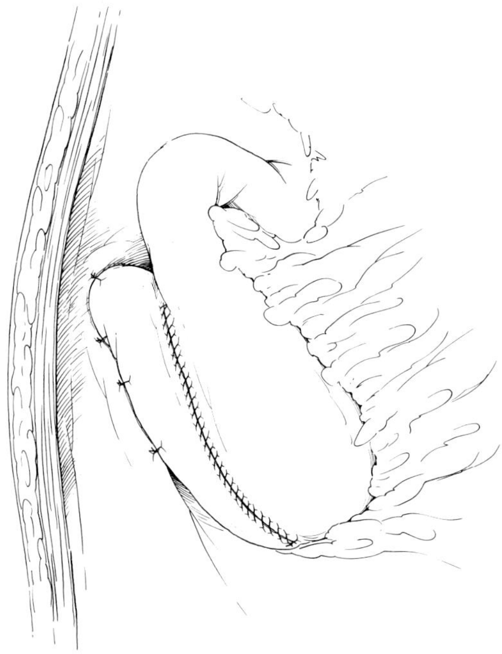

Fig. 10-10. Outflow tract is brought through the abdominal wall. Silk sutures are used to anchor the pouch to the parietal peritoneum.

Before bringing the outflow tract through the abdominal wall, the pouch is rendered heart-shaped by pushing the lateral "ears" into the leaves of the mesentery. Four 3-0 silk anchoring sutures are passed from the pouch to the parietal peritoneum surrounding the stoma site (Fig. 10-10). The outflow tract is passed through the abdominal wall defect, and the anchoring sutures are tied. A closed suction drain is placed in the right gutter, lateral to the pouch. The end of the drain is brought out through a separate abdominal wall stab wound.

The stoma is matured before the abdominal wound is closed. The exteriorized ileum is trimmed until the cut edge is flush with the skin. The ileal edge is anchored to the dermis with interrupted 3-0 long-term absorbable sutures. An ileostomy catheter introduced through the stoma should enter the pouch without difficulty.

A crosspiece is fashioned from a 3-inch segment of 32 Fr rubber tubing by cutting 1 cm holes in the middle of the opposing walls. The crosspiece is used to anchor the ileostomy catheter to the abdominal skin. The ileostomy cathe-

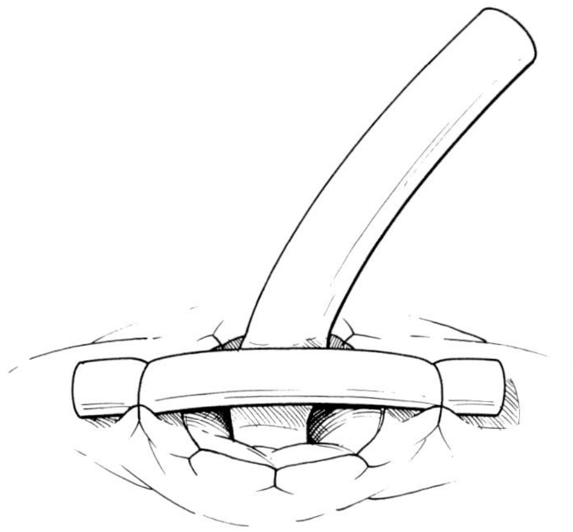

Fig. 10-11. Procedure is completed. Stoma, matured flush to skin level, is just above the pubic hairline. A No. 28 ileostomy catheter has been placed in the pouch and fixed firmly in place with a rubber collar sutured to the skin.

ter is passed through the holes in the crosspiece and then inserted into the pouch. The catheter's position within the pouch is ascertained by palpation. The catheter is held in this position, and the crosspiece is brought to skin level. The crosspiece is then sutured to the abdominal wall skin (Fig. 10-11). The abdominal wound is closed and dressed in standard fashion.

Postoperative Management

Hourly irrigation of the pouch with 20 ml of normal saline instilled through the catheter is performed for the first 24 hours after surgery. Continuous gravity drainage is maintained between irrigations. On the second day the frequency of irrigation is reduced to every 2 hours. This irrigation schedule is continued for 2 weeks. During this period it is imperative that the ileostomy tube remain within the reservoir. Utmost care must be exercised during dressing changes to prevent its dislodgment.

Bowel function usually returns by the fourth or fifth postoperative day. Progressive refeeding begins at that time. The diet should exclude undigestible fruit, nuts, and vegetable material so that plugging of the catheter is avoided.

At the end of the second postoperative week, continuous drainage is discontinued. The catheter remains in the pouch but is occluded with a plastic button. Evacuation of the pouch by "uncorking" the catheter is performed every hour during the daytime. The catheter is returned to gravity drainage at night. The interval between pouch evacuations is progressively lengthened by 15 minutes per day over the remainder of the hospital stay. The maximal interval between evacuations should not exceed 2 hours during this time. Continuous nighttime drainage is maintained until the patient is ready to be discharged.

Patients with uncomplicated courses leave the hospital at the end of the third postoperative week. The patient is taught the technique of pouch intubation before discharge. At the time of discharge the patient is instructed to empty the pouch every 2 hours while awake and once during the night. The dietary exclusion of fruits, nuts, and vegetables should be maintained. The patient is cautioned to avoid straining or pushing to speed evacuation of the reservoir. If repetitive coughing or sneezing, similar to that caused by a cold or allergy, should ensue, the patient is advised to resume continuous reservoir intubation, button occlusion of the catheter, and periodic evacuation at 2-hour intervals. A follow-up appointment is arranged for 2 weeks after discharge.

At the first postoperative visit, usually 5 weeks after surgery, the wound and the stoma are inspected. Most patients will report that continence is perfect for feces and gas and that intubations are uncomplicated. If all is proceeding smoothly, the patient is instructed to omit the nighttime evacuation. Gradually, fiber can be reintroduced into the diet. The interval between evacuations is increased by ½-hour increments every 2 to 3 weeks. The maximum time between intubations should not exceed 5 hours. The patient is reminded to avoid straining while emptying the pouch and that continuous intubation is recommended during periods of prolonged coughing or sneezing for the first 6 months.

Functional Results

The vast majority of patients are satisfied with the outcome of their surgery.[30-34] Although surgical revision of the nipple valve may be required, ultimately more than 90% of patients are perfectly continent or do not require the use of an ostomy management system.[5,27,28,34-36] Most patients evacuate the pouch three or four times daily. The stoma is usually covered with a small dressing between intubations. The flush stoma does not interfere with clothing or physical activities.[30-34] Full-term pregnancy and uncomplicated vaginal delivery are possible in women with continent stomas.[37] Patients whose standard ileostomies were converted to reservoir ileostomies viewed their quality of life as substantially better.[32,33]

Complications

Creation of a continent ileostomy is associated with a variety of early and late complications.* Some problems, such as adhesive small bowel obstruction, are not unique to the complex stoma but are common to all major intra-abdominal procedures. Others are specific to the reservoir and valve of the continent stoma. Of the latter, hemorrhage, pouch leakage, and ischemia of the outflow tract or valve tend to occur in the early postoperative period. Most late complications particular to the continent ileostomy involve the nipple valve. These include valve slippage, fistula, and prolapse. The reservoir itself is prone to a form of mucosal ileitis termed "pouchitis."†

Most authors have reported a lowered complication rate as experience with the procedure and technical modifications have evolved. However, an overall reoperation rate of 12% to 66% has been reported in large series.[5,27,35,36] In more recent studies the incidence of reoperation is approximately 25%. This rate is compared to a reported reoperation rate of 18% to 23% for large series of standard ileostomies.[38,39]

Early complications

Hemorrhage. Hemorrhage from the reservoir usually is noted at approximately the seventh postoperative day.[28] The indwelling catheter returns bloody fluid spontaneously or after irrigation. Bleeding is occasionally brisk, and transfusion may be required. The site of bleeding is most often one or more of the pouch suture lines.

This complication usually can be managed nonoperatively in the hemodynamically stable patient. Bleeding often will cease spontaneously if the pouch can be maintained free of old blood. This state is best achieved through frequent saline irrigations. The addition of norepinephrine to the irrigation fluid is helpful. Systemic vasopressin has been used successfully in extreme cases.[14,28] Fiberoptic or rigid ileoscopy should be avoided because of the risk of perforation. Surgical exploration to control hemorrhage is almost never required. When laparotomy is necessary, excision of the pouch and creation of a standard ileostomy is recommended by some.[28]

Suture-line dehiscence. Suture-line dehiscence is rare and usually can be avoided by scrupulous operative technique and careful postoperative management. This complication occurs in about 2% of cases.[5,35] The patient presents with the symptoms and signs of localized or free visceral perforation.

*References 5, 6, 27, 28, 34-36.
†References 5, 6, 27, 28, 35, 36.

Fluid resuscitation and systemic antibiotics are almost always indicated.[28] Leakage during the first postoperative week is often poorly contained and frequently leads to generalized peritonitis. In this situation reexploration for drainage and proximal diversion is necessary. Excision of the reservoir is almost never indicated. Between the second and fourth weeks, localized abscess and pouch-cutaneous fistula are more common.[28] This complication usually can be managed without laparotomy.

Fistula. The reservoir ileostomy is prone to two distinct types of fistulas: internal and external. External fistulas cause an abnormal communication between the pouch and the skin (Fig. 10-12). Internal fistulas traverse both limbs of the intussuscepted valve, causing communication between the lumen of the pouch and the lumen of the valve (Fig. 10-13). Either type of fistula can appear as an early or late complication.

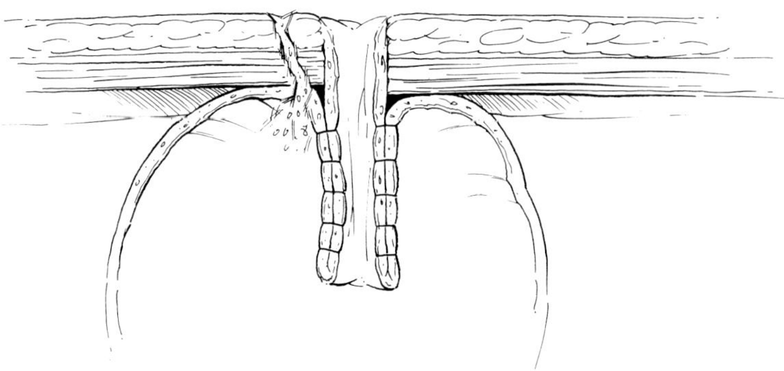

Fig. 10-12. Pouch-cutaneous, or external, fistula.

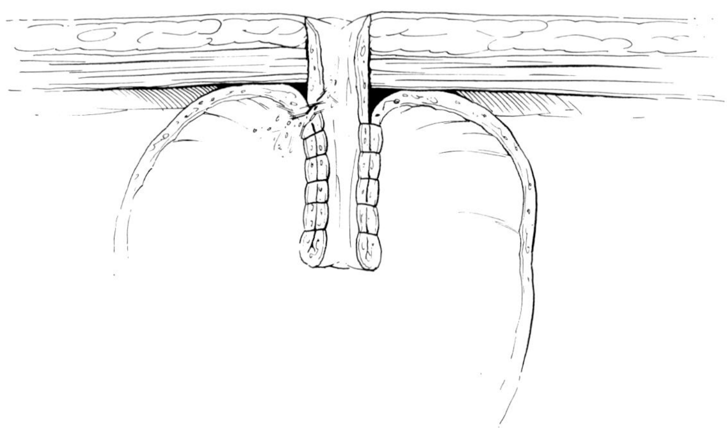

Fig. 10-13. Nipple-valve, or internal, fistula.

Early postoperative fistula formation occurs in approximately 2% of cases.[5,35] Pouch-cutaneous, or external, fistulas are somewhat less common than fistulas involving the nipple valve. An early external fistula tends to arise from the region of the confluence of the reservoir suture lines near the base of the nipple valve. Typically, it is manifest during the second or third postoperative week as either a localized peristomal abscess or cellulitis. Spontaneous or surgical drainage leads to an enterocutaneous fistula.

This complication usually is managed without laparotomy. Systemic antibiotics and sump drainage of the reservoir are indicated.[28] A collection, if present, is drained by incision or percutaneous catheter. In most instances healing is complete within 2 to 3 weeks. Total parenteral nutrition and octreotide are useful therapeutic adjuncts that can speed fistula closure.

Early nipple-valve, or internal, fistulas also present during the second or third postoperative week. These fistulas appear to be caused by pressure necrosis of the tissue under one of the silk sutures placed through the full-thickness of both segments of the intussuscepted valve.[28] Leakage of intestinal contents around the ileostomy catheter is the common presentation. The magnitude of leakage will depend on the size of the fistulous tract and its proximity to the base of the valve. Larger tracts nearer the base of the nipple will cause a greater volume of leakage.

This complication is managed nonoperatively in the immediate postoperative period. An initial trial of antibiotics and continuous sump drainage of the reservoir is warranted. Drainage of intestinal contents around the catheter is controlled by placing a standard ileostomy appliance around the intubated stoma. A small percentage of early nipple fistulas will heal completely within 1 to 2 weeks without further intervention. Others, especially those located near the tip of the valve, may shrink to a point at which continence is only minimally affected when the catheter is removed. These valve fistulas are best left alone unless the patient is intolerant of the volume of leakage.

Fistulas that result in symptomatic incontinence and do not close by 4 to 6 weeks from the initial surgery usually will require operative repair. These fistulas are then managed in the same fashion as nipple fistulas that appear as late complications.

Ischemia. Compromise of the blood supply to the distal portion of the ileum causes ischemia of the outflow tract, the valve, or both. Compression or disruption of the intussuscepted mesentery of the nipple valve is usually the cause. A valve longer than 5 cm, excessive fattiness of the valve mesentery, and overvigorous suturing or stapling of the valve at its mesenteric borders predispose to ischemia by compression.[28] Direct damage to the vasculature of the valve may occur during removal of mesenteric fat.

Ischemia usually becomes manifest within 48 hours of surgery. Dusky discoloration of the stoma, bleeding around the catheter, and bloody returns with irrigation are the hallmarks of poor distal vascularity. Fever and pain are common, especially with tissue necrosis. Frequent irrigation of the ileostomy catheter, administration of systemic antibiotics, and close observation are the best early treatments.[28] Ischemia caused by mesenteric edema may resolve without additional therapy. Progression of the ischemic process can result in necrosis of the outflow tract, the valve, or both.

Outflow tract problems. Chronic ischemia of the outflow tract leads to stenosis of the stoma segment, usually at skin level. Continence is almost always maintained. The problem becomes manifest when the patient begins intubation of the pouch. Progressively increasing difficulty with catheter insertion is the common presentation. This complication is best managed by a 1- to 2-month trial of continuous pouch intubation. The catheter is capped with a plastic button, and the reservoir is emptied intermittently. If the problem persists after this period, elective operative repair by double Z-plasty is recommended.

Ischemic necrosis of the outflow tract causes separation at the mucocutaneous junction and ileal "retraction" by dissolution of the distal bowel. The subcutaneous tissues at the stoma site are exposed, usually resulting in peristomal cellulitis. Sump suction of the reservoir and administration of systemic antibiotics are indicated for early management.[28] Healing usually will occur without immediate surgery, although stricture is almost certain to follow. Continence is maintained unless the valve is also affected.

Stoma revision can be delayed until the pouch has healed completely, usually 2 to 3 months after the initial surgery. The patient can maintain patency at skin level either by continuous intubation or with an infant's pacifier placed in the stoma site between intubations.[28] Stoma revision by double Z-plasty is recommended.

Valve necrosis. Further progression of outflow tract ischemia results in valve loss by ischemic necrosis. This complication occurs in less than 2% of cases.[5,35,36] The patient usually will experience pain and fever. Blood clots, necrotic debris, and sutures or staples may return with reservoir irrigation. Leakage of intestinal contents around the catheter will occur as tissue loss results in valve shortening. When valve necrosis is identified, sump suction of the reservoir and systemic antibiotics should be instituted. Immediate operation is rarely indicated because healing, albeit with incontinence, usually occurs spontaneously.[28]

Revisional surgery often can be delayed until the pouch has healed completely.[28] The ileostomy catheter is left in the reservoir throughout the hospital period and for the 2 to 3 months following discharge. Leakage is controlled by the addition of a standard ostomy device fitted around the intubated stoma. Later, 2 to 3 months after the initial surgery, the patient is readmitted to the hospital for revision. Creation of a new valve involves "turning the pouch."[40]

Late complications

Valve slippage. The most common late postoperative complication of the Kock ileostomy is desusception or slippage of the nipple valve.* Early experiences with the procedure were complicated by valve desusception in 40% to 50% of cases.[1,5,36] With advances in valve stabilization techniques and increasing experience, the incidence of desusception has fallen to 3% to 12%.[5,27-29,35] Most of the patients in this group will require surgical revision of the valve. One quarter of them will require a second revision.[35]

Considerable effort has been devoted to the development of techniques for improving valve stability. Destruction of the serosa, thinning of the mesentery, and suture or staple fixation of the valve are currently standard modifications of Kock's original technique.[1,27,41] Circumferential silk sutures placed from the pouch to the outflow tract also have contributed to reduction in the rate of valve slippage.

Additional work has focused on supporting the valve at the junction of the pouch and the outflow tract. The earliest efforts involved encircling the base of the valve with a strip of fascia[19] or polypropylene mesh.[20,35,42] These techniques reduced the incidence of valve slippage but contributed to a much higher rate of fistula formation.[23,35] Substitution of other synthetic materials, including Mersilene, Teflon, and Gore-Tex, also has resulted in an unacceptably high incidence of fistula formation.[43]

More recently, a limb of ileum, in continuity with the reservoir, has been used as a "living collar" to buttress the valve.[29] Over a short follow-up period, this approach yielded a valve slippage rate somewhat lower than that of "conventional" techniques. However, long-term results have not been published. Anchoring the valve to the pouch wall also has been suggested as a means of improving valve stability.[44]

Desusception is most likely to occur within the first postoperative year.[27,35] The problem usually begins with dehiscence of the opposing mesenteries within the intussuscepted valve[1] (Fig. 10-14). The nipple desuscepts asymmetrically, causing disproportionate "lengthening" of the mesenteric wall of the outflow tract. The intact antimesenteric portion of the valve is

*References 5, 6, 27-30, 35, 36.

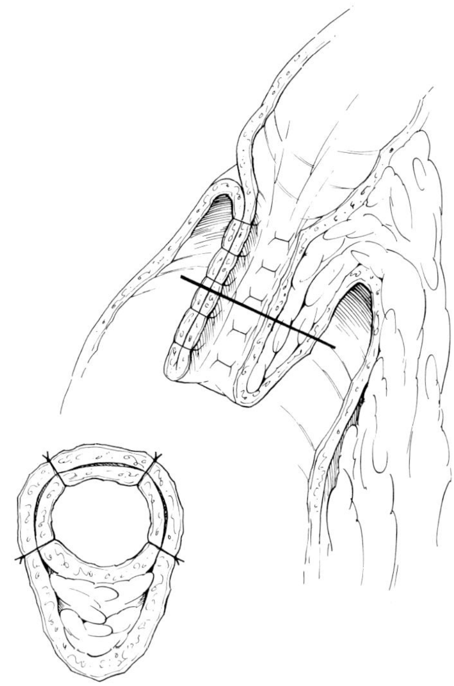

Fig. 10-14. Nipple desusception begins at the site of the opposing mesenteries.

pulled toward the longer mesenteric wall, angulating the valve mechanism (Fig. 10-15). Asymmetrical "unrolling" of the valve initially causes difficulty with intubation. Further desusception leads to valve shortening and incontinence.

Progressive desusception with resulting angulation often leads to complete inability to intubate the pouch. Therefore intestinal obstruction is a common emergency presentation.[5,27] Initial management is directed at relieving obstructive symptoms. Pouch intubation can be accomplished by fiberoptic or rigid ileoscopy using a pediatric gastroscope or an 11 mm rigid sigmoidoscope.[25,45,46] A guidewire or the shaft of a long cotton-tipped swab is left in the pouch, and the endoscope is removed. An ileostomy catheter is threaded over the guide and is taped in place.

At the first episode of valve dysfunction, a trial of prolonged reservoir intubation is warranted. This trial often stabilizes the valve, allowing it to become fixed in the new position. The patient is instructed to leave the catheter taped in place for 2 to 3 weeks. The end of the catheter is occluded with a plastic button, which is removed to empty the pouch. At the end of this period intubation resumes as before. If difficulty in intubation persists, surgical revision is indicated.

OPERATIVE TECHNIQUE. A standard antibiotic preparation is administered

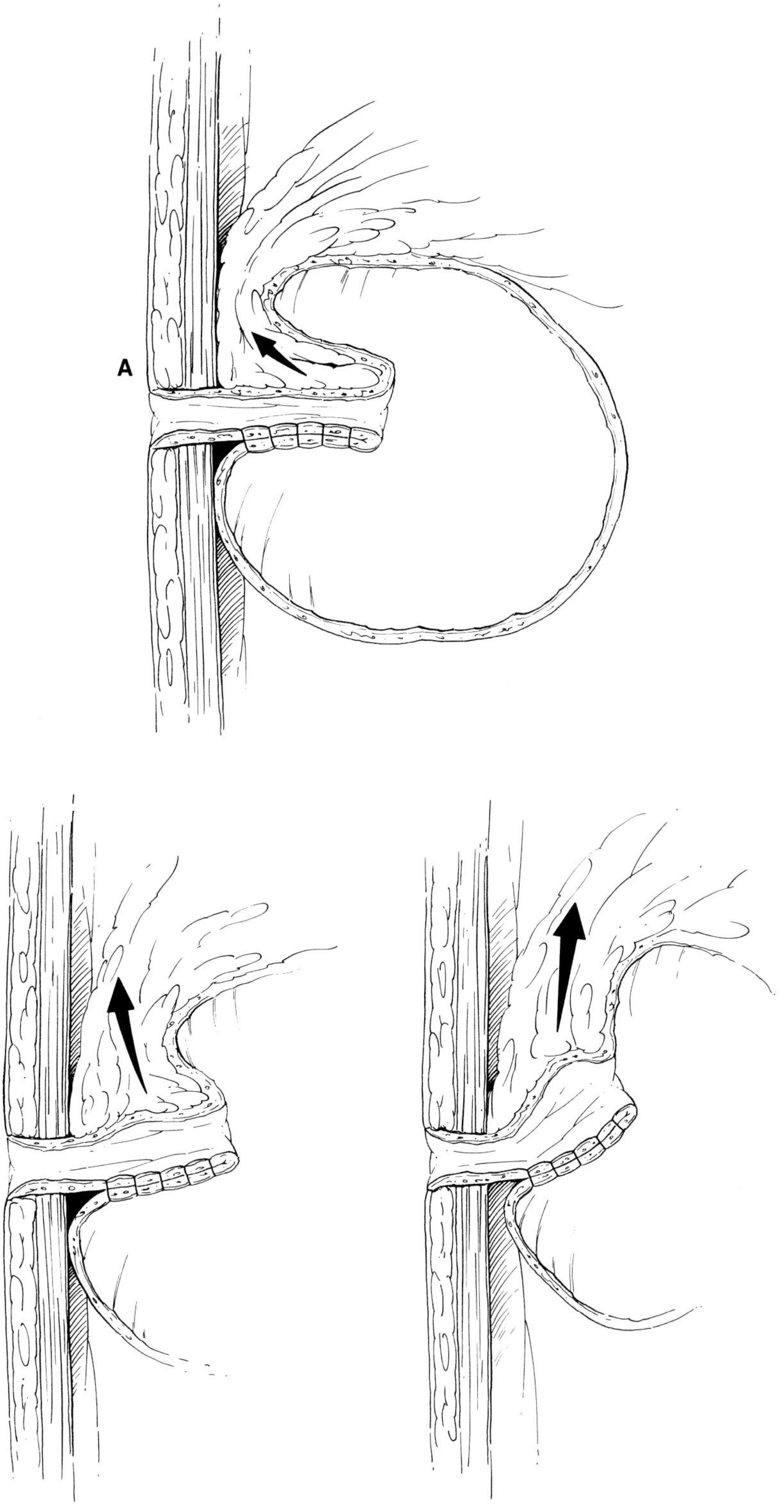

A

B

C

Fig. 10-15. Progressive desusception of the valve causes angulation of the valve and outflow tract.

before surgery. Valve revision usually is possible through a circumstomal incision. The outflow tract is dissected free of the skin, subcutaneous tissue, and fascia. Medial and lateral extensions of the peristomal incision in the skin and fascia may be necessary for pouch mobilization. The reservoir is carefully removed from the abdominal wall and delivered through the surgical wound.

Valve repair. The partially desuscepted valve often can be reintussuscepted by gentle inward pressure. If successful reduction can be achieved, opening the reservoir is not necessary. The intussusception is maintained by suturing the pouch to the outflow tract as in gastric fundoplication. The ileostomy catheter should be inserted into the reservoir prior to placement of these sutures so that the outflow tract is not narrowed. Four or five sutures of 3-0 silk usually will suffice.

Once the valve has been stabilized, the outflow tract is matured in the usual fashion at the old abdominal wall site. The ileostomy catheter is fixed in place as already described. If there is any question about the adequacy of the valve, it should be inspected by opening the pouch along its anterior wall. If a new valve is necessary, pouch "turnaround" is performed.

Valve reconstruction. The 20 cm length of small bowel immediately proximal to the pouch is mobilized. Remnants of the outflow tract and valve are excised from the intact pouch with electrocautery (Fig. 10-16, *A*). The pouch is opened from this point for another 10 cm along its antimesenteric aspect.

The new valve is created by orthograde intussusception of the proximal inflow tract. The afferent ileum is transected with electrocautery 15 cm from its junction with the reservoir (Fig. 10-16, *B*). The proximal 10 cm of the inflow tract is prepared for intussusception by removing the mesenteric fat, abrading the serosal surface, and placing silk sutures, as previously described. A Babcock clamp is passed into the inflow tract to grasp the ileum approximately 5 cm from the reservoir. The bowel is intussuscepted and fixed by sutures and staples as for the original procedure. The catheter is inserted into the pouch, and a collar of pouch is sewn to the new outflow limb with 3-0 silk sutures.

The reservoir is rotated 90 degrees on its axis, which brings the new outflow tract to an anterolateral position. The cut end of the proximal ileum is anastomosed to the pouch at a convenient location by use of the circular stapling instrument. The reservoir walls are reapproximated and closed with two layers of running 3-0 long-term absorbable sutures (Fig. 10-16, *C*). The afferent limb is occluded with a noncrushing intestinal clamp, and the ileostomy tube is inserted through the new valve. The pouch is tested for continence by insufflating air and removing the catheter.

Four 3-0 silk sutures are placed from the pouch to the parietal peritoneum near the stoma aperture prior to exteriorization of the new outflow tract. The outflow tract is then brought through the old stoma opening in the abdominal

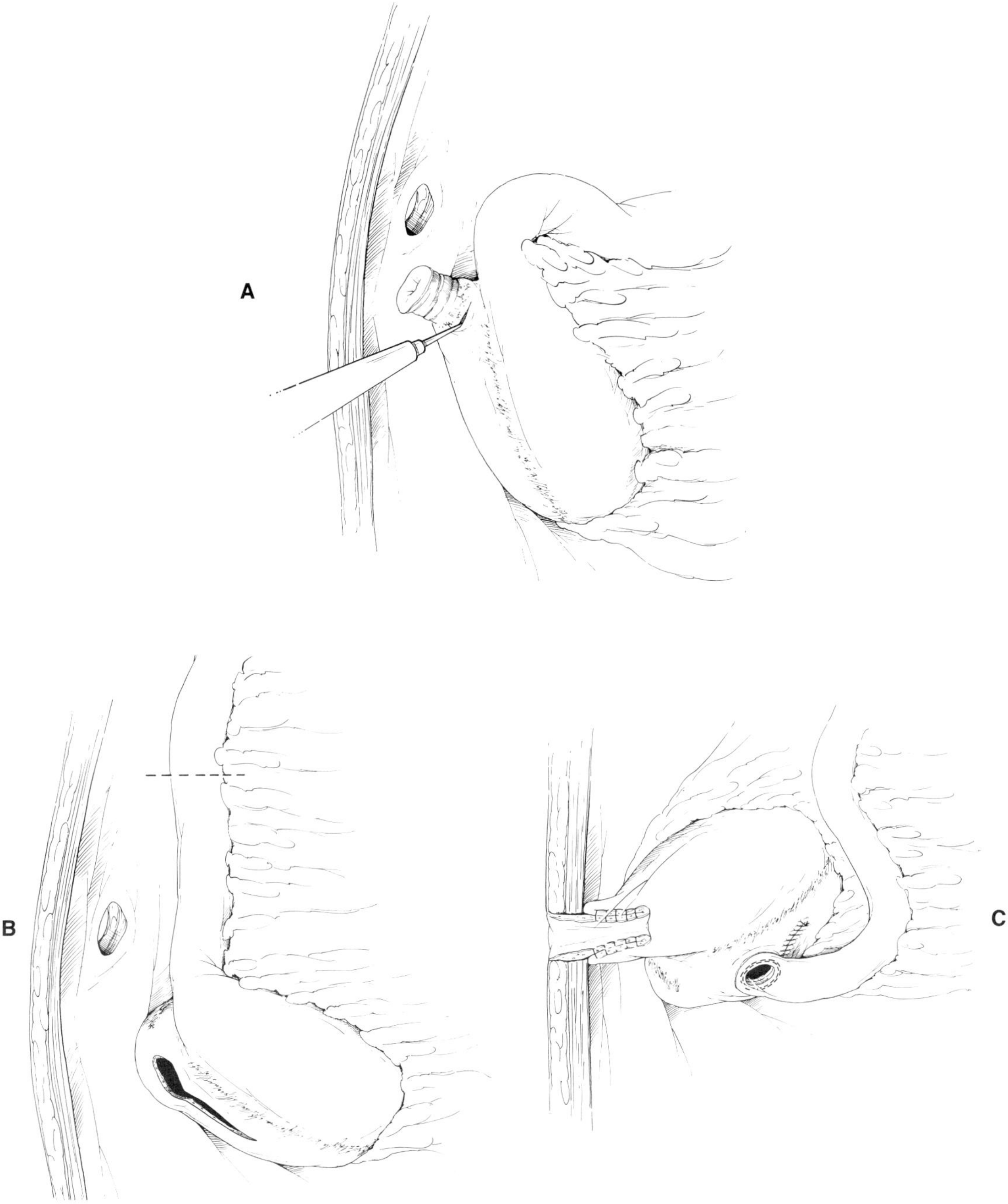

Fig. 10-16. **A,** Outflow tract is removed from the abdominal wall and excised with electrocautery. **B,** Reservoir is opened at the site of the old valve. Proximal bowel is divided 15 cm from the reservoir, and this segment is used to create a new valve. **C,** New nipple valve is created from the proximal bowel in the usual fashion. Cut end of the proximal bowel is anastomosed to the pouch by using the circular stapler. Stapler is introduced through the pouch opening. When the anastomosis is complete, the defect in the pouch is closed with a double layer of running 3-0 absorbable sutures.

wall, and the fixation sutures are tied. A closed suction drain is placed in the right gutter lateral to the pouch. The drain end is brought out at a distance from the stoma. The fascia that is medial and lateral to the stoma opening is reapproximated with heavy long-term absorbable sutures. The outflow tract is trimmed flush with the skin, and the stoma is matured with 3-0 long-term absorbable sutures. The ileostomy catheter is left in the reservoir and connected to dependent drainage.

Fistula. On average, most late fistulas will occur 2 years from the time of initial surgery.[36] Nearly all late fistulas are related to the presence of a foreign body, either a silk suture or plastic mesh.[44] The exception to this general rule occurs in the patient with Crohn's disease. These patients are five times more likely to develop a fistula than patients with colitis or polyposis.[35]

An external fistula usually presents with evidence of cutaneous sepsis. Peristomal cellulitis or subcutaneous abscess usually precedes frank fistulization. Once the tract has been established, leakage of intestinal contents ensues. Pouch-cutaneous fistula is an uncommon late complication, occurring in approximately 3% of cases.[5] Fiberoptic ileoscopy is often helpful in establishing the diagnosis and estimating the chance of nonoperative closure.[45] If the cause of the fistula is a foreign body, the foreign body must be removed either operatively or endoscopically before the pouch will heal. If the offending agent (usually a silk suture) can be removed endoscopically, treatment by continuous pouch intubation and administration of oral antibiotics for 2 to 4 weeks usually will produce closure of the defect. If the foreign body cannot be retrieved or if the fistula does not close, operative removal by excision with primary closure of the pouch is indicated.

Late internal fistulas of the nipple valve occur more frequently and are more troublesome than external fistulas.[35] Leakage of intestinal contents through the unintubated stoma is the common presentation of this complication. The size of the fistula and its location along the length of the valve will determine the degree of incontinence. Leakage is generally greater when the fistula lies near the base of the valve. The fistula does not affect ease of reservoir intubation.

Operative revision is indicated when the amount of leakage inconveniences the patient. Dozois et al.[27] recommend complete nipple revision by pouch rotation in all cases of fistula. We have found such revision often to be unnecessary, especially when the fistula lies at the base of the valve. However, we agree that if the fistula is not readily accessible or if the repaired valve is unsuitable for any reason, then creation of a new valve by using the afferent ileum is indicated.

OPERATIVE TECHNIQUE. The pouch is approached through a peristomal incision. The outflow tract is freed circumferentially. The wound is enlarged by medial and lateral incisions 2 to 3 cm long. The pouch is removed from the abdominal wall and delivered into the wound. The valve is exposed by opening the pouch along its antimesenteric wall.

The nipple fistula is identified. Any foreign body, if present, is removed. A small rim of normal ileum around the foreign body also is excised. The nipple is desuscepted to a point a few millimeters beyond the fistula. This step is relatively easy if the fistula is located at the base of the nipple. The edges of the fistula on both ileal walls are freshened and closed with 3-0 long-term absorbable sutures. The intussusception is restored, with care taken to avoid overlapping the suture lines. The pouch is closed with running 3-0 long-term absorbable sutures. An ileostomy catheter is placed within the pouch, and valvular competence is ascertained.

The outflow tract is brought through the old stoma site. The medial and lateral incisions in the fascia are repaired with heavy long-term absorbable sutures. The skin incisions medial and lateral to the stoma site are closed with fine nylon. The stoma is matured with 3-0 long-term absorbable sutures. The catheter is secured to the abdominal wall with the crosspiece arrangement described earlier. Gravity drainage is instituted.

Skin-level stenosis. Stenosis of the peristomal skin occurs in 8% of patients.[35] Patients suffering this complication find insertion of the ileostomy catheter difficult, painful, and accompanied by modest bleeding. We have found that double Z-plasty of the peristomal skin offers the most satisfactory long-term results.

OPERATIVE TECHNIQUE. The scar at the mucocutaneous junction is excised circumferentially. The subcutaneous outflow limb is mobilized completely to the level of the fascia. Slightly curved 1.5 cm tangential skin incisions are made at opposite points on the stoma circumference. The skin edges are undermined through the creation of two rotational flaps. The ileal walls opposing the skin incisions are divided longitudinally for a distance of 1.5 cm on each side (Fig. 10-17, *A*). The skin flaps are rotated into the groove cut on either side of the ileum (Fig. 10-17, *B*). The two Z-plasties are completed by suturing the full thickness of the ileal wall to the dermis of the flaps. The revision is completed by fixing the remainder of the ileal circumference to the skin with interrupted 3-0 absorbable sutures (Fig. 10-17, *C*).

Prolapse. Prolapse of the intact nipple valve is uncommon, occurring in less than 3% of cases.[35] There seems to be a greater tendency toward prolapse in patients who have undergone previous nipple revision.[28] Continence is generally maintained between episodes of prolapse.

We have found that prolapse is most often associated with an overly large fascial stoma defect. Increased intra-abdominal pressure during exercise or late pregnancy can precipitate nipple extrusion. Reduction usually can be accomplished by gentle manual pressure. Iced witch hazel compresses may be used to reduce stoma edema, facilitating reduction after long-standing

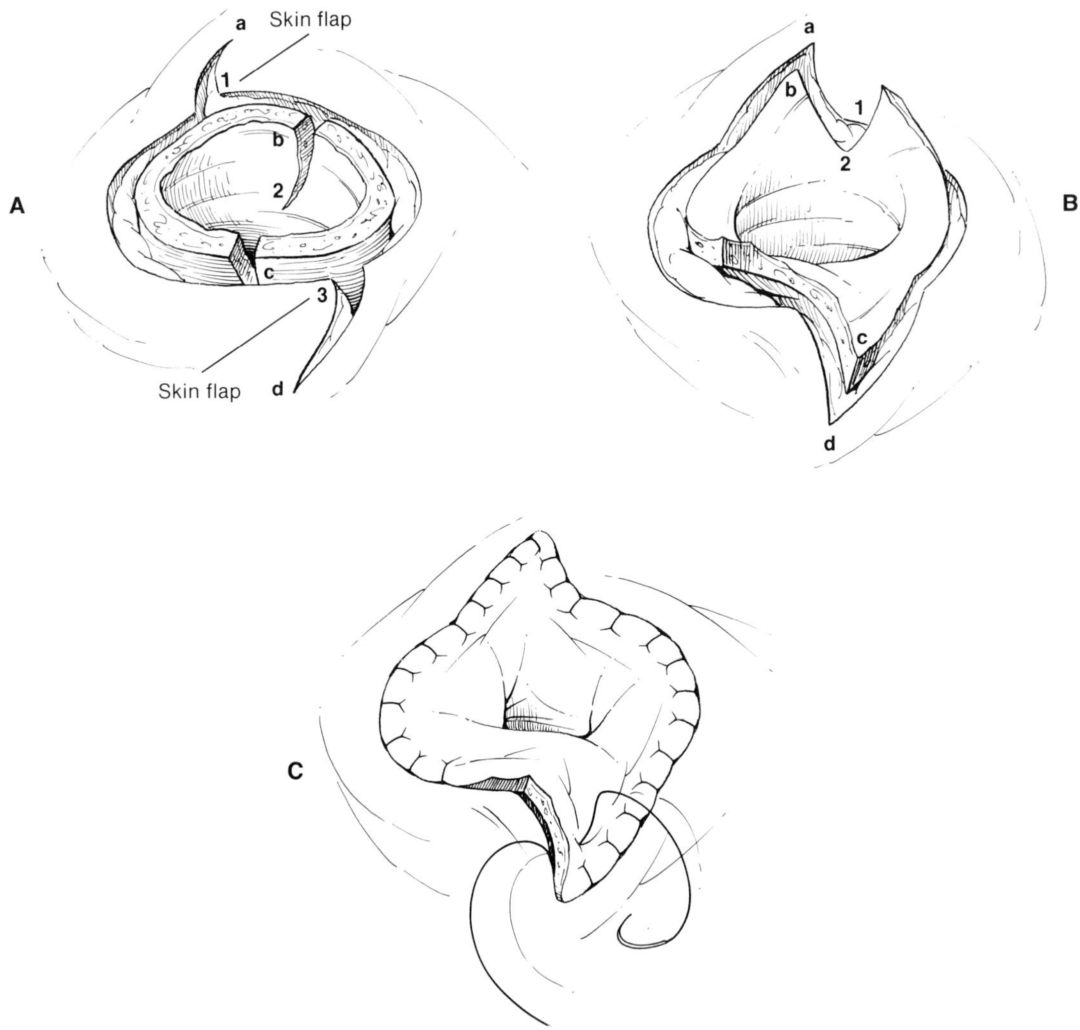

Fig. 10-17. **A,** Skin incisions are made on opposing sides of the stoma. Corresponding incisions are made in the ileum. Skin between *a* and *1* and *d* and *3* is mobilized to create two flaps. **B,** Skin flaps are rotated into the grooves cut in the ileum; *b* is brought to *a,* and *1* is brought to *2;* similarly, *c* is brought to *d.* **C,** New mucocutaneous junction is sewn with interrupted 3-0 absorbable sutures.

prolapse. Once the edema has been reduced, the reservoir usually can be intubated without difficulty.

Nonoperative management of nipple valve prolapse usually involves continuous pouch intubation for 2 to 4 weeks. A recent report described "stiffening" of the outflow tract by transcutaneous electrocauterization and suture. This technique was used successfully in four of eight cases.[47]

Prolapse that occurs during pregnancy is managed best by continuous intubation after valve reduction.[34] The tube is left in place throughout labor and delivery. If cesarean section is indicated, the extracorporeal portion of the catheter is draped laterally with a sterile adhesive sheet. Midline incision usually is required. Operative delivery proceeds according to obstetric principles, with care exercised to avoid injury to the reservoir.

Recurring episodes of valve prolapse generally require revisional surgery. We have found that relocation of the reservoir and stoma to a new site, usually the midline or the left lower quadrant, yields better results than attempts at fascia repair.

OPERATIVE TECHNIQUE. The stoma and outflow tract are mobilized through a peristomal incision. The incision is extended medially and laterally, if necessary, and the abdominal cavity is entered. The pouch is carefully mobilized from the anterior abdominal wall. If doubt exists concerning the viability of the outflow tract, the creation of a new valve by means of pouch rotation is warranted.

The new stoma site is determined by comfortable placement of the outflow tract. When possible, transrectus placement on the opposite side is preferable. A circle of skin at the new site is excised. Dissection is continued into the abdominal cavity. The outflow tract is brought through the new stoma site, and the reservoir is fixed to the anterior abdominal wall. The fascia defect at the old stoma site is closed with heavy long-term absorbable sutures. The wound is covered with sterile towels, and the stoma is matured with 3-0 absorbable sutures.

Pouchitis. The syndrome of reservoir mucosal ileitis, or "pouchitis," has been reported to occur in from 5% to 43% of patients with a reservoir ileostomy.[6,27,28,35,48] Pouchitis appears most characteristically as a change in the nature and quantity of the ileostomy effluent.[49] High-volume (>1000 ml/day), thin, and occasionally bloody returns are common. Intubation may become more difficult, and catheter-induced bleeding may ensue. The syndrome also may include abdominal cramps or pain, arthralgia, fever, and malaise.[50] Pouchitis appears to occur almost exclusively in patients whose initial diagnosis was mucosal ulcerative colitis.[27,28,35] More than half of the patients who develop pouchitis present with their first episode within 6 months of surgery.[51]

The patient presenting with these symptoms for the first time warrants thorough investigation. A careful history and physical examination are performed. Assay of the ileostomy effluent for enteric pathogens and toxins and fiberoptic ileoscopy also are indicated. Typically, ileoscopy reveals mucosal edema, friability, and granularity.[46] The presence of aphthous ulcerations strongly suggests the possibility of Crohn's disease.[50] Biopsy may suggest an alternate diagnosis, or it may show only mild, nonspecific inflammation or even normal mucosal histology.[52] Crohn's disease of the reservoir and infectious enteritis can mimic pouchitis. We have encountered subacute addisonian crisis and hyperthyroidism misdiagnosed as reservoir ileitis.[28]

The cause of pouchitis is unknown. Factors implicated as contributory or causative include pouch stasis, ischemia, altered bacterial flora, bacterial metabolites, and ileal mucosal metaplasia.[53] None of these possible causes has been proven. Resolution of the inflammatory process with treatment by the administration of antibiotics favors a bacterial cause. It is intriguing to consider the possibility that pouchitis, "backwash ileitis," and ulcerative colitis share a common, albeit unknown, cause.

Patients with pouchitis generally respond quickly to the oral administration of metronidazole.[54] Since pouchitis tends to recur in susceptible individuals,[52] each subsequent episode does not require the same investigation as the first. Rather, antibiotic therapy should be started empirically according to the symptoms. The occasional patient will fail to respond to antibiotic therapy. In this situation steroids administered via catheter or systemically may be of value.[49] Very rarely, unremitting pouchitis, recalcitrant to all modes of medical therapy, may prompt the patient to seek removal of the reservoir.[49]

CONTINENT COLOSTOMY

Encouraged by the impressive improvement in patient comfort and life-style obtained with the continent ileostomy, investigators have attempted to achieve similar results with a continent colostomy. Despite intense efforts, this quest has not yet been successful.

A variety of factors has made a reliable, safe, and simple continent colostomy difficult to achieve. The typical permanent colostomy is fashioned from the end of the sigmoid or descending colon. Colostomy output is usually semisolid or solid, foul-smelling, and often accompanied by gas. The nature of colostomy stool and the differing pattern of motor function of the colon render useless many of the continence-preserving approaches used with ileostomies. Furthermore, most patients who require permanent end colostomy suffer from invasive rectal carcinoma. This disease affects an older patient population and carries an uncertain prognosis. A continent colostomy that requires repeated surgical revision or intricate stoma maintenance may not be well accepted by these patients.

Irrigation

Colostomy continence achieved by the irrigation technique was introduced in the 1920s, mainly in response to the dearth of effective pouching systems available at the time.[55] Colostomy irrigation is essentially an enema delivered via the stoma. The irrigating fluid stimulates colonic evacuation in a predictable and reproducible fashion. In many patients irrigation done every day or every other day is all that is required to keep the stoma free of leakage between irrigations.[56-58] Between irrigations, a stoma cap or a gauze pad is worn over the stoma.

Indications and patient selection. Only left-sided colostomies are amenable to control by irrigation. Right-sided or transverse stomas generally will have an output that is too liquid to achieve adequate results. Other relative contraindications to irrigation include parastomal herniation, stoma prolapse, and a predisposition to diarrhea related to either the underlying disease process (e.g., inflammatory bowel disease) or ongoing treatment (e.g., chemotherapy or radiotherapy).[59] In general, children and infants are not good candidates because of increased risk of perforation and lack of attention span.

Although the contraindications to this method are few, irrigation is not appropriate for everyone. The patient must be generally healthy and must possess the manual dexterity and motivation to learn and to apply the technique. Uninterrupted access to the bathroom for at least 1 hour on irrigation days also is required. Even under ideal circumstances, all patients will not achieve continence.[56-58]

Technique. Irrigation should be performed at approximately the same time of day on alternate or third days. The patient should be comfortable with the technique, relaxed, and unhurried. Many patients will choose to perform irrigation while seated in front of the toilet.

The water bag should be filled with no more than a quart of lukewarm tap water. Often a pint of water will yield optimal results. The bag should be suspended at shoulder level within the patient's view. After air has been evacuated from the system, the tubing is clamped and the cone tip is attached.

The irrigating sleeve is placed around the stoma. The long end of the sleeve is placed in the toilet. The cone is lubricated and is inserted into the stoma via the short arm of the sleeve. Gentle pressure allows the tip to occlude the stoma. The clamp is opened and the water is allowed to slowly enter the colon. The entire volume is instilled over 3 to 5 minutes. The infusion should be stopped momentarily if cramping occurs.

After infusion, the cone is removed and the short arm of the sleeve is clipped. The long arm of the sleeve is left in the toilet until the initial return of water and stool has ceased. This action will usually take about 15 minutes. Next, the sleeve is rinsed clean but left in place. The patient then can leave the bathroom or can perform other tasks, if desired. Stool may continue to drain for the next 30 to 50 minutes. With time the patient will recognize when the colon is empty. When there is no further drainage of stool, the sleeve is rinsed and removed. The peristomal skin is cleaned, and a "security pouch," cap, or pad is applied.

Results. Irrigation provides colostomy continence in 30% to 60% of patients.[56-58] Patients report improvement in their sense of security and self-confidence and their ability to function in work and social settings.[57,60] The time spent on stoma management and the cost of equipment are similar to those expended by patients who use natural evacuation.[57,58] Neither age nor diagnosis prevents successful mastery of the technique.[61] Complications are distinctly uncommon.[57-59]

Barrier Devices

Despite good results with colostomy irrigation, many patients find the technique cumbersome and time-consuming. Also, continence is not always perfect between irrigations. In an effort to provide stoma continence more easily, various devices have been designed for temporary stoma occlusion. These methods were intended to provide reliable continence without the need for irrigation or at least to improve continence in the interval between irrigations.

Magnetic cap. The first of these devices was the magnetic stoma cap.[62,63] This three-part system consisted of an implantable, samarium-cobalt magnetic ring, a mushroom-shaped cap, and a three-layer filter-washer used between the skin and the cap (Fig. 10-18). The cap contained a magnetic ring and center pin. The patient centered the washer at the stoma and occluded the colostomy by inserting the pin in the lumen. The cap was held in place by magnetic attraction. The cap was removed when the patient wished to evacuate. Irrigation was used as an adjunct in some patients.

Despite early enthusiasm for the magnetic cap, it yielded disappointing results. Achievement of continence occurred in only 14% to 50% of patients.[64-67] Local infection, erosion of the ring through the skin, and late skin necrosis were the most common complications. The device is no longer commercially available.

Balloon plug. The balloon plug, a device based on the same principle as the magnetic cap, was described in 1984.[68] This device consisted of an implantable silicone ring and an inflatable silicone balloon. The ring was sutured to the parietal peritoneum at the stoma aperture. The colon was brought through the ring and matured at skin level. The stoma was occluded by luminal insertion and inflation of the balloon. The patient deflated the balloon to evacuate the bowel.

Although continence was achieved with this device, patient acceptance was only fair. Complications such as fistula, bowel necrosis, and stoma erosion were also noted. The balloon plug is no longer available for clinical use.

A

B

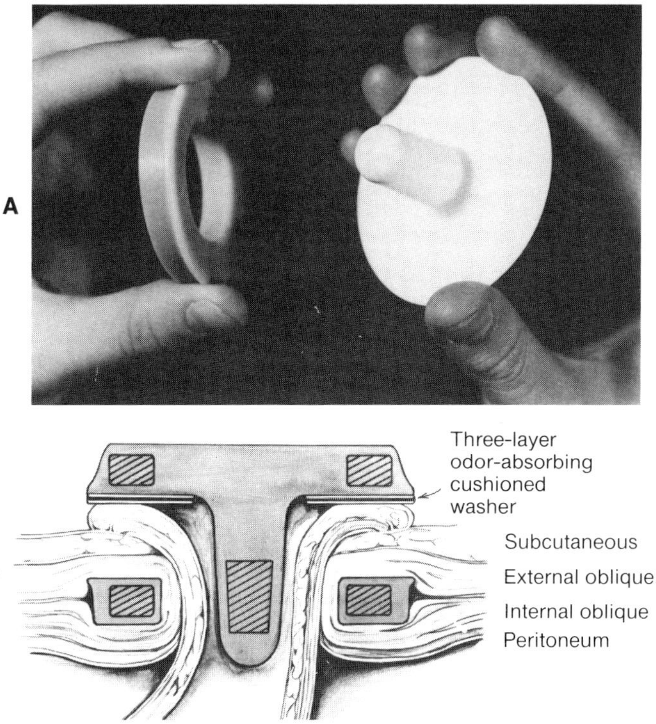

Fig. 10-18. Magnetic stoma cap.

Polyurethane plug. Interest in the use of one- and two-piece, disposable, polyurethane colostomy plug systems has recently resurfaced.[69,70] The device consists of a polyurethane foam cone that is held in a cylindrical shape by polyvinyl alcohol film. The cylinder is inserted into the stoma and held in place by a flange (two-piece system) or by an adhesive/filter base (one-piece system). The moisture in the colon causes the film to dissolve, allowing the polyurethane to assume its original conical shape. The cone occludes the intestinal lumen, preventing leakage of mucus and stool. Gas escapes through the filter system without noise or odor.

The most recent reports of the use of these devices showed acceptable levels of continence, with most patients reporting no significant odor, noise, discharge, or leakage when the plug was in place.[69] Patient acceptance of the technique was excellent.[69,70] Most patients with a colostomy in both studies were concurrently using irrigation techniques. The patients who were not using irrigation were able to confine bowel movements to evening hours when the plug was not in use. They were also satisfied with the device.[69]

Use of the plug appears to be best suited to those patients whose bowel action can be predicted reliably, either by irrigation or "natural" technique. Between bowel movements, the plug serves to control odor, noise, and mucus and to minimize fecal leakage. The interval between irrigations can be prolonged in selected patients.[70]

Other techniques. Other barrier techniques have been tried with varying degrees of success. An implantable hydraulic sphincter has been used to achieve continence to a small number of patients.[71] However, infectious complications occurred in half of these patients. Kock attempted to use a valve similar to the type used in the continent ileostomy.[72] Emptying the bowel through catheter irrigation was so time-consuming that the procedure was abandoned after use in only five patients.

SUMMARY

Perfect, simple, and safe stoma continence has yet to be achieved. Ileostomy continence has come closest to this ideal through modifications of Kock's technique of reservoir ileostomy. The price of excellent continence with this method has been a significant rate of complication and reoperation. Acceptable colostomy continence has been achieved through the use of stoma irrigation. Despite the simplicity and safety of this technique, it is not perfectly reliable. The ideal substitute for the anal sphincter remains elusive.

REFERENCES

1. Kock NG. Historical perspective. In Dozois RR. Alternatives to Conventional Ileostomy. Chicago: Year Book, 1985, pp 133-145.
2. Kock NG. Intra-abdominal "reservoir" in patients with permanent ileostomy: Preliminary observations on a procedure resulting in fecal "continence" in five ileostomy patients. Arch Surg 99:223-231, 1969.
3. Kock NG. Continent ileostomy. Prog Surg 12:180-201, 1973.
4. Cohen Z, Stone RM. Continent reservoir ileostomy. I. Early experience and evolution of the surgical technique. Can J Surg 23:259-262, 1980.
5. Kock NG, Myrvold HE, Nilsson LO, Philipson BM. Continent ileostomy: The Swedish experience. In Dozois RR. Alternatives to Conventional Ileostomy. Chicago: Year Book, 1985, pp 163-175.
6. Dozois RR, Kelly KA, Beart RW Jr, Beahrs OH. Improved results with continent ileostomy. Ann Surg 192:319-324, 1980.
7. Failes D. The Kock continent ileostomy: A preliminary report. Aust N Z J Surg 46: 125-130, 1976.
8. Nilsson LO, Kock NG, Lindgren I, et al. Morphological and histochemical changes in the mucosa of the continent reservoir 6 to 10 years after its construction. Scand J Gastroenterol 15:737-747, 1980.
9. Gadacz TR, Kelly KA, Phillips SF. The continent ileal pouch: Absorptive and motor features. Gastroenterology 72:1287-1291, 1977.

10. Philipson BM, Kock NG, Jagenburg R, Ahren C, Norlen L, Robinson JW, Menge H. Functional and structural studies of ileal reservoirs used for continent urostomy and ileostomy. Gut 24:392-398, 1983.
11. Philipson BM, Kock NG, Robinson JWL, Menge H, Mirkovitch V. Function and structure of the mucosa of continent ileostomy reservoirs in dogs. Gut 16:132-136, 1975.
12. Bokey EL, Hayward PJ, Johnson SE, Pheils MT. Experiments in the development of a continent ileostomy: A simplified technique without a reservoir in dogs. Surgery 90:459-463, 1981.
13. Pemberton JH, van Heerden JA, Beart RW Jr, Kelly KA, Phillips SF, Taylor BM. A continent ileostomy device. Ann Surg 197:618-626, 1983.
14. Gelernt IM, Bauer JJ, Salky BA, Kreel I. The continent ileostomy. In Jirsch DW. Frontiers in General Surgery. Lancaster, England: MTP Press, 1982, pp 313-330.
15. Beahrs OH, Bess MA, Beart RW Jr, Pemberton JH. Indwelling ileostomy valve device. Am J Surg 141:111-115, 1981.
16. Fendel EH, Fazio VW. Construction of a continent ileostomy using a porcine aortic valve. A preliminary report. Dis Colon Rectum 25:21-23, 1982.
17. Orangio GR, Bronsther B, Abrams M, Wise L. A new type of continent ileostomy. Results of an animal study. Dis Colon Rectum 27:238-243, 1984.
18. Salmon R, Bloch P, Loygue J. Magnetic closure of a reservoir ileostomy. Dis Colon Rectum 23:242-243, 1980.
19. Bokey L, Fazio VW. The mesenteric sling technique. Cleve Clin Q 45:231-236, 1978.
20. Cohen Z. Evolution of the Kock continent reservoir ileostomy. Can J Surg 25:509-514, 1982.
21. Barnett WO. New approaches for continent ostomy construction. J Miss State Med Assoc 28:1-3, 1987.
22. Thompson JS, Williams SM. Fistula following continent ileostomy. Dis Colon Rectum 27:193-195, 1984.
23. Cohen Z. Current status of the continent ileostomy. Can J Surg 30:357-358, 1987.
24. Martin LW, LeCoultre C, Schubert WK. Total colectomy and mucosal proctectomy with preservation of continence in ulcerative colitis. Ann Surg 186:477-479, 1977.
25. Parks AG, Nicholls RJ, Belliveau P. Proctocolectomy with ileal reservoir and anal anastomosis. Br J Surg 67:533-538, 1980.
26. Dozois RR. Ulcerative colitis: Surgical alternatives. In Fazio VW. Current Therapy in Colon and Rectal Surgery. Toronto: BC Decker, 1990, pp 166-174.
27. Dozois RR, Kelly KA, Beart RW Jr, Beahrs OH. Continent ileostomy: The Mayo Clinic experience. In Dozois RR. Alternatives to Conventional Ileostomy. Chicago: Year Book, 1985, pp 180-191.
28. Gelernt IM, Gorfine SR. Management of postsurgical problems. In Gitnick G. Inflammatory Bowel Disease: Diagnosis and Treatment. New York: Igaku-Shoin, 1991, pp 451-460.
29. Barnett WO. Current experiences with the continent intestinal reservoir. Surg Obstet Gynecol 168:1-5, 1989.
30. McLeod RS, Fazio VW. Quality of life with the continent ileostomy. World J Surg 8:90-95, 1984.
31. Gerber A, Apt MK, Craig PH. The improved quality of life with the continent ileostomy. J Clin Gastroenterol 6:513-517, 1984.
32. Kock NG, Darle N, Kewenter J, et al. The quality of life after proctocolectomy and ileostomy: A study of patients with conventional ileostomies converted to continent ileostomies. Dis Colon Rectum 17:287-292, 1974.

33. King SA. Quality of life: The continent ileostomy. Ann Surg 182:29-32, 1975.
34. Sjodahl R, Lemon E, Nystrom PO, Olaison G. Complications, surgical revision and quality of life with conventional and continent ileostomy. Acta Chir Scand 156:403-407, 1990.
35. Fazio VW, Church JM. Complications and function of the continent ileostomy at the Cleveland Clinic. World J Surg 12:148-154, 1988.
36. Jarvinen HJ, Makitie A, Sivula A. Long-term results of continent ileostomy. Int J Colorectal Dis 1:40-43, 1986.
37. Ojerskog B, Kock NG, Philipson BM, Philipson M. Pregnancy and delivery in patients with a continent ileostomy. Surg Gynecol Obstet 167:61-64, 1988.
38. Morowitz DA, Kirsner JB. Ileostomy in ulcerative colitis: A questionnaire study of 1803 patients. Am J Surg 141:370-375, 1981.
39. Pemberton JH, Phillips SF, Dozois RR, Wendorf LJ. Current clinical results. In Dozois RR. Alternatives to Standard Ileostomy. Chicago: Year Book, 1985, pp 40-50.
40. Kock NG. Present status of the continent ileostomy: Surgical revision of the malfunctioning ileostomy. Dis Colon Rectum 19:200-206, 1976.
41. Cranley B, McKelvey ST. The Kock ileostomy reservoir: An experimental study of methods of improving valve stability and competence. Br J Surg 68:545-550, 1981.
42. Kock NG, Myrvold NE, Nilsson LO, et al. Construction of a stable nipple valve for the continent ileostomy. Ann Chir Gynaecol 69:132-143, 1980.
43. Bauer JJ, Gelernt IM, Salky BA, Kreel I. Unpublished data, 1978.
44. Myrvold HE. The continent ileostomy. World J Surg 11:720-726, 1987.
45. Waye JD, Kreel I, Bauer JJ, Gelernt IM. The continent ileostomy: Diagnosis and treatment of problems by means of operative fiberoptic endoscopy. Gastrointest Endosc 23:196-198, 1977.
46. Church JM, Fazio VW, Lavery IC. The role of fiberoptic endoscopy in the management of the continent ileostomy. Gastrointest Endosc 33:203-209, 1987.
47. Gottlieb LM, Handelsman JC. Treatment of outflow tract problems associated with continent ileostomy (Kock pouch): Report of six cases. Dis Colon Rectum 34:936-940, 1991.
48. Bonello JC, Thow GB, Manson RR. Mucosal enteritis: A complication of the continent ileostomy. Dis Colon Rectum 24:37-41, 1981.
49. Zuccaro G, Fazio VW, Church JM, et al. Pouch ileitis. Dig Dis Sci 34:1505-1510, 1989.
50. Phillips SF. Altered physiology. In Dozois RR, ed. Alternatives to Conventional Ileostomy. Chicago: Year Book, 1985, pp 146-159.
51. Hulten L. Pouchitis—Incidence and characteristics in the continent ileostomy. Int J Colorectal Dis 4:208-210, 1989.
52. Kelly DG, Phillips SF, Kelly KA, et al. Dysfunction of the continent ileostomy: Clinical features and bacteriology. Gut 24:193-201, 1983.
53. Nivatvongs S. Ulcerative colitis. In Gordon PH, Nivatvongs S, eds. Principles and Practice of Surgery for the Colon, Rectum, and Anus. St. Louis: Quality Medical Publishing, 1992, pp 667-715.
54. McLeod RS, Taylor DW, Cohen Z, Cullen JB. Single-patient randomized clinical trial: Use in determining optimum treatment for patients with inflammation of Kock continent ileostomy reservoir. Lancet 1:726-728, 1986.
55. Smith D. Status of colostomy. JAMA 99:1129-1130, 1932.
56. Jao SW, Beart RW Jr, Wendorf LJ, Ilstrup DM. Irrigation management of sigmoid colostomy. Arch Surg 120:916-917, 1985.

57. Williams NS, Johnston D. Prospective controlled trial comparing colostomy irrigation with "spontaneous-action" method. Br Med J 12:107-109, 1980.
58. Laucks SS II, Mazier WP, Milsom JW, Buffin SE, Anderson JM, Warwick MK, Surrell JA. An assessment of colostomy irrigation. Dis Colon Rectum 31:279-282, 1988.
59. Goode PS. Colostomy irrigation. In Broadwell DC, Jackson BS. Principles of Ostomy Care. St. Louis: CV Mosby, 1982, pp 369-380.
60. Terranova O, Sandei F, Rebuffat C, Maruotti R, Bortolozzi E. Irrigation vs. natural evacuation of left colostomy: A comparative study of 340 patients. Dis Colon Rectum 22:31-34, 1979.
61. Venturini M, Bertelli G, Forno G, Grandi G, Dini D. Colostomy irrigation in the elderly. Effective recovery regardless of age. Dis Colon Rectum 33:1031-1033, 1990.
62. Feustel H, Hennig G. Kontinente Kolostomie durch Magnetverschluss. Dtsch Med Wochenschr 100:1063-1064, 1975.
63. Bauer JJ, Wertkin MG, Gelernt IM, Kreel I. A continent colostomy: The magnetic stoma cap. Am J Surg 134:334-337, 1977.
64. Goligher JC, Lee PW, McMahon MJ, Pollard M. The Erlangen magnetic colostomy control device: Technique of use and results in 22 patients. Br J Surg 64:501-507, 1977.
65. Alexander-Williams J, Amery AH, Devlin HB, et al. Magnetic continent colostomy device. Br Med J 1:1269-1270, 1977.
66. Kewenter J. Continent colostomy with the aid of a magnetic closing system: A preliminary report. Dis Colon Rectum 21:46-51, 1978.
67. Khubchandani IT, Trimpi HD, Sheets JA, Stasik JJ Jr, Balcavage CA. The magnetic stoma device: A continent colostomy. Dis Colon Rectum 24:344-350, 1981.
68. Prager E. The continent colostomy. Dis Colon Rectum 27:235-237, 1984.
69. Cerdan FJ, Diez M, Campo J, Barbero MA, Balibrea J. Continent colostomy by means of a new one-piece disposable device: Preliminary report. Dis Colon Rectum 34:886-890, 1991.
70. Soliani P, Carbognani P, Piccolo P, Sabbagh R, Cudazzo E. Colostomy plug devices: A possible new approach to the problem of incontinence. Dis Colon Rectum 35:969-974, 1992.
71. Heiblum M, Cordoba A. An artificial sphincter: A preliminary report. Dis Colon Rectum 21:562-566, 1978.
72. Kock NG, Myrvold HE, Philipson BM, Svaninger G, Ojerskog B. Continent cecostomy. An account of 30 patients. Dis Colon Rectum 28:705-708, 1985.

11 OSTOMY TAKEDOWN

David A. Rothenberger and Michael P. Spencer

Although the indications for temporary fecal diversion have changed over recent decades, diverting stomas continue to play a crucial role in the management of benign conditions and malignant disease. The advent of restorative proctocolectomy, extended low anterior resection, coloanal anastomosis, and preoperative adjuvant radiotherapy have increased the use of temporary stomas. A prospective review of 2000 colorectal anastomoses by Fielding et al.[1] noted that 15.8% received a protective stoma. Temporary colostomies are used less frequently today, but temporary ileostomies seem to be used more often. A recent review of 350 stoma takedowns performed by members of the Division of Colon and Rectal Surgery of the University of Minnesota revealed that ileostomies outnumbered colostomies by a ratio of 5:1.

Stoma takedown has received little attention compared to stoma placement, construction, care, and physiology. The morbidity associated with ileostomy and colostomy closure varies considerably, with reported anastomotic leakage rates from 0% to 23%.[2-5] Even greater variation exists in the incidence of post-takedown obstructive symptoms and wound infection.[2-5] Our series of 350 randomly selected stoma takedowns revealed an 11% major complication rate (anastomotic leak, obstruction, or anastomotic stricture requiring exploration) and a 13% minor complication rate (partial small bowel obstruction, wound infection, and prolonged ileus) for ileostomy takedown. Colostomy takedown in our series was associated with a 9% major and a 20% minor complication rate.

Despite the current trend toward primary repair of selected colon injuries and performance of ileal pouch procedures without proximal ileostomy in selected patients, temporary diversion will continue to play a critical role in general, trauma, and colon and rectal surgery.[6-8] The use of stomas and their takedown, however, require careful consideration and meticulous surgical technique. It is hoped that a comprehensive approach to stoma closure and a thorough review of the options regarding surgical techniques will minimize overall morbidity.

TIMING OF PROCEDURE

Before a stoma closure is considered for any patient, the rationale for diversion must be reevaluated. Has the stoma served its purpose? It is understandable that most patients are anxious to proceed with closure of a temporary ostomy and often coerce the surgeon to schedule this "minor operation" sooner than originally planned. Usually, this choice is a major mistake because performing takedown too soon can result in a difficult and tedious dissection with later major complications requiring reoperation and rediversion. The guiding principle to follow is that takedown of a stoma is an elective operation and thus should be performed only when the patient's medical condition is optimal. It is especially critical that infectious processes have resolved, that nutrition has been restored, that anemia has been corrected, and that the use of medications such as corticosteroids has been discontinued or minimized. We prefer to wait approximately 8 to 12 weeks before takedown, but in ideal situations a takedown may be done as early as 6 weeks after initial stoma construction.

If the patient should require an urgent exploration before this time (most frequently for adhesive small bowel obstruction), takedown may be considered. Careful assessment and inspection of the diverted limb are mandatory in this situation. If contamination is encountered at the time of laparotomy or if the patient's overall health is less than optimal, takedown usually should be deferred. Delay of stoma takedown very rarely has any adverse affect; in general, the longer one waits, the easier the takedown becomes.

PREOPERATIVE ASSESSMENT

Clinical evaluation of the patient before takedown is essential. A history of severe irritable bowel symptoms, chronic diarrhea, or anal incontinence should raise concerns about the wisdom of proceeding with takedown of a temporary stoma. Similarly, the presence of a weak sphincter or signs of other intestinal dysfunction should alert the clinician to potential problems that might arise after takedown. Whether or not to obtain preoperative manometry or other physiologic evaluation of anal sphincteric competence should be considered before a commitment to restorative surgery is made.

Radiographic or endoscopic studies may be required to evaluate the integrity of the diverted bowel and to identify any strictures, fistulas, or leaks. The proximal bowel, especially in a colostomy takedown, also may need endoscopic or radiographic assessment to exclude other pathology. Imaging studies are helpful in delineating the preoperative anatomy, particularly for those patients who have had stoma complications such as hernia, prolapse, and obstructive symptoms or those patients referred for takedown from another institution.

The review of prior operative reports provides useful information about stoma construction and any technical complications encountered during the initial surgery. It is essential to know if the ostomy to be taken down is a loop, a divided loop, or an end stoma. If an end stoma is present, the clinician must know whether the proximal end of the defunctioned limb is located at the stoma site within the subcutaneous tissue, at the stoma site but intraperitoneally, or at some site other than the stoma. If an extraperitoneal colostomy was constructed, a more difficult dissection during its mobilization can be anticipated.

PREOPERATIVE PREPARATION

The day before the operation the patient is given a lavage or cathartic bowel preparation. Increasingly, this is performed on an outpatient basis; thus it is important that patients be properly instructed about how to take the preparation and maintain adequate hydration. Consideration also is given to flushing the diverted limb, particularly in patients with a loop stoma. Enemas also are useful in patients with complete diversion because the irrigation helps to flush mucous plugs that are frequently present in the rectum. We use a combination of oral and intravenous prophylactic antibiotics for colostomy takedowns, but we use only intravenous antibiotics for ileostomy takedowns. Several studies have demonstrated no significant difference in infectious complications in patients receiving combination therapy vs. oral antibiotics alone.[9]

Because the incidence of deep venous thrombosis increases with pelvic surgery, patients must be evaluated perioperatively for this condition. Patients undergoing multiple procedures within a short time are probably at increased risk for deep venous thrombosis. Use of subcutaneous heparin and/or sequential compressive devices may be warranted in such patients. We routinely use sequential compression devices on a prophylactic basis for all pelvic surgery and the majority of other abdominal cases, including ostomy takedowns. This technique provides the additional benefit of providing extra padding and protection from compressive neuropathy, which is a concern for those patients placed in the modified lithotomy position.

OPERATIVE TECHNIQUES

Ileostomy Takedown

Ileostomy closure most often is performed with the patient in the supine position. However, the modified lithotomy position is used if there is any

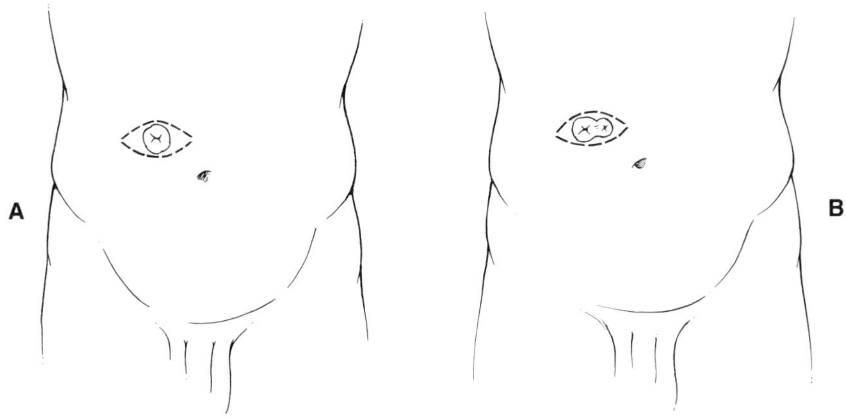

Fig. 11-1. Elliptical incision for end, **A,** and loop, **B,** stomas.

possibility of the need to perform a transanal stapled anastomosis (i.e., with takedown of an end ileostomy after total colectomy and Hartmann's pouch construction. The techniques used for such a takedown are similar to those for takedown of an end colostomy and are discussed later in this chapter).

The stoma opening is closed with a 3-0 suture to prevent intraoperative spillage before abdominal skin preparation is done. The takedown of a loop ileostomy, divided-loop ileostomy, and an end ileostomy with the proximal end of the defunctioned limb nearby usually can be accomplished through a parastomal incision. We generally use an elliptical transverse incision that is extended approximately 2 cm beyond the stoma in both directions. The incision is kept as close to the mucocutaneous junction as possible, generally within 2 mm (Fig. 11-1). Sharp dissection is used through the dermis, after which cautery is used to cut down at right angles to the anterior rectus fascia. The subcutaneous dissection is completed medially and laterally to expose the circumference of the bowel as it exits the muscle (Fig. 11-2, *A* and *B*). This technique minimizes the risk of injuring the bowel as it traverses the subcutaneous tissues and is particularly useful in the obese patient since it provides wider exposure. It is also beneficial in end- and divided-loop ileostomies since the distal limb may be located in a subcutaneous position (Fig. 11-2, *C*). Keeping the ellipse of skin on the terminal bowel until the anastomosis is performed provides a good handle for traction, thus minimizing trauma to the bowel.

The remainder of the dissection is carried out sharply, with the bowel freed from its fascial, muscular, and peritoneal attachments. Meticulous care must be exercised at this time to avoid serosal injury. There is usually at least one site where the bowel is loosely fixed to the abdominal wall, allowing

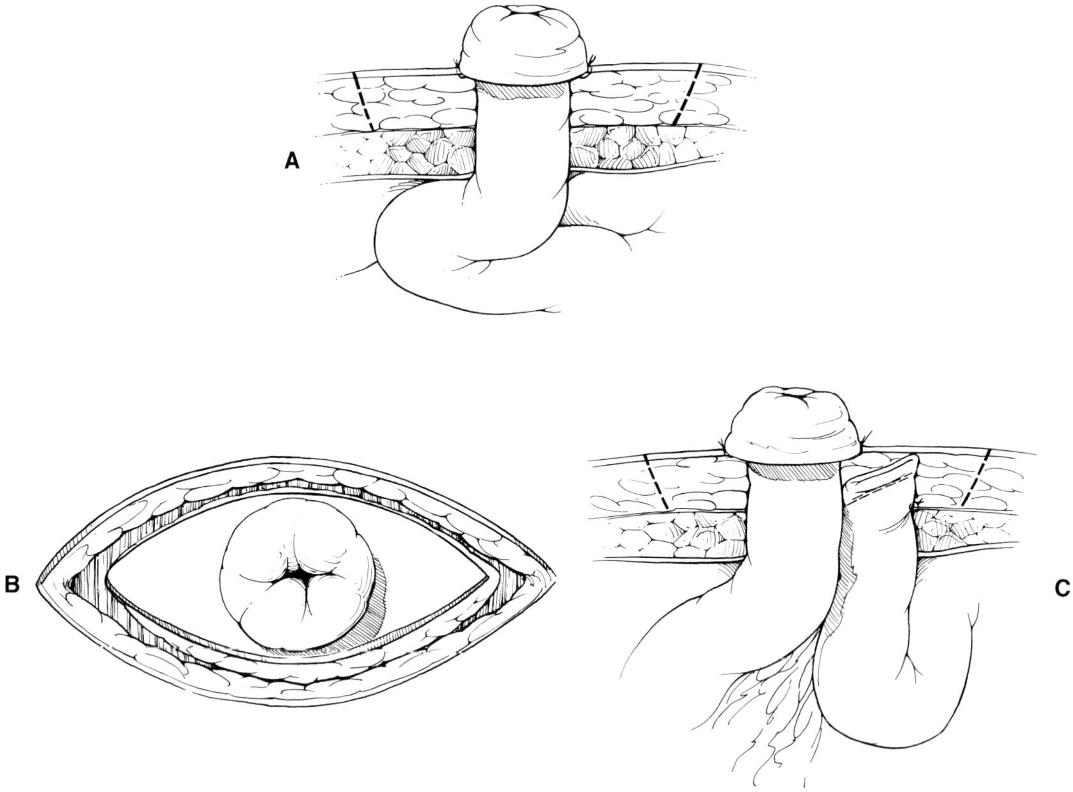

Fig. 11-2. Demonstration of lateral mobilization and preservation of integument with **A,** lateral view, **B,** anterior view, end stomas and, **C,** divided-loop stomas.

insertion of a finger into the abdominal cavity. At this point the stomal defect can be circumscribed with a finger to identify any potentially troublesome adhesions and direct the remainder of the mobilization. If difficulty is encountered in freeing the bowel from intra-abdominal attachments, the incision can easily be extended laterally or medially through the rectus muscle. In our review fewer than 1% of all ileostomy takedowns required a midline incision and formal laparotomy to afford proper exposure. After the mobilization of both the proximal and distal limbs, the anastomosis can be completed.

The choice of ostomy closure dictates the next step. If the antimesenteric bowel wall defect created with a loop ileostomy can be closed, the remainder of the subcutaneous attachments and integument must be sharply excised from the terminal bowel. The edges of the defect may need to be freshly excised if scarring is excessive. The defect is closed with a handsewn technique by placing sutures at the sides of the defect to align it transversely (Fig. 11-3, *A*). Multiple interrupted sutures are used to complete the anastomosis. A stapling technique also can be used for closure (Fig. 11-3, *B*).

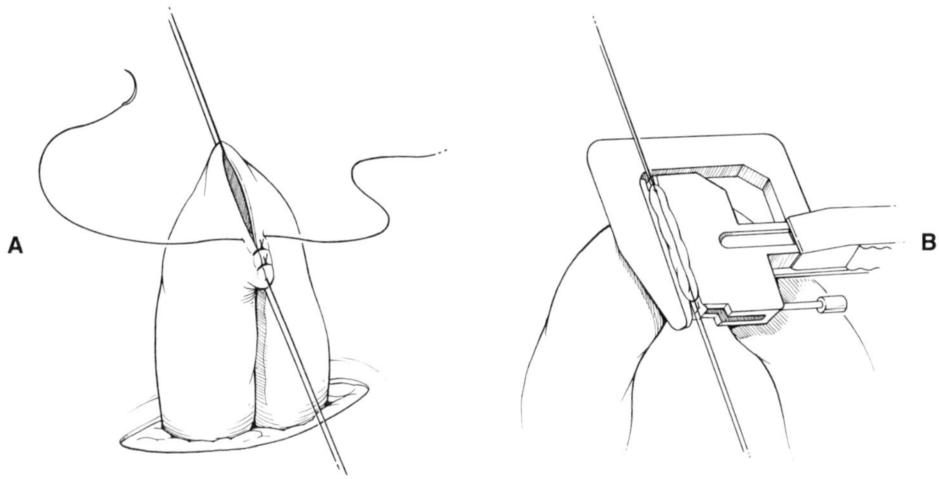

Fig. 11-3. Handsewn, **A**, and stapled, **B**, closure of loop ileostomy.

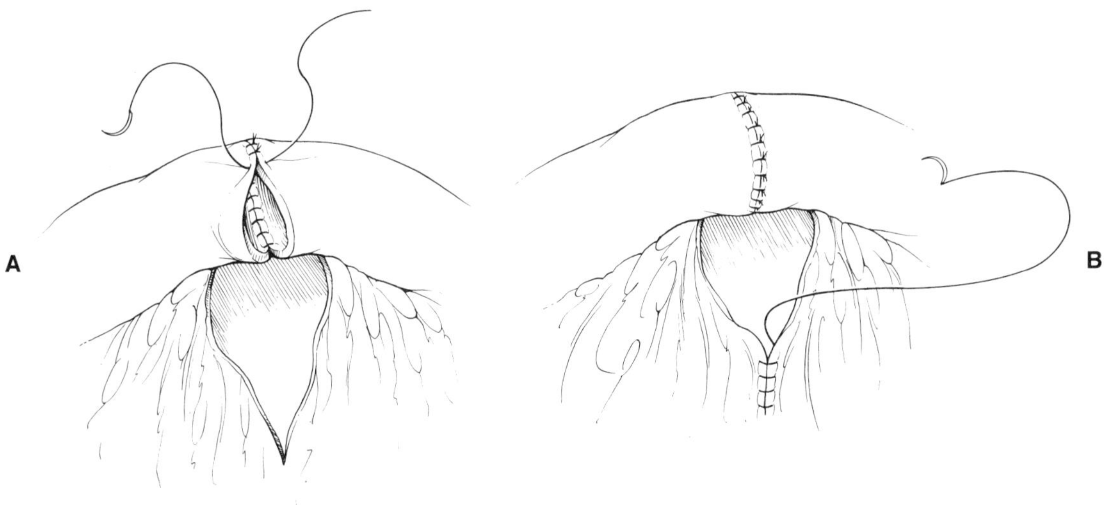

Fig. 11-4. Interrupted handsewn end-to-end anastomosis, **A**, with closure of adjacent mesentery, **B.**

If the terminal bowel is unsuitable for anastomosis or simple closure of the defect, the skin and terminal subcutaneous attachments need not be excised at this time. A handsewn end-to-end anastomosis can be carried out by dividing a sufficient amount of mesentery from the distal and proximal limbs and then transecting the terminal stoma before anastomosis (Fig. 11-4). If the anastomosis will be stapled, keeping the terminal bowel with its ellipse of skin is useful for traction. An enterotomy is made along the antimesenteric

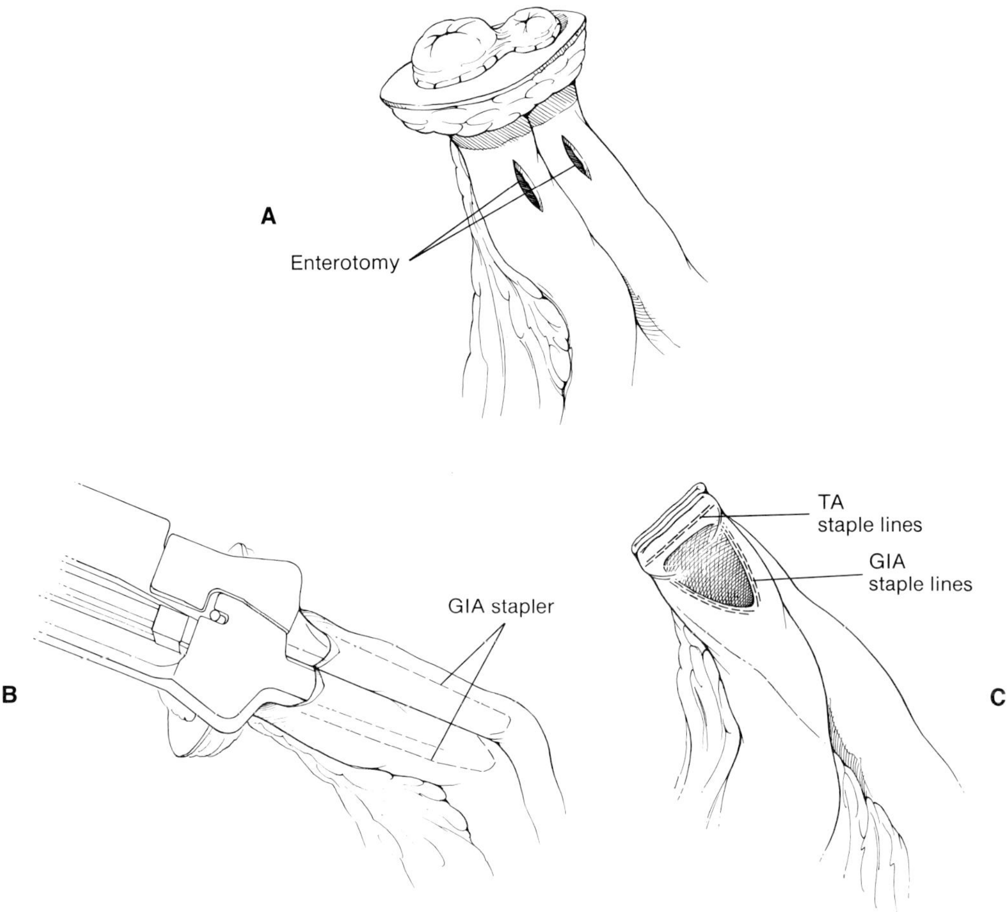

Fig. 11-5. Stapled functional end-to-end anastomosis. **A,** Enterotomy. **B,** GIA stapler inserted. **C,** TA and GIA staple lines with completed anastomosis.

border of each limb (Fig. 11-5, *A*). A linear stapler is inserted (Fig. 11-5, *B*). Care is taken to ensure that the mesentery is free before the stapler is fired. A second firing of a linear or a TA stapler, with the stapler placed just ahead of the enterotomies, completes the anastomosis (Fig. 11-5, *C*). The previous staple line also should be distracted to avoid stenosis. The remainder of the bowel, including the enterotomies and the ellipse of skin, is excised after the stapler has been fired. In the 297 ileostomy takedowns reviewed in our series, there was no significant difference between handsewn vs. stapled or end-to-end vs. functional end-to-end anastomoses.

After completion of the anastomosis, the bowel is placed back into the abdominal cavity, after which the abdomen is irrigated with saline solution. The wound is closed with a single layer of absorbable suture (e.g., Maxon or

PDS) in the anterior fascia. The skin usually is approximated with staples (less often with interrupted subcuticular sutures). We do not routinely use drains; however, they may be useful when contamination is encountered or when a concomitant parastomal hernia is repaired, creating a large subcutaneous space. Although our 13% incidence of seroma and subcutaneous wound infection after ileostomy closure may seem relatively high, this complication is easily remedied by removing one or more staples or sutures to provide adequate drainage.

Postoperative care is routine. The need for using nasogastric suction varies.

Colostomy Takedown

Placing the patient in a modified lithotomy position is almost always preferred for takedown of sigmoid or descending colostomies because this position provides the clinician excellent access to the perineum for a transanal stapled anastomosis. The supine position works well for takedown of most transverse colostomies, which generally involve a loop-type stoma. Their takedown is similar to that of a loop ileostomy and is not discussed further here.

After the ostomy has been closed with a 3-0 suture to prevent intraoperative spillage of feces, the abdomen is prepared and draped. The prior abdominal incision (usually midline) is used most frequently for colostomy takedown since mobilization of both the proximal colon and the distal colorectum is necessary. After abdominal exploration and freeing of the terminal colon from any intraperitoneal attachments, a small ellipse of skin is incised around the stoma. The incision is made as close to the mucocutaneous junction as possible and is carried down to the fascia. The bowel is freed from the muscular and peritoneal attachments by using sharp dissection. Meticulous dissection is required to avoid serosal damage. At this point the ellipse of skin is freed from the terminal bowel and is excised in preparation for the anastomosis. Alternatively, a small segment of colon involved in the stoma is resected by dividing its mesentery and transecting the colon between clamps.

The distal bowel, which is often the upper rectum, is mobilized and prepared for the anastomosis in the usual fashion. It is important to select a suitable portion of bowel that is well vascularized and preferably free from diverticular or inflammatory disease for the anastomosis. If a stiff, noncompliant portion of sigmoid was left behind at the initial operation, it is wise to resect this area.

The anastomosis can be completed with either a stapled or handsewn technique. Our review revealed no statistically significant difference between the two techniques. Two options are available for stapling the anastomosis. A functional end-to-end anastomosis can be completed as depicted in Fig. 11-5 with the use of GIA and TA staplers. This approach is suitable for high anastomoses. The circular end-to-end stapler is the type most commonly used and works especially well for distal anastomoses. However, a single-layer interrupted technique, as depicted in Fig. 11-4, can work just as effectively for most colostomy takedowns. It is our policy to assess the integrity of all low colonic anastomoses via proctoscopy. Not only is the anastomosis visualized, for confirmation of the anastomotic level and viability of the bowel, but a good check is provided for hemostasis, which can be controlled by placing additional full-thickness sutures if needed. To ensure the integrity of the anastomosis, the distal bowel is insufflated with air after the pelvis has been filled with saline solution. If an air leak is noted, the bowel can be reinforced with additional sutures to rectify the problem. The postoperative care is routine.

SUMMARY

Stoma takedown frequently is given little attention in many teaching institutions and is relegated to the junior residents and staff because it is thought to take little preparation "and is a straightforward procedure." Although this often is true, the patient who is not given a thorough preoperative assessment is rendered a great disservice. As with any other operative procedure, preparation is critical. A thorough knowledge of the patient's history and present anatomy minimizes unexpected findings and potential complications. A successful takedown is imperative for ileal-pouch patients and others who have undergone complicated anal reconstructive procedures since complications can jeopardize the eventual outcome of the primary procedure. Diverting stomas continue to play a role in general surgery, and it is critical that surgeons have a consistent, comprehensive approach to stoma takedown. New techniques are presently being developed, with the laparoscope used to assist in mobilization and reanastomosis (see Chapter 13). The surgeon must maintain an accurate account of complication rates after takedown procedures to make optimal decisions about the use of diverting stomas and to inform patients better about their potential morbidity. This information also will prove useful in a comparison of the complication rates of traditional takedown methods to new techniques such as laparoscopic takedown.

REFERENCES

1. Fielding LP, Stewart-Brown S, Hiner R, et al. Covering stoma for elective anterior resection of the rectum: An outmoded operation? Am J Surg 147:524-530, 1984.
2. Knox A, Birkett F, Collins C. Closure of colostomy. Br J Surg 58:668-672, 1971.
3. Freund H, Raniel J, Muggia-Sulam M. Factors affecting the morbidity of colostomy closure. Dis Colon Rectum 25:712-715, 1982.
4. Metcalf AM, Dozois RR, Beart RW Jr, et al. Temporary ileostomy for ileal pouch–anal anastomosis: Function and complications. Dis Colon Rectum 28:300-303, 1986.
5. Roy PH, Sauer WG, Beahrs OH. Experience with ileostomies. Evaluations of long-term rehabilitation in 487 patients. Am J Surg 119:77-85, 1970.
6. Sugarman HJ, Newsome HH, DeCosta G, et al. Stapled ileoanal anastomosis for ulcerative colitis and familial polyposis without a temporary diverting ileostomy. Ann Surg 213:606-619, 1991.
7. Everett WG, Pollard SG. Restorative proctocolectomy without temporary ileostomy. Br J Surg 77:621-622, 1990.
8. Demetriades D, Rabinowitz B, Sofianos C, et al. The management of colon injuries by primary repair or colostomy. Br J Surg 72:881-883, 1985.
9. Wolff BG, Beart RW Jr, Dozois RR, et al. A new bowel preparation for elective colon and rectal surgery. Arch Surg 123:895-900, 1988.

SELECTED READINGS

Alexander-Williams J. Loop ileostomy and colostomy for faecal diversion. Ann R Coll Surg Engl 54:141-148, 1974.

Demetriades D, Pezikis A, Melissas J, et al. Factors influencing the morbidity of colostomy closure. Am J Surg 55:594-596, 1988.

Farnell MB, Worthington S, Mucha P, et al. Closure of abdominal incisions with subcutaneous catheters. Arch Surg 121:641-647, 1986.

Fasth S, Hulten L. Loop ileostomy: A superior diverting stoma in colorectal surgery. World J Surg 8:401-405, 1984.

Garber H, Morris D, Eisenstat T, et al. Factors influencing the morbidity of colostomy closure. Dis Colon Rectum 25:464-470, 1982.

Kelly KA, Pemberton JH, Wolff BG, et al. Ileal pouch–anal anastomosis. Curr Probl Surg 29:57-131, 1992.

Parks S, Hastings P. Complications of colostomy closure. Am J Surg 149:672-675, 1985.

Schwartz S, Ellis H. Maingot's Abdominal Operations, 8th ed, vol 2. Norwalk, Conn.: Appleton-Century-Crofts, 1990.

Todd G, Kutcher L, Markowitz A. Factors influencing the complications of colostomy closure. Am J Surg 137:748-751, 1979.

12 METHODS OF URINARY DIVERSION

Daniel P. Dalton

Supravesical diversion of the urinary tract to the abdominal wall, with bowel used as a conduit, was introduced in the 1950s by Bricker[1] and Gilchrist et al.[2] The concepts described by these pioneers in urinary diversion (i.e., Bricker's ileal conduit and Gilchrist et al.'s use of the ileocecal segment) remain the basis of most cutaneous urinary diversions used today. The recent introduction of continent urinary diversion, bladder substitution, and intermittent catheterization and the recognition of long-term complications of ileal conduits in the pediatric population have led to a decrease in the use of the standard ileal conduit. This procedure remains, however, a mainstay in the care of adult patients who require urinary diversion.

Cutaneous urinary diversion is used most commonly in patients with pelvic malignancy. Bladder carcinoma is the most common lesion, but occasionally patients with urethral, prostatic, colonic, or gynecologic cancer require diversion, as does the occasional patient with a pelvic sarcoma. Severe radiation damage to the pelvic viscera and recalcitrant fistulas are occasional entities necessitating diversion. The advent of intermittent catheterization, enterocystoplasty, and the artificial urinary sphincter has rendered urinary diversion a procedure of last resort in patients with neurologic disorders. Certain congenital anomalies (e.g., bladder exstrophy) require urinary diversion, as does the rare patient with interstitial cystitis, intractable incontinence, or severe pelvic injury.

TECHNIQUES WITH INCONTINENT STOMAS

Although various segments of bowel have been used as urinary conduits, the terminal ileum and the ileocecal segment are the most commonly used. When nonrefluxing ureteroenterostomies are desired or previous radiation therapy has damaged the small bowel, colonic conduits are used.

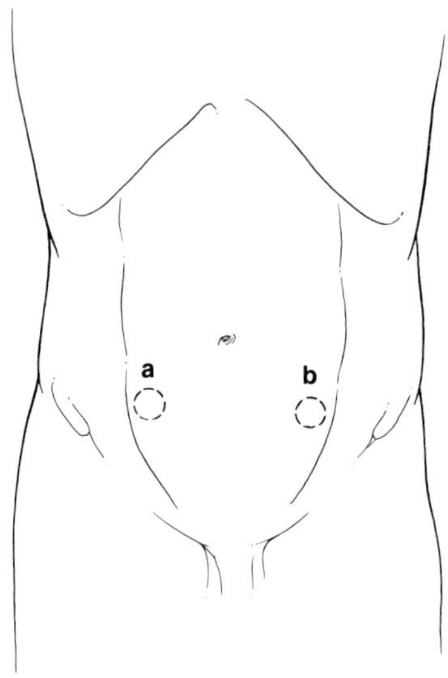

Fig. 12-1. Selection of stoma site should take into consideration factors such as body habitus, scars, and planned bowel segment. Typical site for ileal conduit (*a*) and sigmoid conduit (*b*).

As with any major surgical procedure, the patient's medical and nutritional status is optimized. Important historical information, such as prior bowel surgery, gastrointestinal illnesses, and prior radiation therapy, must be carefully sought, because significant alteration of the procedure may be necessary in certain settings. I perform a mechanical and oral antibiotic bowel preparation on all patients and initiate prophylactic systemic antibiotics before surgery. Intravenous hydration is initiated the evening before surgery, as are antithrombotic precautions (i.e., elastic stockings and intermittent compression boots). Preoperatively the ET therapist introduces the patient to collection devices, and various acceptable stoma sites are marked (Fig. 12-1).

Ileal Conduit

A midline incision is made and exploratory laparotomy is performed. Primary procedures (i.e., cystectomy) are performed first. The ureters are isolated as they cross the iliac vessels; they are carefully mobilized and divided several centimeters above the bladder. If malignancy is present, frozen-section analysis of the proximal margins is performed. The end of the proximal ureter is secured with catgut sutures or hemoclips to allow slight ureteral dilatation and to prevent continuous soiling of the pelvis with urine (Fig. 12-2). If not already done, appendectomy is performed.

Attention is then directed to preparing the ileal segment. The mesentery of the terminal ileum is transilluminated, and the ileocolic artery is identified. The distal end of the loop should be 10 to 15 cm proximal to the ileocecal junction (Fig. 12-3). A stay suture is placed. A segment of ileum that has at least two vascular arcades supplying it and is of sufficient length to reach the abdominal wall is identified. If a Turnbull-type stoma is to be constructed, an additional 8 to 10 cm of ileum should be used.[3] A second stay suture marks the proximal extent of the loop, and the mesentery is examined again to ensure adequate blood supply. The mesentery is then divided at right angles to the bowel in standard fashion. To provide greater mobility of the distal segment, the mesentery should be divided to a greater degree, with care taken not to injure a major vascular arcade.

After the ends of the proposed ileal segment are cleared of attached mesentery and fat, the bowel is divided so that a slightly shorter antimesenteric border results. The isolated loop is brought down toward the pelvis, and the proximal stay suture is removed so that the distal end of the segment is easily identifiable to allow isoperistaltic placement of the conduit. A standard ileo-ileostomy is performed according to the preference of the surgeon, although the use of stapling techniques shortens operative time. The mesentery is closed with 3-0 chromic suture (Fig. 12-4).

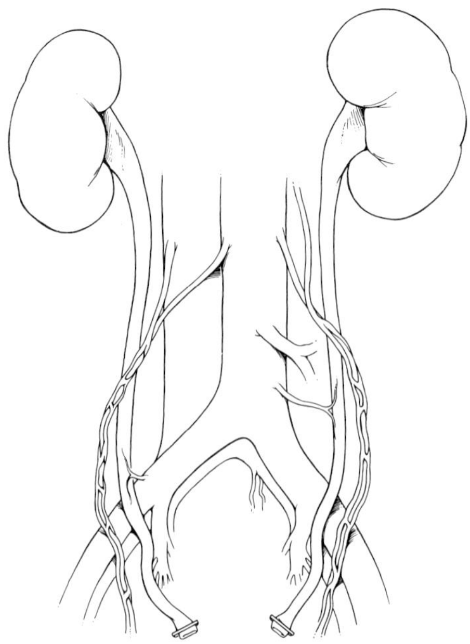

Fig. 12-2. Following division and frozen-section analysis (if indicated), the ureters are temporarily occluded to allow dilatation.

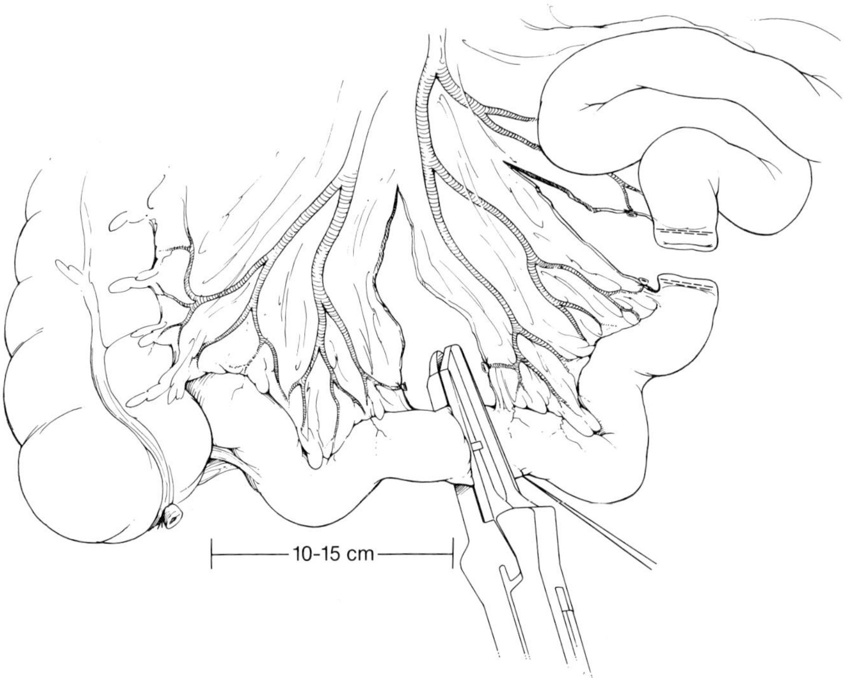

Fig. 12-3. In isolation of the ileal loop, distal end of loop should be 10 to 15 cm proximal to ileocecal junction.

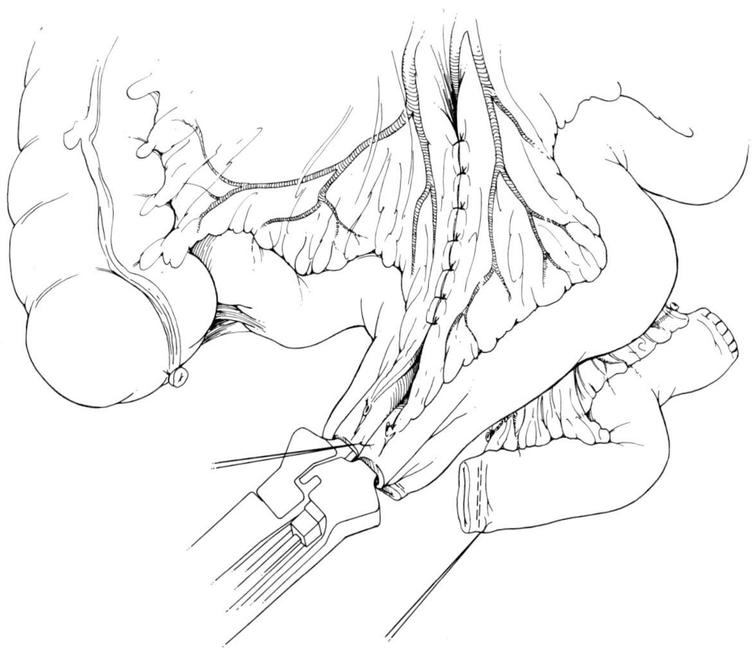

Fig. 12-4. After standard ileoileostomy is performed, mesentery is closed with 3-0 chromic suture.

The ileal segment is irrigated, and, if necessary, the proximal end is closed in a watertight fashion with absorbable suture. The left ureter is delivered under the sigmoid mesentery, with care taken to avoid sharp angulation. The ureteroileal anastomosis then can be constructed, with either an end-to-side or a conjoined technique used[4] (Fig. 12-5, *A-B*). I generally place indwelling ureteral stents, although this is not a universal practice.[5] Nonrefluxing ureteroileostomies have been described[6] (Fig. 12-5, *C*). The proximal end of the conduit may be secured to the presacral area with absorbable suture.

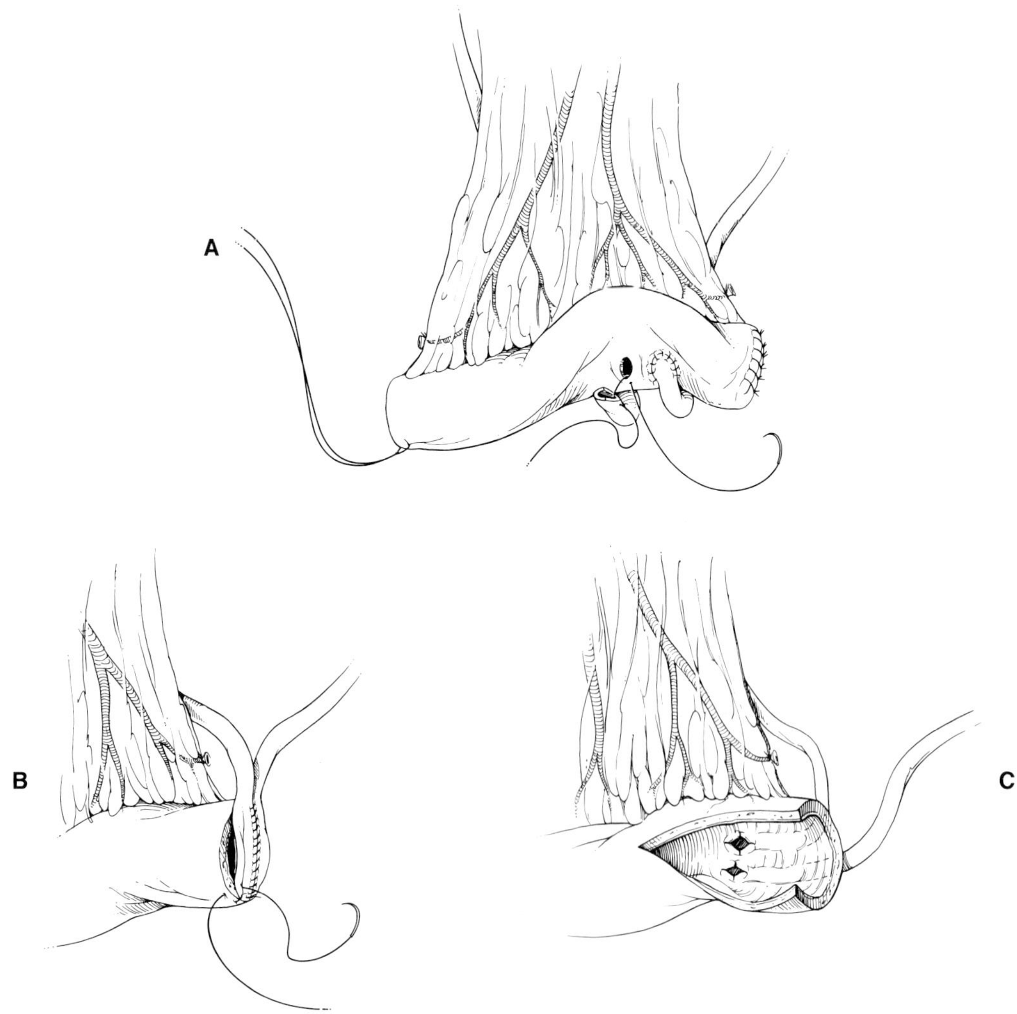

Fig. 12-5. Methods of constructing ureteroenterostomies. Careful mucosa-to-mucosa apposition with fine absorbable suture is done. **A,** End-to-side anastomosis. **B,** Conjoined ureteroileal anastomosis. **C,** Nonrefluxing ureteroileostomies.

Careful attention is paid to the creation of the abdominal wall stoma. The skin and the underlying subcutaneous tissue are removed circumferentially down to fascia at the previously marked stoma site (Fig. 12-6, *A*). I use the end of a 20 ml syringe plunger to mark the amount of skin to remove. A cruciate incision is made in the anterior rectus fascia, and four separate 2-0 chromic sutures are placed at the four points of the incision (Fig. 12-6, *B*). The fibers of the rectus muscle are separated, and the posterior sheath and the peritoneum are opened bluntly with a clamp (Fig. 12-6, *C*). This opening should freely

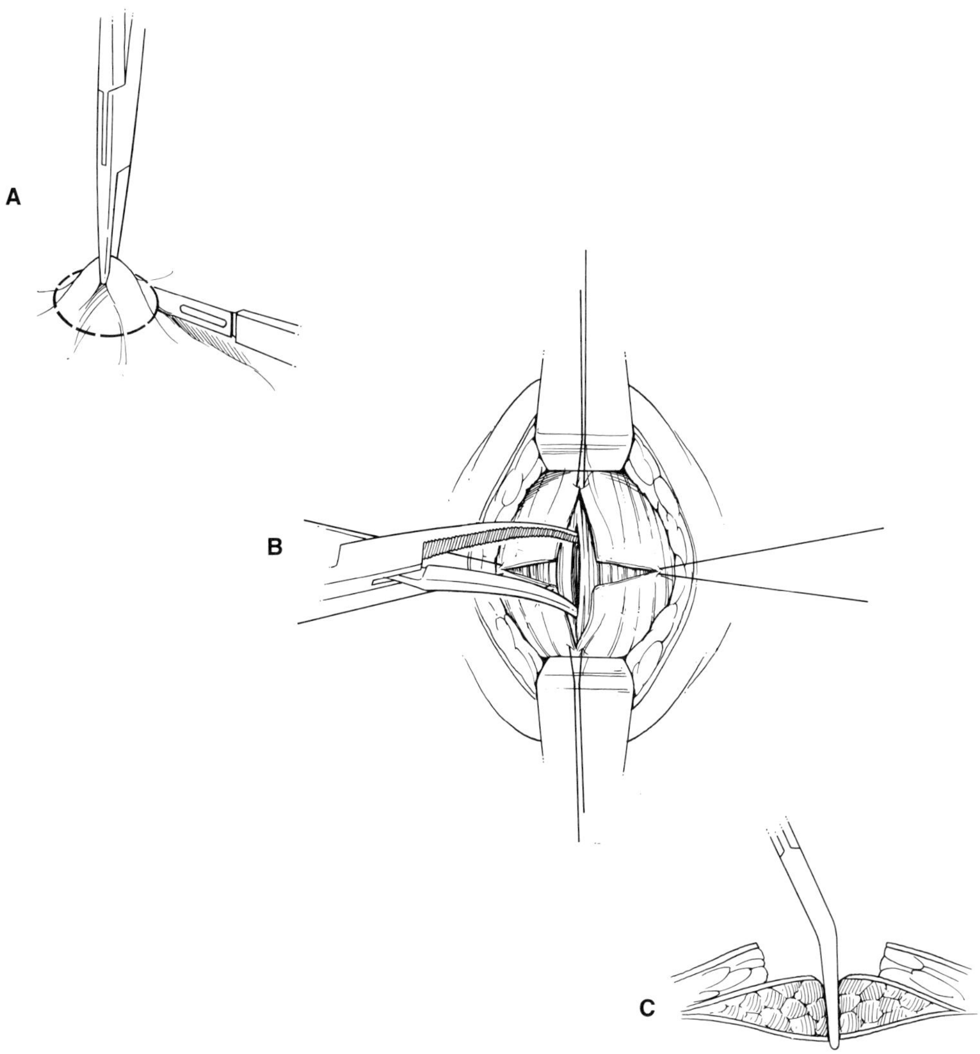

Fig. 12-6. Preparation of stoma site.

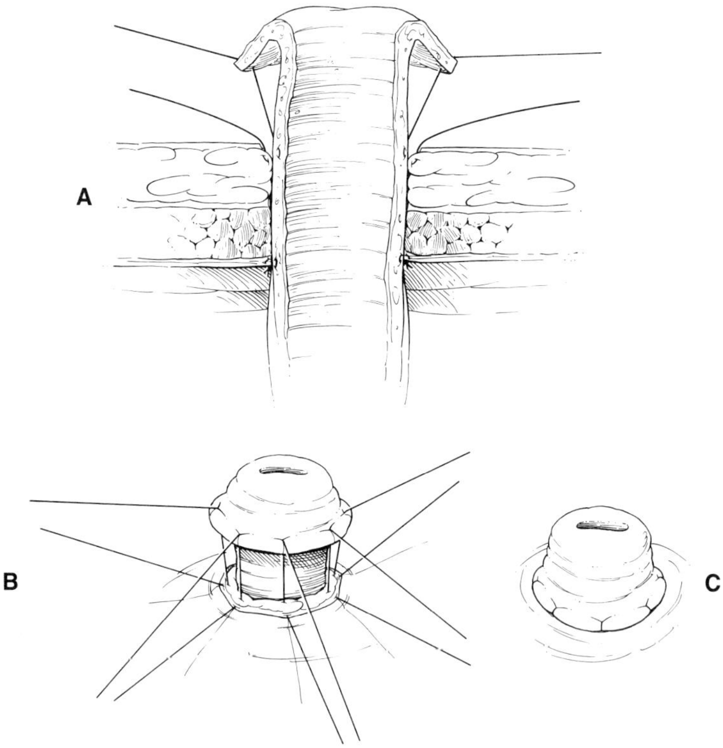

Fig. 12-7. Creation of nipple-type stoma.

admit two fingers. The previously marked distal end of the ileal loop is delivered through the abdominal wall; it should rest without tension 3 to 4 cm above the skin (Fig. 12-7, *A*). The conduit is secured to the anterior fascia with the previously placed chromic sutures, and a protruding, nipple-type stoma is created.[7] To create the nipple stoma, four quadrant 2-0 chromic sutures are placed sequentially through conduit seromuscular tissue, the full-thickness distal margin of conduit, and the subcuticular layer of skin (Fig. 12-7, *B*). After all sutures have been placed, they are tied. Interrupted 3-0 chromic sutures are placed to seal bowel mucosa to skin (Fig. 12-7, *C*). A finger is placed carefully in the stoma to determine that narrowing or angulation is not present at the fascial level, and a collecting device is applied. Before closing, several 3-0 chromic sutures can be placed to secure the conduit to the posterior fascia. Alternatively, particularly in obese individuals, a Turnbull-type loop stoma can be constructed[3] (Fig. 12-8).

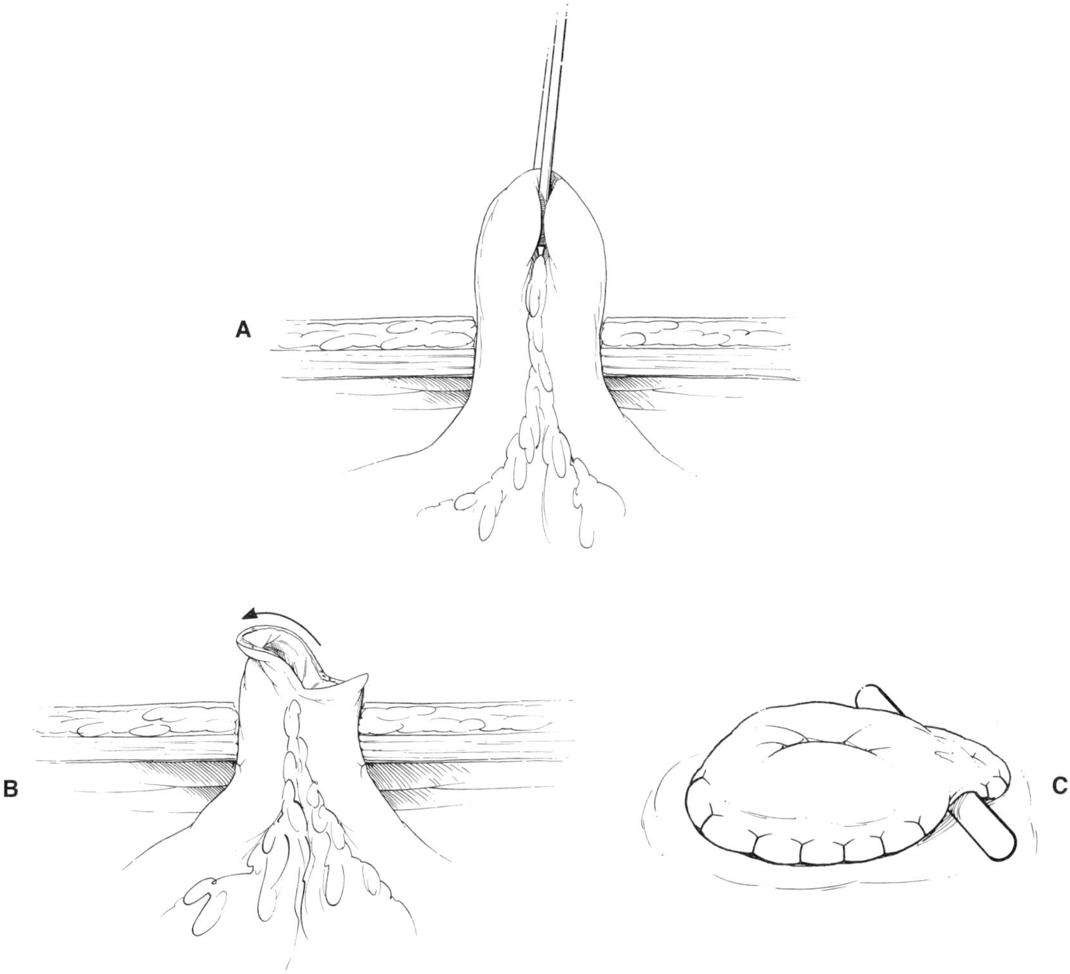

Fig. 12-8. Turnbull-type loop stoma. After closure of the distal conduit, the loop of ileum is delivered (**A**) and opened (**B**). Bowel is secured to the anterior fascia, and the mucosa is approximated to the skin with absorbable suture. **C**, Occasionally, placement of a rod is helpful to prevent early stoma retraction, although it is usually unnecessary.

Jejunal Conduit

Jejunal conduits have a high incidence of metabolic and electrolyte abnormalities; therefore their use has been abandoned by most urologic surgeons unless no other bowel segment is available. The inefficiency of the jejunal mucosa in absorbing sodium gives rise to the classic "jejunal conduit syndrome,"[8,9] consisting of hyponatremic, hypochloremic, hyperkalemic metabolic acidosis.

Complications and long-term results with ileal conduits. The reported rates of perioperative morbidity range from 20% to 50%; mortality rates, from 1% to 13%.[10-20] Hampel et al.[21] have reviewed the pertinent literature (Tables 12-1 and 12-2). Superficial wound infections occur in 5% to 10% of cases, and fascial dehiscence has been reported in approximately 3%. I routinely use retention sutures, prophylactic antibiotics, and hyperalimentation in an attempt to avoid these problems. Complications such as atelectasis, small bowel obstruction, and thromboembolic disease occur with a frequency similar to that of other major intra-abdominal procedures.

The immediate postoperative problems unique to the ileal conduit and other methods of urinary diversion are urinary extravasation and loop necrosis. Mild leakage of urine from the ureteroileal anastomosis occasionally occurs. It is recognized clinically by an increase in drain output with a high blood urea nitrogen (BUN) and creatinine content. This problem is usually a self-limited situation that resolves in 2 to 4 days. Rarely, however, massive leakage occurs, accompanied by anuria, large drain output, and urinoma formation. A loopogram should be performed immediately to document the location of the leak, and a catheter should be left in the conduit and attached to dependent drainage. If marked drainage persists, distal ureteral necrosis or dehiscence of the proximal conduit must be considered as possibilities. Percutaneous drainage of one or both kidneys can be performed; if a stent is not already in place, placement of one in an antegrade fashion can be attempted. Most major leaks can be managed in this way in conjunction with maintenance of nutritional status, treatment of infection, and patience. Reoperation with reconstruction of the anastomosis and, occasionally, the entire conduit sometimes is necessary, but it is extremely difficult because of the severe inflammatory changes involved. The havoc wreaked by postoperative urinary extravasation underscores the importance of adhering strictly to basic surgical principles in constructing the conduit.

Loop necrosis is both disastrous and avoidable. It occurs in less than 1% of cases[14,17] and has not occurred at all in several large series.[18,20] An adequate blood supply and avoidance of torsion and tension on the mesentery should prevent this calamity. When loop necrosis does occur, the stoma appears dusky and the patient may become acidotic. Prompt recognition of this complication and reconstruction of the conduit are mandatory.

Late complications unique to ileal conduit and other forms of urinary diversion include deterioration in renal function, nephrolithiasis, recurrent febrile urinary tract infections, obstruction of the ureteroenteric anastomosis, loop stenosis and other stoma complications, electrolyte abnormalities, nutritional deficiencies, and, perhaps, carcinogenesis[21] (see Table 12-2).

Long-term follow-up of children with ileal conduits reveals a significant degree of deterioration of renal function seemingly directly related to time.[10-13,15,16,19] The longest follow-up was that reported by Pitts and

Table 12-1. Early complications of ureteroileal conduit diversion*

Reference	No. of Patients	Peri-operative Mortality	Intestinal Obstruction	Intestinal Fistula	Wound Infection	Wound Dehiscence	Uretero-ileal Leakage	Loop Necrosis	Acute Pyelo-nephritis	Total Complications
Jaffe et al. (1968)[14]	543	6.6	5.5	1.1	7.6	2.6	2.6	0.2	2.8	38.1
Schmidt et al. (1973)[18]	178	3.4	6.2	1.1	6.2	3.4	2.4		2.8	33.7
Remigailo et al. (1976)[17]	152	0.7	0.7		7.2	3.3	2.6	0.7		19.7
Malgieri et al. (1978)	136	3.7	4.4		21.3		8.1			55.9
Sullivan et al. (1980)[20]	336	13.7		5.4	20.2		3.3		19.2	
Heath & Eckstein (1984)[13]	144	1.4	4.9	2.1	3.5	4.9	3.5	5.6		22

*From Hampel N, Bodner D, Persky Z. Ileal and jejunal conduit urinary diversion. Urol Clin North Am 13:2, 215, 1986.

Table 12-2. Late complications of ureteroileal conduit diversion*

Reference	No. of Patients	Intestinal Obstruction	Pyelo-nephritis	Renal Deterioration (yr)	Ureteroileal Obstruction	Stoma Stenosis	Renal Calculi	Total Complications	Years Follow-Up (mean)
Jaffe et al. (1968)[14]	543	6.5		7	3.7	5.5			1-14
Schmidt et al. (1973)[18]	178	6.2	21.9	17.7	7.9	18.9	10.7	81	1-10 (4)
Remigailo et al. (1976)[17]	152	10.6	8.6		4	12.6	2.6	68.2	1-9 (2)
Pitts & Muecke (1979)[16]	242		10.7	(0-5) 6 (6-10) 13 (10-15) 19	9.1	14	5.8	38.8	1-20 (6.2)
Sullivan et al. (1980)[20]	336	14.9			7.5	5.1	4 (Lt. 13.4) (Rt. 2.6)		5-21
Heath & Eckstein (1984)[13]	144	3.5		(<10) 6.4 (>19) 19	2.1	25	5.5	28	>6.9

*From Hampel N, Bodner D, Persky Z. Ileal and jejunal conduit urinary diversion. Urol Clin North Am 13:2, 216, 1986.

Muecke,[16] which revealed deterioration of renal function in 35% of patients who were followed up for 16 to 20 years. Recurrent infection, reflux, nephrolithiasis, and anatomic obstruction all play a potential role and should be sought and treated. Because most patients with ileal conduits have asymptomatic bacteriuria, the presence of reflux is particularly bothersome. A classic study by Richie et al.[22] demonstrated an 83% incidence of pyelonephritis in refluxing units as compared to 7% in nonrefluxing ones. As a result, when children or young adults require urinary diversion, a method incorporating reliable nonrefluxing ureteroenteric anastomosis is generally used.

Up to 10% of patients develop nephrolithiasis. Dretler[23] theorized that the mixture of urea-splitting organisms and high-conduit residual urines with its resultant acidosis is the primary cause. I treat asymptomatic bacteriuria only when a likely urea-splitting organism is found (e.g., *Proteus mirabilis*). Furthermore, a kidney-ureter-bladder (KUB) study should be performed on the patient every 1 to 2 years to identify early stone formation.

Obstruction of the ureteroileal anastomosis occurs in approximately 5% of patients and is due to either ischemia, localized fibrosis, radiation change, or recurrent tumor. This condition can occur silently and emphasizes the need for performing serial loopograms or renal ultrasounds. When an obstructed segment is identified and the initial procedure was performed for a malignancy, its recurrence must be ruled out with cytologies and brushings of the anastomosis. In the past open procedures with reconstruction of the anastomosis were used in those patients with benign strictures. More recently, endourologic treatment with balloon dilatation and cold-knife incisions has been attempted[24] (Fig. 12-9).

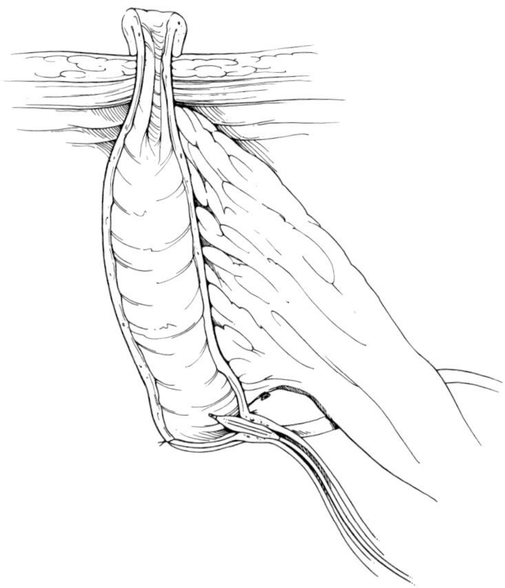

Fig. 12-9. Endourologic management of ureteroenteric structures is becoming the treatment of choice, although open repair or chronic stenting are still required for failures.

Stoma stenosis has been reported in up to 25% of cases, but it probably has an incidence closer to 5%.[13] Use of a protruding nipple stoma and the Turnbull loop stoma in obese patients should keep the incidence low. Nevertheless it does occur and may be a source of significant morbidity. When repair is necessary, simple interposition of a segment of skin may suffice, although advancement of the conduit and reconstruction of the stoma may be required (Fig. 12-10). Stenosis of the conduit itself also may occur as a result of long-standing infections and fibrosis and require reconstruction.[25]

Peristomal hernias, stoma prolapse, chronic intestinal fistulas, and peristomal skin complications are dealt with elsewhere in this text and are not discussed here.

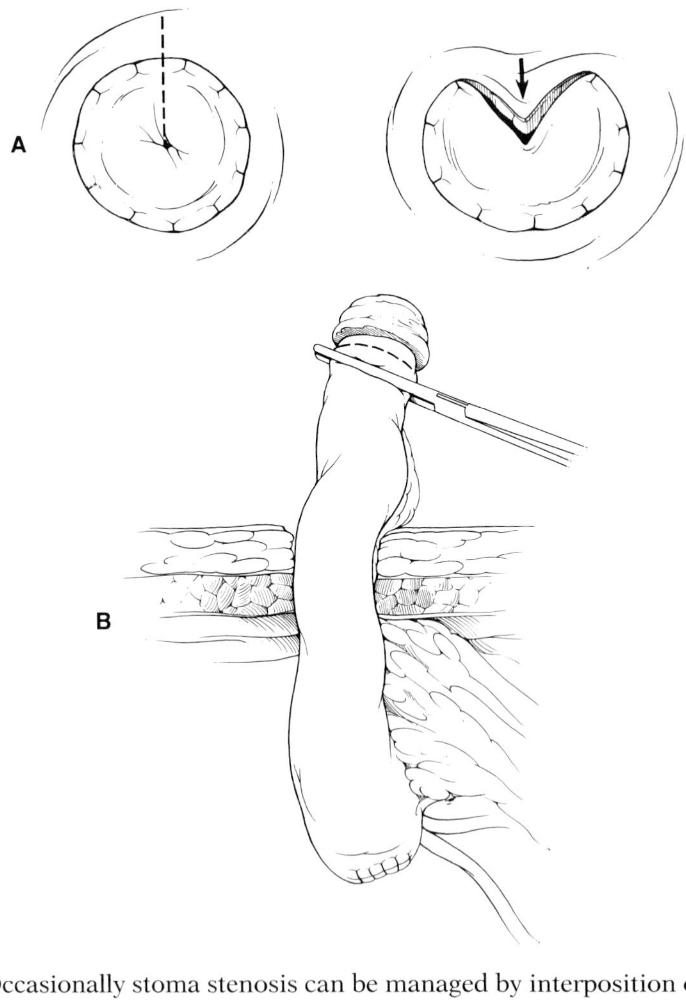

Fig. 12-10. Occasionally stoma stenosis can be managed by interposition of full-thickness skin **(A)**. Severe cases require total reconstruction **(B)**, although simple advancement of the conduit may suffice.

When urine comes in contact with bowel mucosa, electrolyte and free-water transfer can occur, resulting in metabolic abnormalities. The ileum plays primarily an absorptive role; therefore patients with ileal conduits can develop a hypernatremic, hypokalemic, hyperchloremic metabolic acidosis.[26] This condition almost always occurs in the presence of renal insufficiency and can be treated with oral alkali. Occasionally a redundant conduit secondary to either stoma stenosis or too long an ileal loop can result in a large amount of residual urine and hyperabsorption. These entities require surgical correction.

Resection of large amounts of ileum can result in bile salt deficiencies and steatorrhea or vitamin B_{12} deficiency and megaloblastic anemia. These conditions do not occur after a simple ileal conduit but may develop in patients with previous small bowel resection or in whom large segments of ileum are used in the construction of urinary reservoirs.[27]

Filmer and Spencer[28] reviewed carcinogenesis in bowel segments used for urinary diversion. There has been only one case of an adenocarcinoma occurring in an ileal conduit. Several cases have been described in patients undergoing ileocystoplasty, suggesting that long contact time between urine and bowel mucosa may play a role in carcinogenesis.

Sigmoid Colon Conduit

Sigmoid colon conduit urinary diversion is used in those circumstances when nonrefluxing ureteroenterostomies are desirable. When total pelvic exenteration is required for locally advanced malignancies, a sigmoid colon conduit obviates the need for an enteroenterostomy.[29] Mogg[30] popularized the sigmoid colon conduit in the 1960s in an attempt to avoid the complications of reflux.

Preoperative preparation is similar to that described for ileal conduits. Again, the stoma site should be selected and marked preoperatively in the left lower quadrant by the ET therapist, who needs to take into account body habitus and scars.

The descending and sigmoid segments of the colon are mobilized from the splenic flexure to the sacral promontory. A segment of sigmoid colon approximately 20 cm long is selected and marked with stay sutures (Fig. 12-11). The mesentery is carefully divided at right angles to the ends of the conduit, with 4-0 silk sutures used for hemostasis. The distal mesenteric division should include the superior hemorrhoidal artery to aid in mobility. After removal of the attached fat and mesenteric attachments, the colon is divided and the conduit is placed to the left. The colon is reapproximated with either a two-layer hand-sewn technique or a stapling technique. The conduit

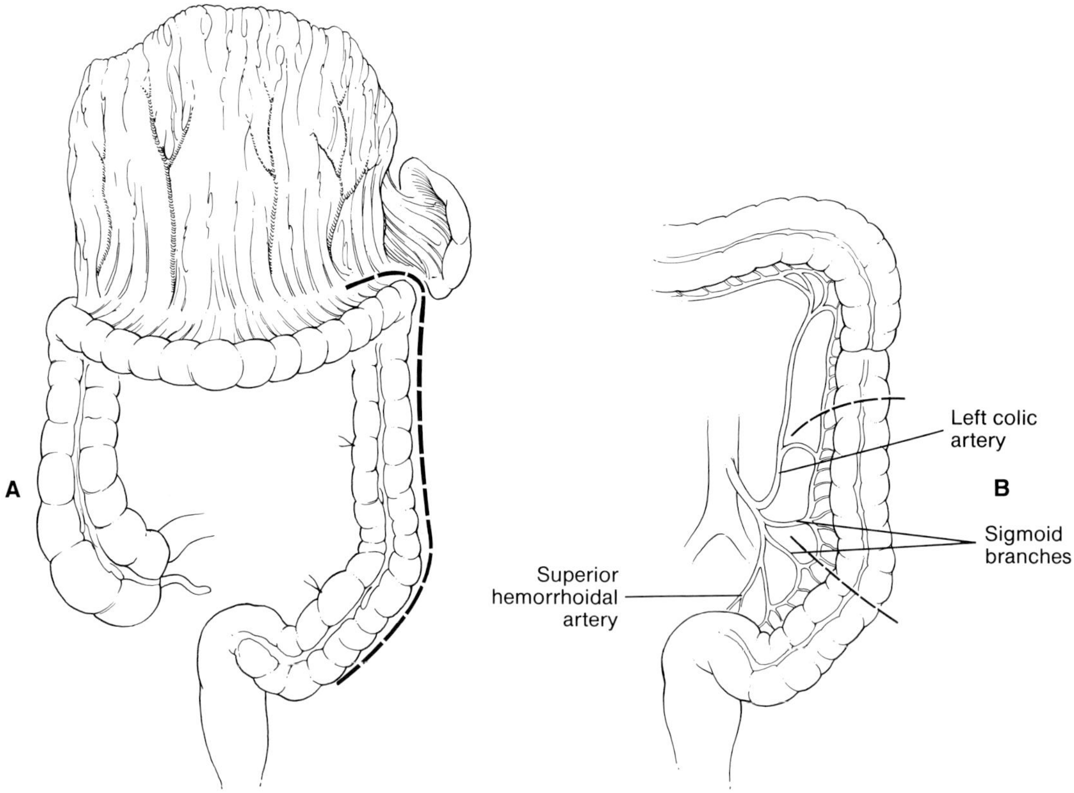

Fig. 12-11. Sigmoid colon conduit. **A,** Segment of sigmoid colon approximately 20 cm long is selected and marked with stay sutures. **B,** Although adequate blood supply should be ensured during creation of the sigmoid conduit, superior hemorrhoidal branch of inferior mesenteric artery may be divided to increase mobility of distal segment.

is irrigated to remove remaining intestinal contents, and the proximal end is closed in a watertight manner with absorbable sutures.

Construction of nonrefluxing ureterocolostomies is performed according to the method described by Leadbetter and Clarke.[31] The right ureter is delivered under the sigmoid colon beneath the parietal peritoneum. Two separate 5 cm incisions are made through the teniae, with care taken to avoid injury to the mucosa (Fig. 12-12, *A*). Submucosal instillation of saline solution or saline with epinephrine (1:100,000) solution may facilitate dissection. Traction sutures of 4-0 silk are placed to aid in retraction, and the mucosa is dissected from the muscular colon wall with fine scissors. The end of each ureter is spatulated and a mucosa-to-mucosa anastomosis is constructed with 5-0 chromic suture (Fig. 12-12, *B*). Stents are used at the surgeon's discretion. The colonic wall is reapproximated with interrupted 4-0 silk sutures, with care taken to avoid obstruction of the ureter at the proximal tunnel (Fig. 12-12, *C*). An additional stabilizing 4-0 chromic suture is placed through the sero-

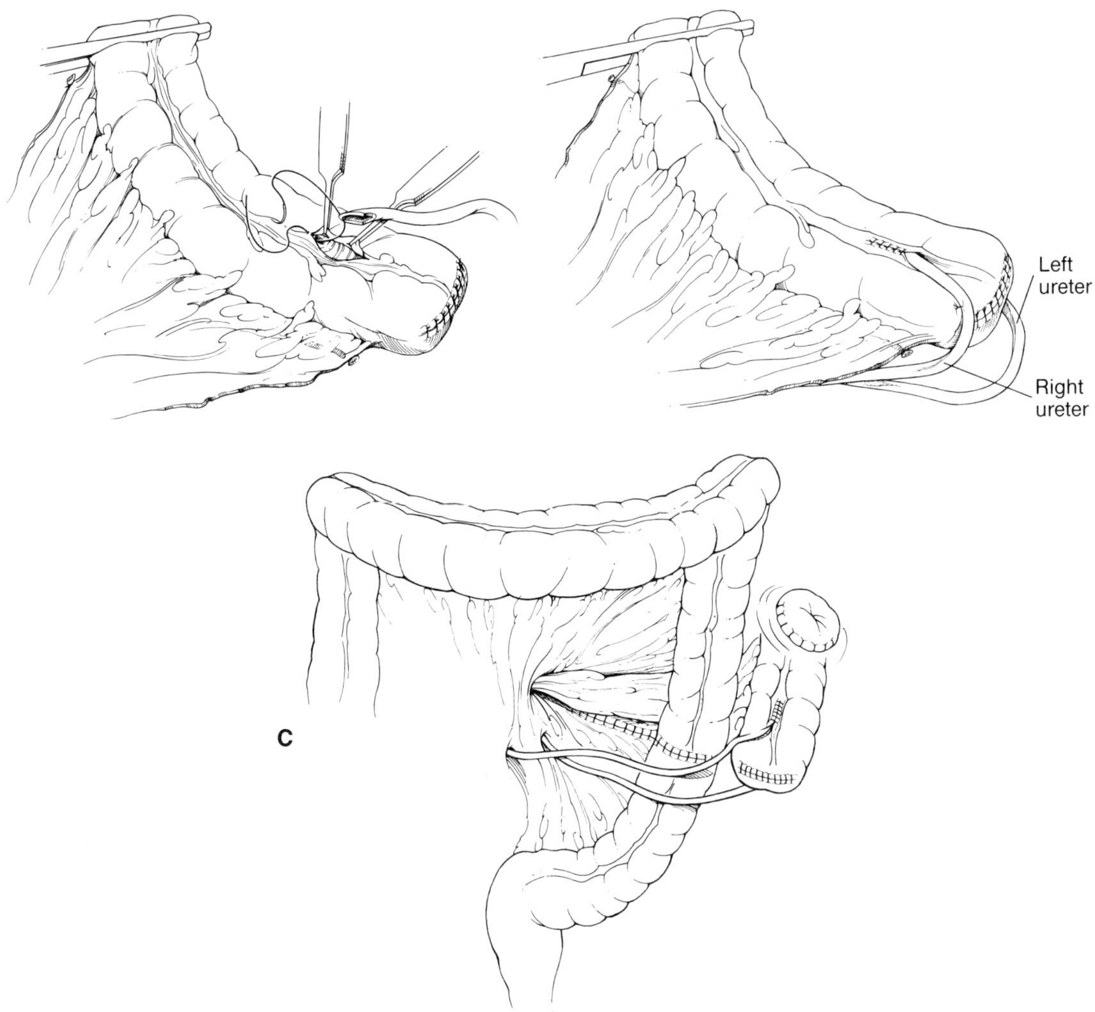

Fig. 12-12. Antirefluxing ureterocolostomies. A 5 cm submucosal tunnel is created for each ureter.

muscular layer of the ureter and the colon 2 to 3 cm proximal to the tunnel. The nipple stoma is created as described for ileal conduits, with the exception of excising a slightly larger circle of skin and subcutaneous tissue to accommodate the colonic segment.

Transverse Colon Conduit

The transverse colon conduit has been popularized by Schmidt.[32] It is used primarily in situations in which pelvic radiation has been given or markedly foreshortened ureters are present. The procedure essentially parallels that of the sigmoid colon conduit with the following exceptions.

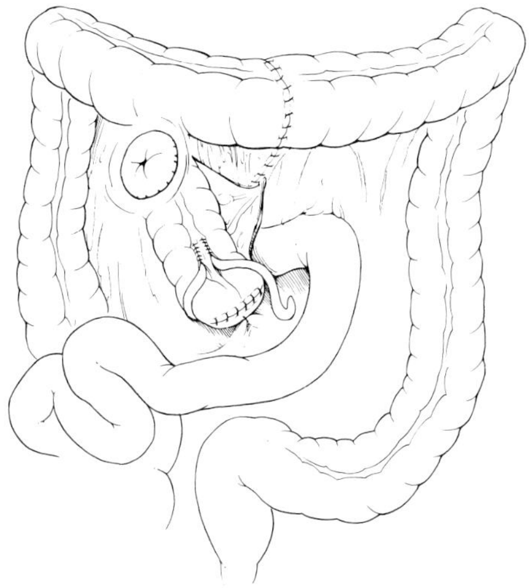

Fig. 12-13. Transverse colon conduit.

The stoma can be placed in any of the four quadrants, allowing more options if significant abdominal wall abnormalities are present. A 10 to 15 cm length of transverse colon is selected, and the greater omentum is dissected from its superior surface. The blood supply is based on the middle colic artery with extensive collateral circulation, making devascularization of the segment unlikely (Fig. 12-13). The conduit is placed below the colon, and colocolostomy is performed according to the surgeon's preference. Colon conduits need not be placed in isoperistaltic fashion because they empty by mass contraction. The end selected as the "nonstomal" end should be closed in a watertight fashion. The ureters are delivered through the posterior peritoneum with avoidance of angulation, and nonrefluxing ureterocolostomies are constructed as described previously. Formation of the nipple stoma is the same as discussed earlier.

Ileocecal Conduit

Gilchrist et al.[2] introduced the ileocecal segment as a urinary conduit in an early attempt at continent diversion. Zinman and Libertino[33] used this ileocecal segment to construct a nonrefluxing conduit. The stoma site is again selected in the right lower quadrant. The conduit is based on the ileocolic vessels, which can be visualized with transillumination of the mesentery (Fig. 12-14). After the right colon has been mobilized, the ileum is divided approximately 10 cm proximal to the ileocecal valve and the colon is divided just proximal to the right colic artery. Bowel continuity is restored according to the surgeon's preference, with the conduit placed to the right of the intact colon.

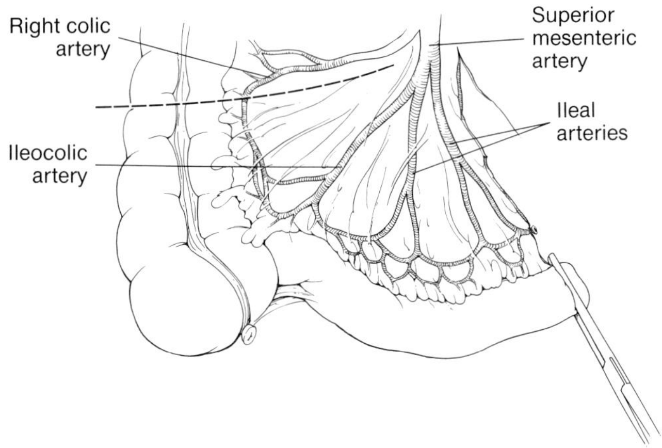

Fig. 12-14. Ileocecal segment showing ileocolic vessels.

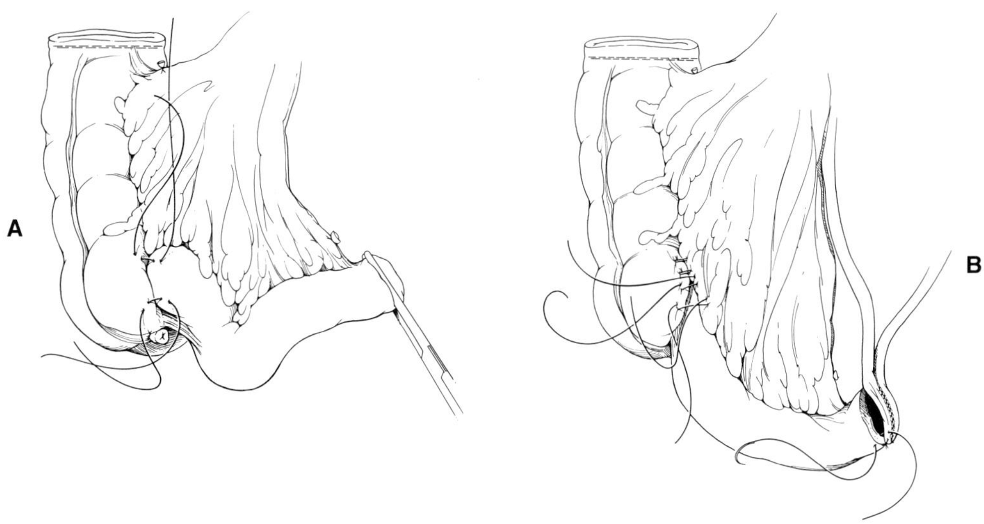

Fig. 12-15. Nonrefluxing ureteral anastomosis is dependent on reinforcement of the ileocecal valve.

The antirefluxing ureterocolostomies depend on reinforcement of the ileocecal valve as described by Zinman and Libertino[33] (Fig. 12-15, *A*). This reinforcement is accomplished by intussusception of the ileum into the cecum and by "wrapping" the redundant cecal wall around the ileum (Fig. 12-15, *B*). Conjoined ureteroileostomies are then constructed, and the standard stoma is made.

Complications and long-term results of colon conduits. The immediate postoperative complications do not differ significantly from those already discussed for the ileal conduit. The presence of nonrefluxing ureteral anastomosis has led to stable renal function in 80% to 90% of patients.[31-33] Nephrolithiasis tends to occur in those patients with failure of the antireflux mechanism or those who develop acidosis from urine absorption. Ureteroenteric anastomotic stricture occurs with a frequency similar to that of ileal conduits and is managed in the same fashion. The incidence of early anastomotic obstruction may be higher because of the tunneling techniques, leading many urologists to use stents in the early postoperative period. Problems such as peristomal hernias and prolapse are handled as described in Chapters 15 and 16, respectively.

Colonic mucosa is efficient at reabsorption of sodium and chloride, although it does so less than the ileum. As with ileal conduits, the presence of renal insufficiency or large amounts of residual urine may lead to hyperchloremic acidosis. A recent review of carcinogenesis in patients with intestinal conduits documented three cases with colon conduits.[28] It is unclear whether this carcinogenesis represents spontaneous colonic primary lesions or lesions induced by urine-borne carcinogens.

CONTINENT RESERVOIRS WITH ABDOMINAL WALL STOMAS

The past decade has seen an explosion in interest in avoiding external collecting devices. Several methods of continent urinary diversion have been described, and modifications are reported frequently. The basic requirements for a successful continent urinary diversion include (1) a large, low-pressure reservoir; (2) absence of reflux; and (3) continence. The basic methodologies are described below, although the reader is referred to the Suggested Readings for sources of detailed descriptions of all the various modifications.

Indiana Pouch

Gilchrist et al.[2] initially used the ileocecal segment in an attempt to provide continent diversion. Their dependence on the unreinforced ileocecal valve led to poor continence rates, and the procedure was not embraced by urologists. At the University of Indiana several modifications were introduced in the 1980s, and these developments led to what has become known as the "Indiana pouch."[34,35] The most important modifications include (1) plication of the ileal segment and ileocecal valve to provide continence and (2) detubularization of the bowel to avoid mass contraction and obtain greater reservoir capacities.

Patient selection is important. The patient must be highly motivated and cooperative in regard to postoperative care and lifelong intermittent catheterization. Some surgeons believe that the need for postoperative radiation therapy or chemotherapy obviates the use of continent diversion for pelvic malignancies, although others use the procedure uniformly.

After mobilization of the terminal ileum and the ascending colon (including the hepatic flexure), 25 to 30 cm of colon and 10 cm of terminal ileum are measured and marked. The mesentery is examined to ensure adequate blood supply, and the bowel is divided. An ileocolostomy is performed according to the surgeon's preference. The bowel is irrigated, and the colon is opened along its antimesenteric border (Fig. 12-16, *A*). The Indiana group now advises tapering the ileum and ileocecal valve before closure of the reservoir (Fig. 12-16, *B*). A 12 Fr catheter is placed, and the ileum is tapered with the use of a GIA stapler. The ileocecal junction and valve are tapered with 3-0 silk Lembert sutures. The 12 Fr catheter is removed, and easy passage of a 16 Fr catheter is ensured. Stented ureterocolostomies are constructed as described previously. To detubularize the reservoir and avoid mass contractions, the

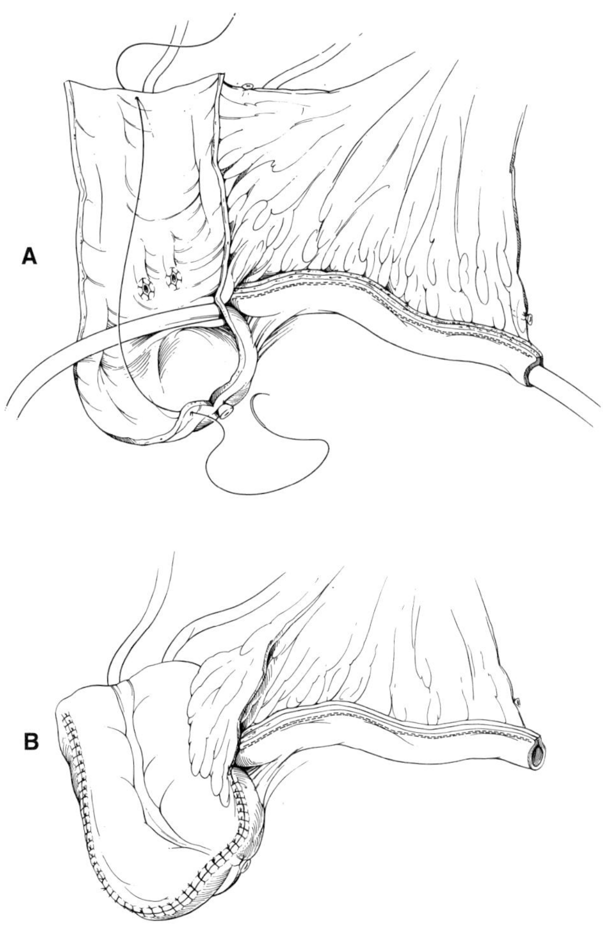

Fig. 12-16. Indiana pouch. **A,** Extended ileocecal segment is isolated, and colon is opened along its antimesenteric border. Nonrefluxing ureterocolostomies and tapering of ileal limb are performed before closure of colonic segment. **B,** Colon is closed in a Heineke-Mikulicz fashion. Flush stoma is constructed, and cecostomy tube is placed for postoperative drainage.

colon is closed with two layers of 3-0 Vicryl suture in a Heineke-Mikulicz fashion. A flush stoma is created in an appropriate location, a cecostomy tube is inserted and delivered through the abdominal wall, and the ureteral stents are brought out through a separate stab incision. Ease of catheterization is documented before closure. Drains are placed dependently.

Mucous secretion poses a problem postoperatively and requires irrigation via the cecostomy tube three or four times a day. After radiographs have confirmed the absence of extravasation and obstruction, the patient is discharged with instructions for home colostomy tube irrigation. Intermittent catheterization is taught 2 to 3 weeks after discharge and the cecostomy tube removed.

In their most recent review the Indiana group reported a 92% continence rate with 4- to 6-hour catheterizations.[35] Approximately 50% of patients require one nocturnal catheterization to remain dry. Approximately 5% of patients required reoperation for either reflux or ureterocolonic obstruction. Since using the stapling technique, only 1 of 35 patients required revision of the efferent limb. Hyperchloremic metabolic acidosis occurs and occasionally requires oral alkali therapy.

Mainz Pouch

Thuroff et al.[36] developed the Mainz pouch coincidentally with development of the Indiana pouch. It differs in the use of a longer segment of ileum (50 cm; Fig. 12-17) and a shorter segment of colon. Continence depends on the construction of a nipple valve as described for the Kock pouch. The reservoir is constructed after detubularization of the colon and ileum along the antimesenteric border. A 10 cm segment of proximal ileum is used to construct the nipple valve. Other aspects are similar to those described previously.

Mitrofanoff Principle

Mitrofanoff[37] first reported the use of the appendix for the construction of a continent stoma that could be catheterized. The appendix is mobilized with preservation of its mesentery, and it may be tunneled into the bladder or the cecal tinea similar to the construction of a nonrefluxing ureterocolostomy (Fig. 12-18). The distal end of the appendix is opened, and a flush stoma is created in a predetermined location. Other structures used to construct a similar stoma include fallopian tubes, ureters, umbilical vein, and ileum.[38]

Tube-Within-a-Tube Continent Stomas

Benchekroun[39] also has described a variation on the use of the ileocecal segment to construct a continent reservoir. Of particular interest is his

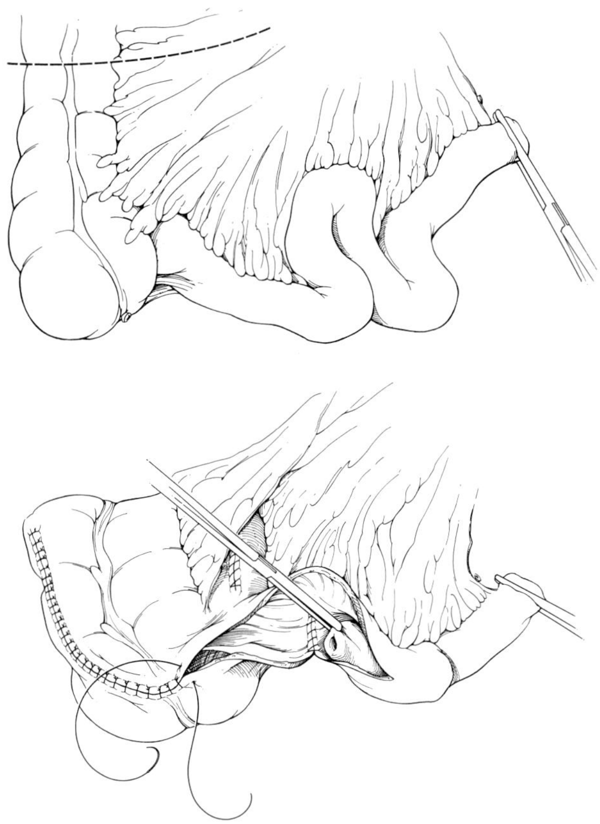

Fig. 12-17. Mainz pouch. A shorter colonic segment and a longer ileal segment as well as reliance on a nipple valve for continence differentiate the Mainz pouch from the Indiana pouch.

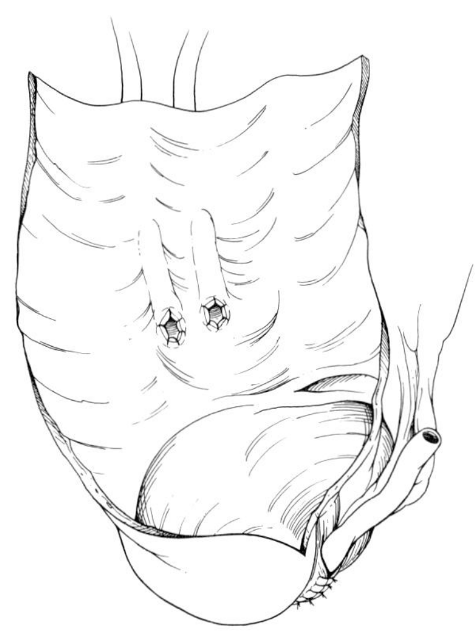

Fig. 12-18. Example of use of a catheterizable appendiceal stoma (Mitrofanoff principle) with a cecal reservoir.

method of constructing the continent stoma (Fig. 12-19). A separate 14 cm segment of ileum is isolated and invaginated. The anterior surfaces are secured with a continuous stitch of 3-0 Vicryl. When attached to the reservoir, the outer, mucosa-lined tube fills with urine, thereby compressing the inner, serosa-lined catheterizable tube and providing continence. Of 160 patients, 142 were continent (27 of them required reoperation to achieve continence).[40]

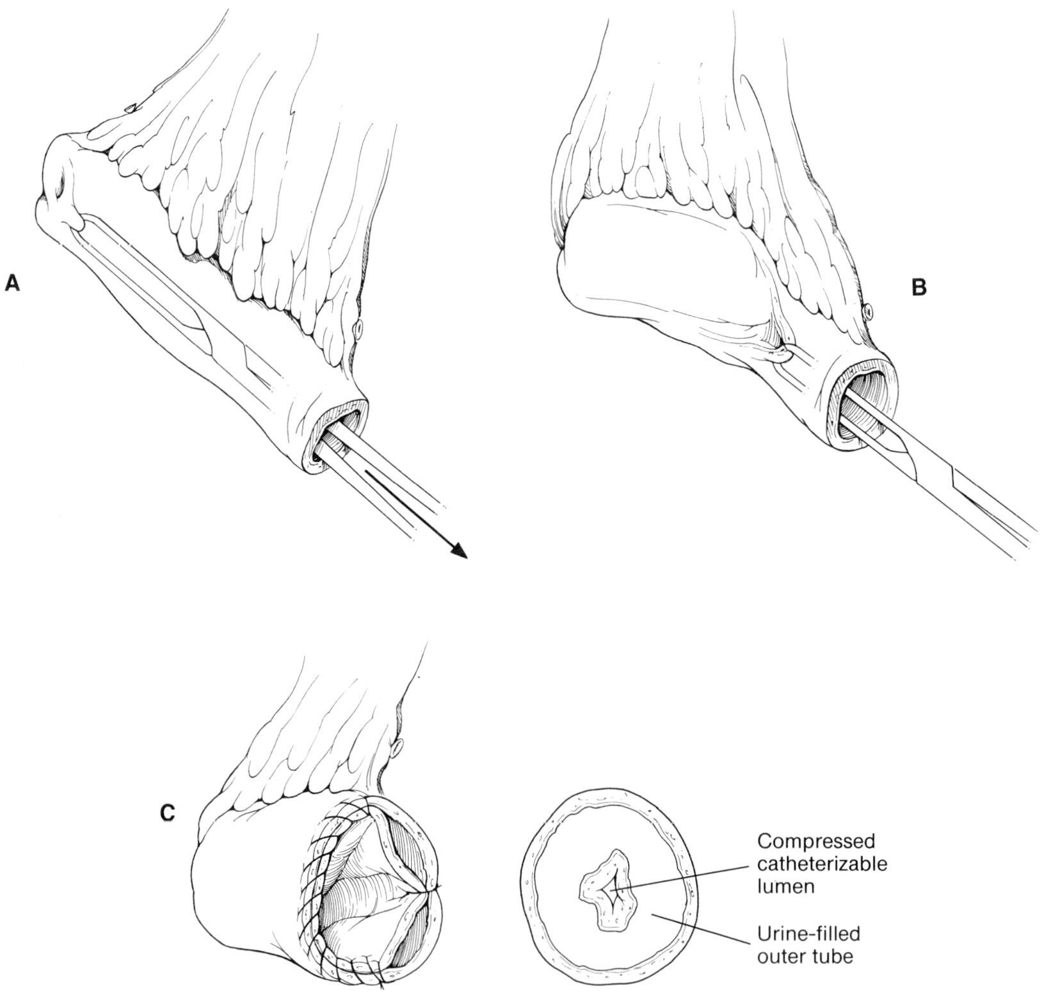

Fig. 12-19. Benchekroun's method of maintaining a continent stoma. **A-B,** Segment of ileum is inverted. **C,** Anterior walls of inverted ileum are approximated. Posterior opening is left to allow urine to enter from the reservoir, thus "squeezing" the inner chamber.

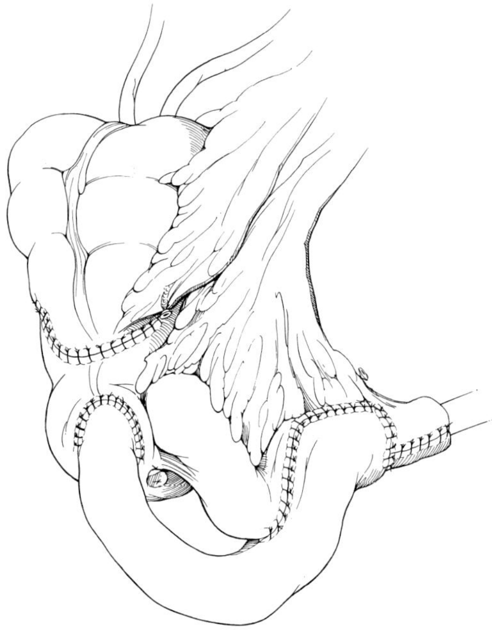

Fig. 12-20. Koff's continent stoma. This method utilizes a separate ileal segment attached to the reservoir and "wrapped" around the catheterizable terminal ileum.

Koff et al.[41] use an imbricated ileal segment similar to that used in the Indiana pouch. It is augmented by a second segment of ileum approximately 10 cm long used to construct a urine-filled external compression chamber (Fig. 12-20). The distal end of the ileal segment is spatulated and wrapped around the imbricated ileal segment. A watertight attachment is achieved with 3-0 Vicryl sutures. The proximal end is attached to the reservoir, allowing the "cuff" to fill with urine and compress the imbricated segment, resulting in continence. Fourteen of 15 patients were continent, with 3 patients requiring reoperation for stoma problems.[42]

Kock Pouch

The continent ileostomy developed by Nils Kock[43] is discussed in Chapter 10. This technique was modified for urinary diversion[44] and ushered in the era of continent urinary diversion. Skinner and associates,[45] at the University of Southern California, popularized the procedure in the United States. Their methods are summarized in the following discussion.

An ileal segment approximately 80 cm long is selected. The distal margin should be approximately 20 cm proximal to the ileocecal valve. The bowel and mesentery are divided, with close attention paid to maintaining the blood supply. An ileoileostomy is performed according to the surgeon's preference.

The ileal segment is marked into four segments: 17, 22, 22, and 17 cm. The two 22 cm segments are placed side by side and opened along their antimesenteric border (Fig. 12-21, *A*), and the back walls are closed with a continuous 3-0 Vicryl suture (Fig. 12-21, *B*).

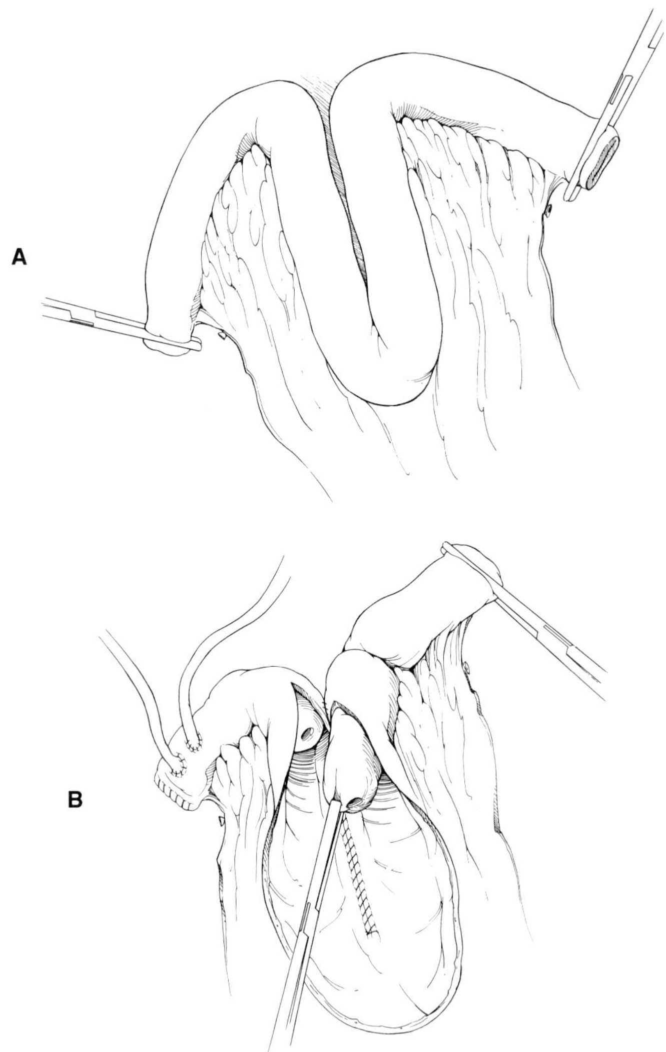

Fig. 12-21. Modification of Kock pouch for urinary diversion. Ureterocolostomies are constructed on afferent limb, and efferent limb is used as a catheterizable stoma. Most reoperations are performed to repair the efferent limb.

Construction of the nipple valves is the crux of the procedure because most reoperations are performed to repair them. The mesentery is separated from the bowel closest to the reservoir for approximately 8 cm, and the bowel is intussuscepted. Boyd et al.[45] currently place a 2 cm strip of Vicryl mesh through a mesenteric window 2 to 3 cm away from the previously made mesenteric opening. They also have begun using a GIA stapler to support the valve by placing two rows of 3.5 mm staples. The distal six staples are removed to prevent stone formation. The back wall of the valve is secured further to the reservoir with a TA-55 stapler, and the tips of the valves are secured to the inside of the reservoir with 3-0 Vicryl suture. In a further attempt to prevent loss of intussusception, the Vicryl mesh is secured to the ileal limb and reservoir.

The pouch is closed in a watertight manner to provide a detubularized pouch. End-to-side ureteroileostomies are constructed on the afferent limb with the aid of stents. A flush stoma is constructed from the efferent limb in a convenient location previously selected by an ET therapist. An additional 1 cm strip of Marlex mesh is used to secure further the mesenteric side of the efferent limb to the posterior rectus fascia. A 30 Fr catheter is left in the efferent limb to provide reservoir drainage, and a drain is placed.

As noted previously, frequent irrigation is necessary to avoid development of a mucous plug. Instruction for self-catheterization is given at approximately 3 weeks.

The most recent data from the University of Southern California state that 11% of patients require revision of the efferent limb to maintain continence.[45] Reflux or ureteroenteric strictures have occurred only 2% to 3% of the time. Vitamin B_{12} levels should be closely monitored.

SIMULTANEOUS DIVERSION OF URINARY AND FECAL STREAM

The standard wet colostomy as described by Brunschwig and Daniel[46] has been generally abandoned because of development of severe electrolyte imbalance, pyelonephritis, and stoma complications. My colleagues and I recently have begun performing a new procedure, the "double-barreled" wet colostomy,[29] which seems to have avoided the majority of these complications. Fortunately, patients needing this procedure are rare and usually have advanced pelvic malignancies or severe radiation damage to the pelvic viscera.

If no colostomy exists, the sigmoid colon is mobilized, and an appropriate portion of the proximal sigmoid is selected as the stoma site (Fig. 12-22). We create the stoma first. A plug of skin and subcutaneous tissue is removed from

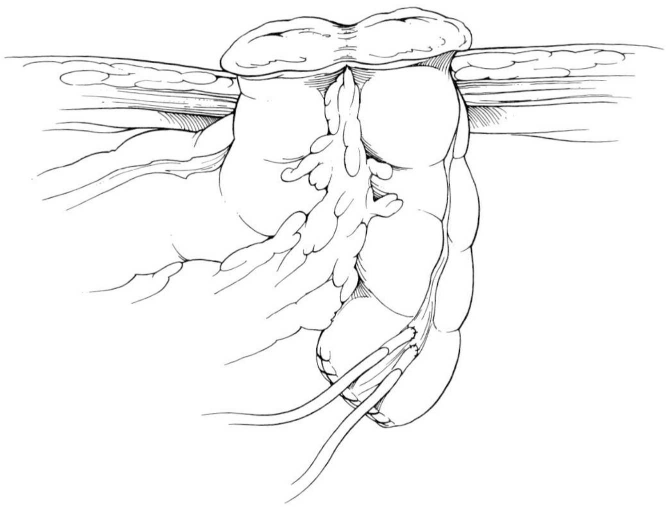

Fig. 12-22. Double-barreled wet colostomy.

the left middle abdomen and the rectus fascia is opened in a cruciate fashion as described previously. The muscle fibers are separated, and a loop of sigmoid colon is delivered. The colon is secured to the anterior fascia to avoid retraction. The colon is opened, and the mucosa is secured to the skin with 3-0 Vicryl suture. The colon is divided with a GIA stapler approximately 15 to 20 cm distal to the stoma, thus forming a "urine limb." The staples are removed from the urine limb, and the colon is closed in watertight fashion with 3-0 Vicryl suture. If severe ureteral dilatation is not present, nonrefluxing ureteroenterostomies are performed; otherwise an end-to-side technique is used.

If a loop colostomy already exists, the urine limb is constructed and ureterocolostomy is performed (see Fig. 12-22). If an end sigmoid colostomy is present, it is taken down and the colon and the splenic flexure are mobilized. The procedure then proceeds as described previously.

Eight of the 10 patients operated on had advanced pelvic malignancies and succumbed to their disease within 2½ years. The two patients with severe radiation damage to pelvic viscera are doing well after approximately 3 years. Upper tract function and/or radiographic appearance remained stable or improved in 9 of 10 patients, with the remaining patient developing malignant ureteral obstruction. There were no episodes of pyelonephritis, but metabolic acidosis occurred in two patients with renal insufficiency. Overall patient acceptance has been excellent.

SUMMARY

Improvements in methods of urinary diversion continue to the benefit of patients requiring these procedures. The ileal conduit remains the gold standard in adult patients, but many alternatives exist. Continent urinary diversion and bladder substitutions continue to grow in popularity and have become the procedures of choice in many clinical situations.

REFERENCES

1. Bricker EM. Bladder substitution after pelvic evisceration. Surg Clin North Am 30: 1511, 1950.
2. Gilchrist RK, Merricks JW, Hamlin HH, et al. Construction of a substitute bladder and urethra. Surg Gynecol Obstet 90:752, 1950.
3. Turnbull RB Jr, Hewitt CR. Loop-end myotomy ileostomy in the obese patient. Urol Clin North Am 5:423, 1958.
4. Wallace DM. Ureteric diversion using a conduit: A simplified technique. Br J Urol 38:527, 1966.
5. Regan JB, Barrett DM. Stented versus non-stented ureteroileal anastomoses: Is there a difference with regard to leaks and stricture? J Urol 134:1101, 1985.
6. Lilfen OM, Camey M. 25 year experience with replacement of the human bladder (Camey procedure). J Urol 132:886, 1984.
7. Brooke BN. Management of ileostomy including its complications. Lancet 2:102, 1951.
8. Clark SS. Electrolyte disturbance associated with jejunal conduit. J Urol 112:42, 1974.
9. Golimbo M, Morales P. Jejunal conduits: Technique and complications. J Urol 113: 787, 1987.
10. Cass AS, Luxenberg M, Gleich P, et al. A 22 year follow-up of ileal conduits in children with a neurogenic bladder. J Urol 132:529, 1984.
11. Dunn M, Roberts JRM, Smith PJB, et al. The long-term results of ileal conduit urinary diversion in children. Br J Urol 51:458, 1979.
12. Arnarson O, Straffon RA. Clinical experience with ileal conduit in children. J Urol 102:768, 1969.
13. Heath AL, Eckstein HB. Ileal conduit urinary diversion in children: A long-term follow-up. J Urol (Paris) 90:91, 1984.
14. Jaffe BM, Bricker EM, Butcher HR. Surgical complications of ileal segment urinary diversion. Ann Surg 167:367, 1968.
15. Middleton AW, Hendrew WH. Ileal conduit in children at the Massachusetts General Hospital from 1955-1970. J Urol 115:591, 1976.
16. Pitts WR, Muecke EC. A 20-year experience with ileal conduits: The fate of the kidneys. J Urol 122:154, 1979.
17. Remigailo RV, Lewis EL, Woodard JR, Walton KN. Ileal conduit urinary diversion: Ten-year review. Urology 7:343, 1976.
18. Schmidt JD, Hawtry CE, Flocks RH, Culp DA. Complications, results, and problems of ureteroileals. J Urol 109:210, 1973.

19. Shapiro SR, Lebowitz R, Cozodny AH. Fate of 90 children with ileal conduit urinary diversion a decade later: Analysis of complications, pyelography, renal function and bacteriology. J Urol 114:289, 1975.
20. Sullivan JW, Gbabstald H, Whitmore WF. Complications of ureteroileal conduit with radical cystectomy: Review of 336 cases. J Urol 124:797, 1980.
21. Hampel N, Bodner D, Persky Z. Ileal and jejunal conduit urinary diversion. Urol Clin North Am 13:2, 207, 1986.
22. Richie JP, Skinner DG, Waisman J. The effect of reflux on the development of pyelonephritis in urinary diversion: An experimental study. J Surg Res 16:256, 1974.
23. Dretler SA. The pathogenesis of urinary tract calculi occurring after ileal conduit urinary diversion. I. Clinical study. II. Conduit study. III. Prevention. J Urol 109:204, 1973.
24. Kramolowsky EV, Clayman RV. Advances in endosurgery: Treatment of ureteral-enteric anastomotic strictures. Urol Clin North Am 15:3, 413, 1988.
25. Mitchell ME, Yoder IC, Pfister RC, et al. Ileal loop stenosis: A late complication of urinary diversion. J Urol 118:957, 1977.
26. Castro JE, Ram MD. Electrolyte imbalance following ileal urinary diversion. Br J Urol 42:29, 1970.
27. Steiner MS, Morton RA. Nutritional and gastrointestinal complications of the use of bowel segments in the lower urinary tract. Urol Clin North Am 18:4, 743, 1991.
28. Filmer RB, Spencer JR. Malignancies in bladder augmentations and intestinal conduits. J Urol 143:671, 1990.
29. Carter MF, Dalton DP, Garnett JE. Simultaneous diversion of the urinary and fecal streams utilizing a single abdominal stoma. The double barrelled wet colostomy. J Urol 141:1189, 1988.
30. Mogg RA. The treatment of urinary incontinence using the colonic conduit. J Urol 97:684, 1967.
31. Leadbetter WF, Clarke BG. Five years experience with ureteroenterostomy by the "combined" technique. J Urol 73:67, 1954.
32. Schmidt JD, Buchsbaum HJ. Transverse colon conduit diversion. Urol Clin North Am 13:2, 233, 1986.
33. Zinman L, Libertino JA. The ileocecal conduit for temporary and permanent urinary diversion. J Urol 113:317, 1975.
34. Rowland RG, Mitchell ME, Bihrle R, et al. Indiana continent urinary reservoir. J Urol 137:1136, 1987.
35. Bihrle R, Foster RS. Continent ileocecal reservoirs: The Indiana pouch. In King LR, Stone AR, Webster GD. Bladder Reconstruction and Continent Urinary Diversion. St. Louis: Mosby–Year Book, 1991, p 308.
36. Thuroff JW, Alken P, Hohenfeller R. The Mainz pouch (mixed augmentation with ileum and zecum) for bladder augmentation and continent diversion. In King LR, Stone AR, Webster GD. Bladder Reconstruction and Continent Urinary Diversion. Chicago: Year Book Medical, 1987, p 252.
37. Mitrofanoff P. Cystostomie continence transappendiculaire dans le traitement des vessies neurologiques. Chir Pediatr 21:297, 1980.
38. Woodhouse CRS. The Mitrofanoff technique for a continent stoma. In King LR, Stone AR, Webster GD. Bladder Reconstruction and Continent Urinary Diversion. St. Louis: Mosby–Year Book, 1991, p 299.
39. Benchekroun A. Continent caecal bladder. Eur Urol 3:248, 1988.

40. Benchekroun A. The ileocecal continent bladder. In King LR, Stone AR, Webster GD. Bladder Reconstruction and Continent Urinary Diversion. St. Louis: Mosby–Year Book, 1991, p 324.
41. Koff SA, Circulli C, Lucero SP, et al. An operation to create a continent catheterizable urinary sphincter from a short intestinal segment. J Urol 138:996, 1987.
42. Koff SA, Wise H. Continent diversion using an ileal segment servomechanism. In King LR, Stone AR, Webster GD. Bladder Reconstruction and Continent Urinary Diversion. St. Louis: Mosby–Year Book, 1991, p 337.
43. Kock, NG. Intra-abdominal "reservoir" in patients with permanent ileostomy: Preliminary observations on a procedure resulting in fecal "continence" in five ileostomy patients. Arch Surg 99:223, 1969.
44. Kock NF, Nilsson AE, Nilsson LO, et al. Urinary diversion via a continent ileal reservoir: Clinical result in 12 patients. J Urol 128:469, 1982.
45. Boyd SD, Skinner DG, Lieskovsky G. Kock pouch: Update of USC technique and results. In King LR, Stone AR, Webster GD. Bladder Reconstruction and Continent Urinary Diversion. St. Louis: Mosby–Year Book, 1991, p 308.
46. Brunschwig A, Daniel W. Pelvic exenteration operations. Ann Surg 151:571, 1960.

SUGGESTED READINGS

Bricker EM. Bladder substitution after pelvic evisceration. Surg Clin North Am 30:1511, 1950.

Of great historical interest, Dr. Bricker's initial description of the ileal conduit differs little from the procedure performed more than 40 years later.

Hampel N, Bodner DR, Persky L. Ileal and jejunal conduit urinary diversion. Urol Clin North Am 13:2, 207, 1986.

An excellent review of the literature pertaining to operative complications and long-term results of ileal conduit urinary diversion.

King LR, Stone AR, Webster GD. Bladder Reconstruction and Continent Urinary Diversion. St. Louis: Mosby–Year Book, 1991.

This well-written, well-illustrated text contains contributions from the pioneers in continent urinary diversion and represents a single resource for understanding all the major procedures.

13 LAPAROSCOPIC-ASSISTED COLOSTOMY

Martin A. Luchtefeld and John M. MacKeigan

Although laparoscopy has been used safely and effectively for decades for diagnostic purposes and minor gynecologic procedures, only in the last several years have laparoscopic techniques gained a much broader application in the fields of general and colorectal surgery. Since the first reports of laparoscopic cholecystectomy in 1987, there has been an overwhelming shift from "open" cholecystectomy to this new technique.[1,2] With the success of this operation, laparoscopic techniques have been applied to an ever-widening field, including colon and rectal surgery.[3,4]

INDICATIONS AND CONTRAINDICATIONS

The indications and contraindications for laparoscopic-aided colostomy or ileostomy are similar to those for open surgery. At this embryonic stage in laparoscopic bowel surgery, not all patients should be considered candidates for an attempt at a laparoscopic approach. Colonic obstruction, peritonitis, and multiple adhesions are all relative contraindications to laparoscopic surgery, but this determination is highly dependent on the level of skill and experience (and patience!) of the surgeon. Pregnancy should be considered a contraindication also at this time, not because laparoscopic surgery is technically impossible with a pregnant patient, but because the full maternal and fetal effects are unknown. As laparoscopic skills and technology evolve and improve, the contraindications are likely to decrease so that they will differ only minimally from those for open surgery.

OPERATIVE TECHNIQUE

The technique for creating a stoma with laparoscopic assistance is not standardized, but certain general principles do apply. Preoperatively the patient should receive stoma instructions and should be marked for a stoma site to ensure optimal placement. The bowel preparation (both antibiotics and mechanical cleansing) should be done as usual. Once adequate anesthesia and a sterile field have been established, the placement of trocars can be done. A port usually is placed in the periumbilical position for the camera. Depending on the surgeon's preference, this first port can be inserted with either an open (Hasson) technique or in a closed fashion after adequate insufflation with a Veress needle. Once the camera has been inserted and there is sufficient pneumoperitoneum, the surgeon can determine where additional ports can be safely inserted. This determination may require some adhesiolysis; in fact, at this point the decision can be made to convert to an open procedure if the adhesions seem to pose great difficulty. Trocar placement is done under the direct vision of the camera and is highly individualized for each surgical team. In general, at least two or three additional ports, sometimes more, are needed. Usually ports are needed on both sides of the abdomen. It is advantageous if one port site can be at the previously marked stoma location so that ultimately there is one less entry into the peritoneal cavity. The authors' preferred location and size of trocars are illustrated in Fig. 13-1, *A*.

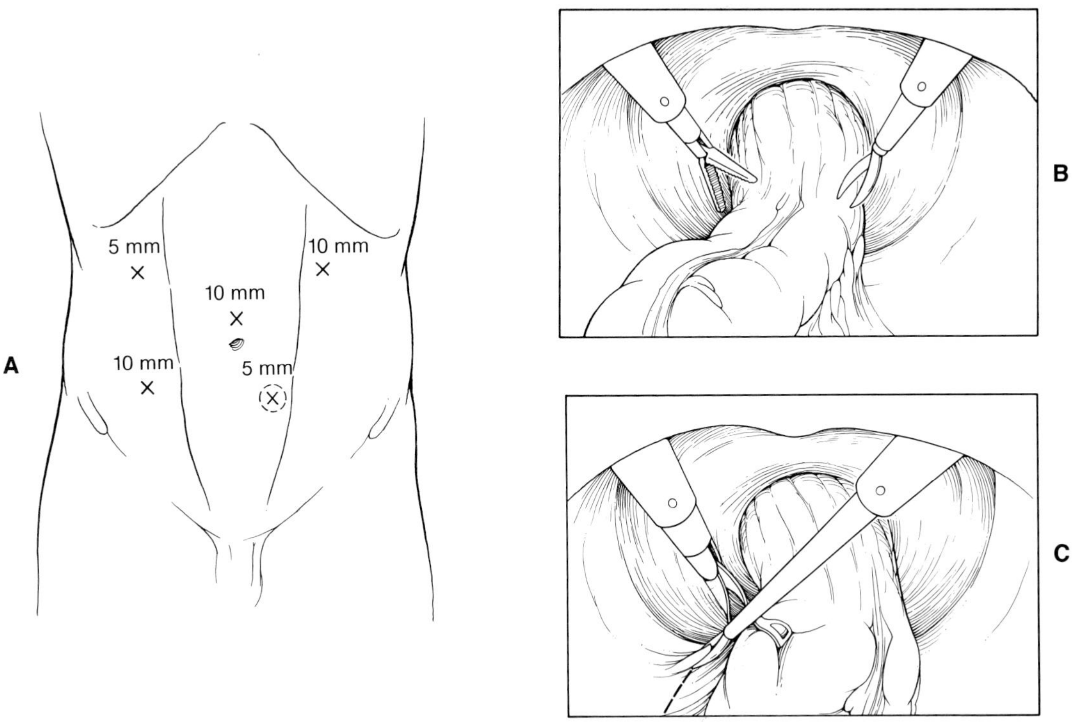

Fig. 13-1. A, Most colonic laparoscopic surgery requires three to five ports. Placing port and location of anticipated stoma (i.e., left lower quadrant) as shown here is advantageous. **B,** Distal sigmoid colon and rectum are grasped with forceps prior to dissection. **C,** Sigmoid colon is grasped with Babcock forceps, and lateral peritoneal reflection is incised.

Once the above maneuvers have been completed, the actual intra-abdominal portion of the procedure can take place. Fig. 13-1, *B-C,* outlines the few basic steps necessary for formation of a loop sigmoid colostomy, but any kind of stoma can be created with laparoscopic assistance. The sigmoid colon is mobilized by incising the lateral peritoneal attachments. This dissection can be carried out as high as necessary, even to include taking down the splenic flexure. Illuminated ureteral catheters can be inserted preoperatively to aid in identification of the ureters if a difficult dissection is anticipated. The adequacy of mobilization can be checked by grasping the proposed loop of bowel and lifting it toward the colostomy site. Once this adequacy has been ensured, the skin is excised in a circular fashion at the stoma site, the fascia is incised, and the loop of bowel is delivered upward through the abdominal wall. This maneuver is facilitated by having a port at the planned stoma site. The mobilized bowel can be grasped with an atraumatic laparoscopic instrument passed through the stoma site port and pulled up flush with the abdominal wall. It is then a simple matter to cut down around the port site and pull the loop of colon onto the skin. The colostomy can be matured in the fashion preferred by the surgeon. The same basic steps and principles apply to formation of a loop ileostomy in a laparoscopic-assisted fashion.

Recently laparoscopic-assisted colon resections have allowed mobilization and resection of colon segments by using the principles of laparoscopy with traditional surgery. Transection of the colon with linear stapling devices, along with transection of portions of mesentery in the same fashion, allows creation of an end colostomy with a closed distal limb. In situations in which the stoma probably will be in place a long time, an end stoma with closure of the rectal stump or even creation of a stoma with mucous fistula can be facilitated laparoscopically.

Colostomy Closure

Loop colostomy or ileostomy closure usually can be performed without a laparotomy (i.e., through a peristomal incision), making laparoscopic assistance unnecessary. However, the situation is different after a Hartmann procedure (sigmoid resection, creation of an end sigmoid colostomy, and closure of the rectal stump). "Hartmann takedown," or reestablishment of intestinal continuity after a Hartmann procedure, traditionally has involved a laparotomy, but it can now be performed laparoscopically (Fig. 13-2).

These laparoscopic procedures usually are difficult because the pathologic condition that led to the colostomy initially (most commonly a complication of diverticular disease or an obstructing cancer) also has resulted in formidable adhesions. Port placement should be individualized; however, commonly the camera is placed periumbilically, and additional ports are

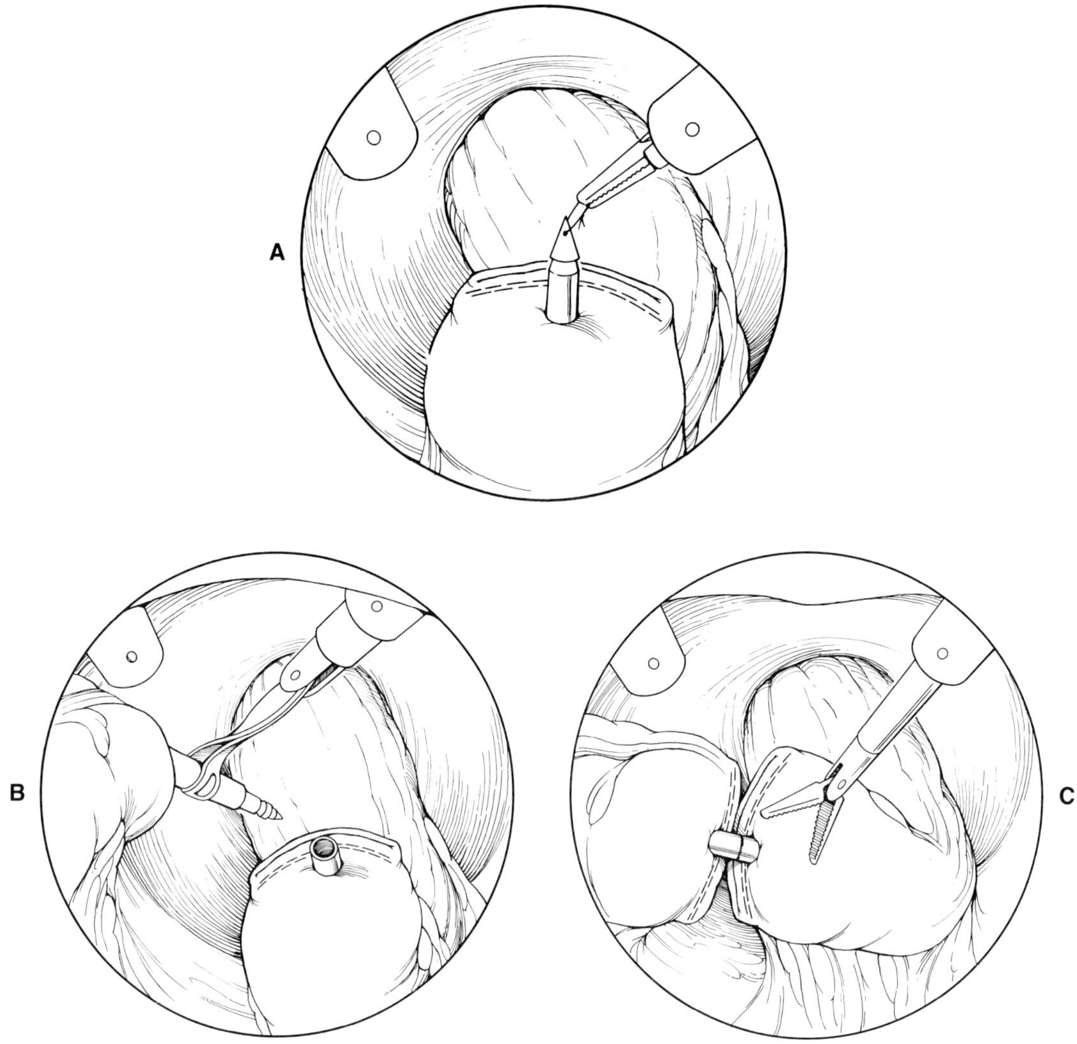

Fig. 13-2. **A,** Rectal stump has been stapled. Spike of an end-to-end stapling device protrudes through rectal stump. Spike is grasped and removed by forceps. **B,** Proximal colon has been joined to rectal stump with anvil. **C,** Triple staple technique allows anastomosis of proximal colon to rectal stump prior to approximation.

placed in the right lower and left lower quadrants. In addition, a suprapubic port may be required.

Adhesions are taken down (often a difficult and time-consuming task), and the rectal stump is identified and cleared of surrounding structures. This procedure may be facilitated by transanal passage of the EEA instrument (United States Surgical Corp., Norwalk, Conn.) or the ILS instrument (Ethicon Endo-Surgery, Cincinnati, Ohio). The colostomy is then freed from the skin and subcutaneous tissues by standard techniques. The EEA or ILS anvil is placed into the proximal colon and the pursestring suture is applied. The proximal bowel is placed into the abdomen and directed toward the pelvis.

The colostomy incision is closed in multiple layers, or, alternatively, it can be closed around a port. Pneumoperitoneum is reestablished, and the spike is brought through the apex of the rectal stump. The spike is removed (EEA), and the ends are mated. The anastomosis is completed in standard fashion, and anastomotic rings are checked. The anastomotic integrity can be checked as in an open procedure. The pelvis is filled with saline solution, the proximal bowel is occluded with an endogauge or bowel clamp, and air is instilled through a sigmoidoscope transanally. Leaks will appear as air bubbles around the anastomosis. Small defects can be repaired with laparoscopic suture techniques; however, major anastomotic defects will require open laparotomy.

POSTOPERATIVE CARE

Laparoscopic colon surgery is new enough that dogmatic statements cannot be made about analgesic needs, length of ileus, or postoperative hospital stay. Early reports indicate that there probably is a beneficial effect in all these areas.[5,6] However, there is justifiable concern that the increased instrumentation and operating room costs may outstrip any savings realized by a shorter hospitalization.

COMPLICATIONS

All the usual complications associated with colostomy formation and closure can be expected when laparoscopic techniques are used. Although the rate of complications with this new approach is not yet known, it is clear from the laparoscopic cholecystectomy data that there is a definite learning curve that results in an increased number of adverse outcomes in the initial series of procedures.[7] Complications more likely to occur or unique to a laparoscopic approach include unrecognized bowel injury, bowel or vascular injury secondary to trocar placement, hypercarbia, and carbon dioxide air embolism.[8-10]

SUMMARY

Laparoscopic-assisted procedures will have a role in colon and rectal surgery in the future, but how extensive that role will be remains unclear. Although this method could be confined to a small niche, it more likely will be the seed for continued evolution of increasingly sophisticated, minimally invasive surgery.

REFERENCES

1. Filipi CJ, Fitzgibbons RJ Jr, Salerno GM. Historical review: Diagnostic laparoscopy to laparoscopic cholecystectomy and beyond. In Zucker KA, ed. Surgical Laparoscopy. St. Louis: Quality Medical Publishing, 1991, p 14.
2. Baird DR, Wilson JP, Mason EM, et al. An early review of 800 laparoscopic cholecystectomies at a university-affiliated community teaching hospital. Am Surg 58:206-210, 1992.
3. Redwine DB, Sharpe DR. Laparoscopic segmental resection of the sigmoid colon for endometriosis. J Laparoendosc Surg 1:217-220, 1991.
4. Lange V, Meyer G, Schardey HM, et al. Laparoscopic creation of a loop colostomy. J Laparoendosc Surg 1:307-311, 1991.
5. Jacobs M, Verdeja JC, Goldstein HS. Minimally invasive colon resection (laparoscopic colectomy). Surg Laparosc Endosc 1:144-150, 1991.
6. Fowler DL, White SA. Laparoscopy-assisted sigmoid resection. Surg Laparosc Endosc 1:183-188, 1991.
7. Southern Surgeons Club. A prospective analysis of 1,518 laparoscopic cholecystectomies performed by Southern U.S. surgeons. N Engl J Med 324:1073-1078, 1991.
8. Kent RB. Subcutaneous emphysema and hypercarbia following laparoscopic cholecystectomy. Arch Surg 126:1154-1156, 1991.
9. DePlater RHM, Jones ISC. Non-fatal carbon dioxide embolism during laparoscopy. Anaesth Intensive Care 17:359-361, 1989.
10. Henning H. The Dallas report on laparoscopic complications. Gastrointest Endosc 31:104-105, 1985.

BIBLIOGRAPHY

Ballantyne G. Laparoscopic Colon and Rectal Surgery. Philadelphia: WB Saunders, 1992.
This text deals exclusively with the laparoscopic approach to multiple colon and rectal procedures.

PART THREE

SPECIAL PROBLEMS

14 ILEOSTOMY AND POUCH DYSFUNCTION

Amanda M. Metcalf

After proctocolectomy patients can expect to have a normal life expectancy. However, loss of the colon's normal absorptive function makes such patients particularly susceptible to salt and water loss. Diarrhea, a disease of a trivial nature in patients with a normal colon, can be life threatening in patients with an ileostomy or ileal pouch. *Diarrhea* in the patient with either a conventional or continent stoma can be defined as a fecal volume of more than 1 L per day. The same definition can be applied to those patients with an ileal pouch–anal procedure, although in such patients frequent evacuation can be an additional complaint or the primary complaint. Ileostomy diarrhea is most often caused by conditions unique to the postoperative state, and they are the focus of the subsequent discussion. However, it must be remembered that diarrhea can be secondary to the same diseases that affect the intact gut.

CONVENTIONAL ILEOSTOMY

Ileal Resection

Resection of even small lengths of terminal ileum can have significant long-term effects on the volume of effluent from a conventional stoma. In addition to a chronically elevated effluent volume, patients have a higher-than-normal output of sodium and potassium. They also may have higher-than-normal fecal concentrations of nitrogen and fat.[1] This phenomenon may be a result of more rapid transit of intestinal content, loss of the portion of the small bowel that is most responsive to mineralocorticoids, or steatorrhea.

Patients who have undergone proctocolectomy are chronically dehydrated and have elevated mineralocorticoid levels. The terminal ileum appears to respond to mineralocorticoids by increasing absorption of sodium and water and excreting potassium.[2] This response of the terminal ileum is believed to account for the adaptive response to colectomy, and this gradual decrease in stomal output in the first few weeks after proctocolectomy is not seen in patients who have undergone an ileal resection. Steatorrhea after resection is probably secondary to the impairment of bile salt absorption from loss of the terminal ileum, with secondary depletion of the bile salt pool. Whatever the precise mechanism, patients who have had an ileal resection will demonstrate high effluent volumes in the early postoperative period that do not decrease over time.

Partial Small Bowel Obstruction

Approximately 10% of patients who undergo proctocolectomy will develop a small bowel obstruction. The risk of this complication is greatest in the first 3 years after surgery and decreases thereafter.[3] Symptoms of bowel obstruction include a significant change in ostomy output, cramping, bloating, nausea, and vomiting. The most common cause is the presence of adhesions. The exact mechanism by which partial obstruction of the small bowel produces increased effluent is not well understood. It has been demonstrated that with complete obstruction, fluid and electrolyte absorption is impaired and fluid secretion is increased proximal to the obstruction.[4] If this phenomenon were present in a partial obstruction, it would explain the increased volume of ileal effluent. Bacterial overgrowth has been demonstrated in patients with partial bowel obstruction, although its role in fluid and electrolyte abnormalities is uncertain.

Recurrent Regional Enteritis

Even a pathologically confirmed diagnosis of ulcerative colitis does not preclude the possibility of regional enteritis (Crohn's disease) as a cause of ileostomy diarrhea. This situation is especially true in patients with ileal pouches of any type. A number of such patients with "pouchitis" postoperatively are ultimately diagnosed months or even years later as having Crohn's disease. Recurrence rates after colectomy for Crohn's disease vary, but longitudinal studies suggest ever increasing rates with time.[5] High-volume output in these patients may be caused by either mucosal disease, with resultant malabsorption of fluid, electrolytes, and nutrients, or partial intestinal obstruction with its attendant pathophysiology.

Peritonitis or Abscess

In the early postoperative period intra-abdominal infection, whether diffuse or localized, can result in increased ileal effluent.[6] The mechanism by which this increase occurs may be analogous to that of partial obstruction in which the bowel adjacent to the area of inflammation has abnormal motility and therefore acts as a functional obstruction.

Gastric Hypersecretion

Gastric hypersecretion is rarely seen after proctocolectomy alone. It occurs more commonly when proctocolectomy is combined with extensive small bowel resection. Acid hypersecretion results in low jejunal pH, impaired micellar solubilization of fat, steatorrhea, and diarrhea.[7]

CONTINENT STOMA OR ILEAL POUCH

Pouchitis or Bacterial Overgrowth Syndrome

Patients with either a continent stoma of the Kock type or with a pelvic ileal reservoir are prone to develop a type of ileostomy dysfunction that is not seen in patients with conventional ileostomies. This syndrome, called either pouchitis or bacterial overgrowth syndrome, may occur in up to 50% of patients who undergo these procedures.[8,9] Clinically it is manifest by increased fecal output, discomfort in the region of the pouch, and bloody effluent. Sometimes it is accompanied by fevers, arthralgias, anorexia, weight loss, and even uveitis. Patients with a continent stoma may have difficulty intubating the pouch, whereas patients with a pelvic pouch can have deterioration in their anorectal function, with urgency and frequency. The precise cause of this syndrome is not known, but most theories center on the phenomenon of bacterial overgrowth in the proximal bowel. Jejunal aspirates in symptomatic patients have revealed increased numbers of anaerobic bacteria compared to the numbers in asymptomatic pouch patients.[10] Small bowel bacterial overgrowth is known to cause both deconjugation of bile salts and vitamin B_{12} malabsorption.[11]

Unconjugated bile salts impair sugar, water, sodium, and potassium transport in the small intestine.[12] Anaerobic bacteria are also capable of binding the vitamin B_{12}–intrinsic factor complex, making it unavailable for absorption.[13] Thus the findings and the response to treatment seem to support the theory of proximal jejunal anaerobic bacterial overgrowth as the causative factor in bacterial overgrowth syndrome. This anaerobic overgrowth is presumably secondary to the prolongation of small bowel transit that has been documented in patients with ileal pouches.[14] Of concern, however, is that some patients initially thought to have pouchitis eventually have been diagnosed with Crohn's disease. Since metronidazole does have some activity against small-bowel Crohn's disease, its efficacy in the treatment of this syndrome may be secondary to this effect. Longer follow-up of patients with pouchitis may provide the answer to this question.

Outlet Obstruction

Patients with a pelvic ileal pouch may develop frequent stools and incontinence secondary to poor emptying of the pelvic pouch. Apparently this result most commonly is related to a mechanical outlet obstruction. In patients with a J-type pouch this most commonly results from a pouch-anal anastomotic stricture.[15] Occasionally incomplete division of the limbs of a J pouch at the apex of the pouch results in a septum that can obstruct defecation. In patients with an S-type reservoir it is usually secondary to elongation of the efferent limb, with kinking of the outflow tract.[16]

CONSEQUENCES OF ILEOSTOMY DIARRHEA

Since even patients with a well-functioning ileostomy have chronic mild dehydration, it is not surprising that severe dehydration can develop very rapidly in the patient with dysfunction. Both total body water and exchangeable sodium will be reduced; thus serum levels of sodium likely will be normal. A secondary potassium deficiency can develop because of renal losses of potassium in an attempt to conserve sodium. Occasionally magnesium and calcium deficiencies are evident in patients with long-standing high ileostomy output. Vitamin B_{12} deficiency is a well-known sequela to ileal resection, and abnormal vitamin B_{12} absorption has been documented in patients with pouchitis. Patients with chronic ileostomy diarrhea are also more likely to develop uric acid or calcium oxalate kidney stones and cholelithiasis.

CLINICAL EVALUATION

History

Knowing the details of the original diagnosis, the type of procedure performed, and the postoperative complications helps in narrowing the differential diagnosis. Symptoms present since surgery suggest ileal resection, chronic obstruction, or a preexisting condition such as lactose intolerance that has been unmasked by colectomy. The volume of stool effluent can be estimated by the number of times patients empty their ostomy device or pouch. The character of stool and the presence or absence of blood can provide clues. The patient's state of hydration can be assessed by inquiring about the frequency and volume of urination and recent weight loss. Associated gastrointestinal symptoms such as cramping, bloating, and difficult evacuation or intubation should be ascertained, as should extraintestinal symptoms of stomatitis, arthritis, or uveitis. Such symptoms are suggestive of partial small bowel obstruction, bacterial overgrowth syndrome, or recurrent Crohn's disease. Any recent or current use of medication, similar diarrhea symptoms in family members or acquaintances, and a history of travel also are pertinent.

Physical Examination

A complete physical examination should be performed, with particular emphasis given to the state of hydration, the abdomen, the appearance of the stoma, the peristomal skin, and the perineum. If the patient has had a pelvic ileal pouch procedure, examination of the perianal skin and a digital examination should be performed. Endoscopic examination through a stoma, if present, or the anus can allow assessment of the small bowel mucosa.

Laboratory Studies

The history and physical examination will dictate the studies that should be obtained. A complete blood count and serum electrolyte, creatinine, and blood urea nitrogen determinations are appropriate in most patients. Quantification of gastric acid secretion and serum gastrin levels may be indicated. Fecal studies for *Campylobacter, Clostridium difficile* toxin, enteric pathogens, and ova and parasites may be appropriate. Quantification of 24-hour fecal volumes, electrolytes, and fat is appropriate in most chronic cases. Contrast examinations of the small bowel and endoscopy are useful to exclude obstruction or recurrent regional enteritis. Anorectal manometry and defecating proctograms may be indicated for patients with pelvic ileal pouches with normal stool volumes and increased defecatory frequency.

MEDICAL MANAGEMENT

Patients in whom a surgically correctable cause for diarrhea has been found should undergo appropriate surgical intervention. In patients with recurrent Crohn's disease initial treatment with immunosuppressive agents active against Crohn's disease should be tried. Patients in whom pouchitis apparently is implicated should receive metronidazole or another broad-spectrum antibiotic such as tetracycline, clindamycin, or ampicillin. A 2-week trial of antibiotics should be tried, and then the antibiotic should be discontinued. Occasionally such patients need long-term low-dose antibiotic therapy to control symptoms. The long-term follow-up and management of such patients should take into account the ever-present possibility of Crohn's disease.

In patients who have high ileostomy output after ileal resection in whom other treatable conditions have been excluded, it is important to quantitate the amount of steatorrhea on a known (70 to 100 g) fat diet. Patients with steatorrhea with an output of more than 15 g of fat per day should be treated with a diet containing 50 to 70 g of fat per day; in more severe cases further reduction to low-fat diets of 40 g per day may be tried, with dietary supplementation with medium-chain triglycerides. Patients also should receive an agent such as loperamide or codeine. If minimal response occurs, opium can be tried. A course of histamine-receptor–blocker therapy might also be tried, especially in patients with steatorrhea.

For the difficult patient scattered case reports note improvements in salt and electrolyte balance with treatment with an orally administered glucose polymer solution (Polycose; Ross Laboratories, Columbus, Ohio). The active absorption of the glucose polymer in this solution in the proximal jejunum is believed to result in an increase in the passive absorption of salt and water.[17] There also have been scattered case reports of good responses to a long-acting somatostatin analog. Investigation has revealed that the effect of somatostatin in such patients is to decrease water secretion and prolong small bowel transit time. Gastric emptying and glucose and nitrogen excretion were not altered in the patients studied, although fat excretion was increased.[18] In addition, there has been a single case report of a case of ileostomy diarrhea in a patient with intestinal pseudo-obstruction that appeared to respond to oral indomethacin, presumably through an antiprostaglandin effect.[19] In patients with truly uncorrectable ileostomy diarrhea and with problems limited primarily to fluid and electrolyte balance, fluid therapy through a permanent indwelling intravenous catheter may be necessary. If a patient with long-term high ileostomy output develops urolithiasis, alkalinization of urine should be considered. Patients who develop symptomatic cholelithiasis would be most appropriately treated with cholecystectomy.

SUMMARY

Most patients with ileostomy dysfunction have an underlying cause that is relatively easy to diagnose and treat. In most instances the cause is related to the underlying disease or the type of surgical procedure that was performed, and the condition can be successfully managed.

REFERENCES

1. Neal OE, William NS, Barker MCJ, et al. The effect of resection of the distal ileum on gastric emptying, small bowel transit and absorption after proctocolectomy. Br J Surg 71:666-670, 1984.
2. Kramer P, Levitan R. Effect of 9-fluorohydrocortisone on the ileal excreta of ileostomized subjects. Gastroenterology 62:235-241, 1972.
3. Watts J, deDombal FT, Goligher JC. Long-term complications and prognosis following major surgery for ulcerative colitis. Br J Surg 53:1014-1023, 1966.
4. Shields R. The effect of experimental obstruction on the intestinal absorption of water, sodium, and potassium. In Smith AN. Surgical Physiology of the Gastrointestinal Tract. Edinburgh: The Royal College of Surgeons of Edinburgh, 1963, p 166.
5. Ritchie JK, Lockhart-Mummery HE. Nonrestorative surgery in the treatment of Crohn's disease of the large bowel. Gut 14:263-270, 1973.
6. Smiddy FG, Gregory SD, Smith IB, et al. Faecal loss of fluid, electrolytes and nitrogen in colitis before and after ileostomy. Lancet 1:14-19, 1960.
7. Cortot A, Fleming RC, Malagelada JR. Improved nutrient absorption after cimetidine in short bowel syndrome with gastric hypersecretion. N Engl J Med 300:79-80, 1979.
8. Kock NG, Darle N, Halten L, et al. Ileostomy. Curr Probl Surg 14:6-52, 1977.
9. Fonkalsrud EW. Endorectal ileo-anal anastomosis with isoperistaltic ileal reservoir after colectomy and mucosal proctectomy. Ann Surg 199:151-157, 1984.
10. Kelly DG, Phillips SF, Kelly KA, et al. Dysfunction of the continent ileostomy: Clinical features and bacteriology. Gut 24:193-201, 1983.
11. Tabaqchali S, Hatz J, Booth CC. Bile salt deconjugation and steatorrhea in patients with stagnant loop syndrome. Lancet 2:12-16, 1968.
12. Gracey M, Burke V, Oshin A. Reversible inhibition of intestinal sugar transport by deconjugated bile salt in vitro. Biochim Biophys Acta 225:308-314, 1971.
13. Gianella RA, Broitman SA, Zamchec N. Vitamin B_{12} uptake in intestinal microorganisms: Mechanisms and relevance to syndrome of bacterial overgrowth. J Clin Invest 50:1100-1107, 1971.
14. Soper NJ, Orkin BA, Kelly KA, et al. Gastrointestinal transit after proctocolectomy with ileal pouch–anal anastomosis or ileostomy. J Surg Res 46:300-305, 1989.
15. Metcalf AM, Dozois RR, Beart RW, et al. Ileal J pouch–anal anastomosis: Clinical outcome. Ann Surg 202:735-739, 1985.
16. Lindquist K, Liljeqvist L, Sellberg B. The topography of ileoanal reservoirs in relation to evacuation patterns and clinical functions. Acta Chir Scand 150:573-579, 1984.
17. Saunders DR, Saunders MD, Sillery JK. Beneficial effects of glucose polymer and an H_2-receptor blocker in a patient with a proximal ileostomy. Am J Gastroenterol 84: 192-194, 1989.
18. Cooper JC, Williams NS, King RF, et al. Effect of a long-acting somatostatin analogue in patients with severe ileostomy diarrhea. Br J Surg 73:128-131, 1986.
19. Keshavarzian A, Isaacs P, McColl I, et al. Idiopathic intestinal pseudoobstruction and contaminated small bowel syndrome—Treatment with metronidazole, ileostomy and indomethacin. Am J Gastroenterol 78:562-565, 1983.

BIBLIOGRAPHY

Gorbach SL. Infectious diarrhea. In Sleiserge MH, Fortran JS. Gastrointestinal Disease. Philadelphia: WB Saunders, 1983, p 925.

Complete description of infectious causes of diarrhea.

Sherman P. Bacterial overgrowth. In Yamda T. Textbook of Gastroenterology. Philadelphia: JB Lippincott, 1991, p 1530.

Concise chapter covering the basic pathophysiology and treatment of bacterial overgrowth.

15 PARASTOMAL HERNIAS

Marc S. Rubin and H. Randolph Bailey

Parastomal hernia, an incisional hernia at the site of an intestinal stoma, has been a recognized complication of stoma surgery for a long time. According to Goligher,[1] "Some degree of herniation around a colostomy is so common that this complication may be regarded as inevitable." Although hernias associated with ileostomy and urostomy are less frequent, they are still common. The potential complications of parastomal hernia can be mild and easily managed or serious and potentially life-threatening. The patient may present with a cosmetic problem, with difficulty managing the stoma (particularly with irrigation), or with any of the usual complications of a hernia. Repair is complex, although infrequently necessary. The poor results with standard local repair have caused surgeons to favor relocation of the stoma or techniques using prosthetic material. Even with these methods, results are often less than ideal. As is almost always the case, the best solution to the problem is prevention. Good preoperative planning and careful attention to technical detail can minimize parastomal herniation.

INCIDENCE AND PREDISPOSING FACTORS

Identifying the incidence of parastomal hernia is difficult. Various authors have reported the frequency as 0% to 100%.[1-14] Table 15-1 lists the incidence in the published series to date. Clearly the rate varies with the type and age of the stoma and with the technique and circumstances of the operation. Patient characteristics and postoperative events also affect the likelihood of hernia development.

Table 15-2 lists identified or suggested predisposing factors for parastomal hernia formation. Despite the long list of things that might make an individual with an ostomy prone to hernia development, only a handful of factors have been studied and found truly instrumental in increasing the risk. Although many factors, such as obesity, steroid use, advanced age, and obstructive pulmonary disease, are likely to play a part in hernia formation, the

Table 15-1. Published series of incidence of parastomal hernia

Author	Year	Stoma Type	Number	Years of Follow-up*	Incidence in >30-day Survivors	Required Operation	Comment†
Birnbaum & Ferrier[15]	1952	End colostomy	569	1-34	27/569 (5%)	—	b,d
Grier et al.[16]	1964	End colostomy	50	5.2	29/50 (58%)	—	c,e,f
Green[17]	1966	Loop colostomy	160	2-7	8/318 (3%)	—	b,d,q
		End colostomy	158				
Watts et al.[18]	1966	End ileostomy for chronic ulcerative colitis (CUC)	151	3.4	3/119 (3%)	0/3	b
Roy et al.[19]	1970	End ileostomy	497	7.4	3/469 (1%)	—	b,g
Burns[20]	1970	Loop colostomy	99	0-21	1/99 (1%)	6/16	b
		End colostomy	219		15/219 (7%)		
Harbach et al.[21]	1971	Urostomy	244	3-15	12/214 (6%)	—	b
Schmidt et al.[22]	1973	Urostomy	178	3-11	8/172 (5%)	6/8	b,h
Saha et al.[23]	1973	Loop colostomy	190	1-7	2/200 (1%)	—	b,d
		End colostomy	10				
Balslev[24]	1973	End colostomy for cancer	546	14.5	62/110 (56%)	9/62	c,e
Kronborg et al.[25]	1974	End colostomy	362	1-10	42/362 (12%)	4/42	b,d
Harshaw et al.[26]	1974	End colostomy for cancer	99	1-8	9/99 (9%)	—	b,d
Marshall et al.[27]	1975	Urostomy	400	2-10	18/400 (5%)	—	b,d,g
Prian et al.[28]	1975	All colostomies	262	0-20	8/262 (3%)	—	b,d,g
Marks & Ritchie[29]	1975	End colostomy for cancer	227	0-6	23/224 (10%)	—	b,i
Raza et al.[30]	1977	End umbilical colostomy	101	2.5	0/101 (0%)	—	b
Abrams et al.[31]	1979	Loop transverse colostomy	202	9-18	4/189 (2%)	—	b
		End sigmoid colostomy	46				
Wara et al.[32]	1981	Loop transverse colostomy	257	0-10	10/212 (5%)	—	b,j

Stothert et al.[33]	1982	Ileostomy	10	0-5	2/42 (5%)	—	b,p
		Transverse colostomy	23				
		Sigmoid colostomy	18				
Eldrup et al.[34]	1982	Transrectus colostomy	77	2.8	1/77 (1%)	—	b,e
		Lateral colostomy	63		12/63 (19%)	—	
Burgess et al.[35]	1984	End colostomy for cancer	124	0-10	6/121 (5%)	1/6	b
Devlin[10]	1988	Ileostomy	102	—	5/102 (5%)	—	s
Phillips et al.[36]	1985	Colostomy	328	1-4	11/243 (5%)	—	b,e,k,l
		Ileostomy	232		8/175 (4%)	—	
Pearl et al.[37]	1985	All stomas	610	—	5/610 (1%)	—	b,d,m
Winkler[3]	1986	All stomas	164	—	42/164 (30%)	—	c,g,n,o
Sjodahl et al.[14]	1988	End colostomy	79	7	7/79 (9%)	4/9	h,e,r
		End ileostomy	45		1/45 (2%)	—	
Phillips et al.[38]	1989	End ileostomy for CUC	70	6	3/70 (4%)	—	b,g
Williams et al.[39]	1990	End ileostomy for inflammatory bowel disease	60	6.5	13/46 (28%)	9/13	c,e
Fleshman & Lewis[40]	1991	Ileostomy	6024	—	4%	50%	a
		Colostomy	7083		11%	—	
		Urostomy	2613		8%	—	

*Single numbers indicate mean follow-up; hyphenated numbers indicate range.

†a Questionnaire
b Chart review
c All patients examined
d Fails to exclude early deaths
e Survivors only
f Nonrandom group of patients selected by fact that they did not irrigate colostomy
g Only considers hernias that required repair
h Five hernias occurred within 1 week of operation
i 32% of patients followed >5 yr had hernias
j 105 were closed during study period
k 141 colostomies were closed during study period
l In group of 100 patients referred for stoma problems, 11 had hernias
m Study of early postoperative complications occurring during the admission at which stoma was created
n Rate in outpatient group was 45%
o Nonrandom group of patients presenting for stoma problem
p Both hernias in proximal colon group
q 86 patients had stoma closed during study period
r Does not identify which hernias required repair
s Method of study unknown

Table 15-2. Factors predisposing to parastomal hernia

Factors	Supporting Studies	Refuting Studies
Patient characteristics		
Obesity	27	—
Advanced age	—	14, 27
Debility/malnutrition	—	—
Malignancy	—	14
Obstructive pulmonary disease	—	—
Urinary outflow disease	—	—
Steroid use	—	—
Factors at operation		
Colonic stoma	14, 33, 40	36
Large trephine size	—	—
Stoma placed in laparotomy incision	1, 17	—
Stoma placed lateral to rectus muscle	14, 15, 16, 34	29, 39
Extraperitoneal technique	—	26, 29
Prior denervation/devascularization of site	—	—
Laparotomy or other incision nearby	—	—
Urgent/emergent operation	32, 33	—
Intestinal distention/edema	—	—
Postoperative factors		
Parastomal infection	—	—
Other abdominal complications	27, 29	—
Postoperative distention/ascites	—	—
Radiation therapy	27	—
Weight gain	—	39
Development of prolapse	—	—
Early or excessive physical exertion	—	—
Long-term survival	14, 25, 29, 39	—

Note: Numbers shown for studies refer to reference list.

evidence is largely anecdotal.[41] One frequent observation is that a permanent colostomy develops a hernia (0% to 58%) more commonly than a permanent ileostomy (0% to 28%) or urostomy (5% to 8%). Only speculation exists about the cause of this difference. Goligher et al.[2] have cited the relatively advanced age and associated muscle weakness in the colostomate, whereas Winkler[3] has noted the tendency of solid stool to enlarge the orifice over time. It is likely that the larger trephine size required to deliver the colon plays a role in the development of a paracolostomy hernia.

Loop stomas apparently are less prone to hernia formation than end stomas. The risk of hernia formation apparently increases with time (36% to

48% of hernias appear within 1 year and 36% to 100% within 2).[25,28,29,42] Since many loop stomas are temporary and are closed in less than 1 year (before a hernia can develop), the true incidence of hernia may be much higher.

Improperly located stomas have a higher incidence of hernia. Goligher[1] and Green[17] discuss at length the many early and late complications associated with bringing a stoma through the laparotomy incision. Goligher[1] notes that "the grosser forms [of paracolostomy hernia] are found in cases where the colon has been brought out in the line of the main incision." Several authors have noted that stomas placed through the rectus muscle have significantly lower incidence of parastomal hernia than those placed lateral to the rectus muscle. Birnbaum and Ferrier,[15] in the largest series in the literature, noted that the incidence was four times greater in lateral colostomies. Grier et al.[16] examined 50 patients, with a mean time of 5.4 years after colostomy, and found hernias associated with only 1 of 10 (10%) transrectus stomas but with 28 of 40 (70%) lateral ones. Eldrup et al.[34] found hernias in 1% and 19% of transrectus and lateral colostomies, respectively, and Sjodahl et al.[14] noted rates of 3% and 26%. Two other series in which this subject was investigated, however, failed to show a significant difference.[29,39]

Goligher,[1] Devlin,[10] and Todd[12] do not believe that creating an extraperitoneal stoma lessens the incidence of parastomal hernia. The literature contradicts this impression. In a series by Harshaw et al.[26] none of 17 extraperitoneal colostomies developed hernias whereas 9 of 82 (11%) transperitoneal ones did. In a series of colostomies by Marks and Ritchie,[29] the figures were 1 of 37 (3%) and 22 of 190 (12%), respectively.

Urgent or emergency surgery has been hypothesized as a risk factor for hernia. This hypothesis is very difficult to study because mortality is high in this group and survivors often have their stoma closed or revised. Wara et al.,[32] nonetheless, found in children a statistically significant increase in herniation and prolapse with urgently created stomas. Stothert et al.[33] also noted a higher rate of hernia in stomas created at emergency surgery. This rate may be related to larger stoma apertures initially created to accommodate the obstructed colon.

Although many technical factors that predispose a patient to parastomal herniation have been documented, patient characteristics and postoperative factors have been less well studied. Many experts cite obesity, advanced age, debility, malignant disease, pulmonary disease, and steroid use as certain culprits; however, only one study[27] has found obesity to be more common in patients with hernia, and none of the other factors has even been examined. Since these factors also are associated with a decrease in life expectancy, their influence on incidence of hernia may be diminished statistically since nonsurvivors are included in most calculations. Similarly, in many series evaluating the incidence of parastomal hernia, the only factors shown to be significantly predisposing are the occurrence of a postoperative abdominal complication (especially wound infection and urinary retention) and the use of postoperative radiation therapy.[27,29] Several authors cite anecdotal experience that parastomal infection and abdominal distention or ascites are commonly followed by hernia formation.

The many reported series of parastomal hernias suffer largely from being retrospective chart-review or questionnaire-type evaluations. Duration and degree of follow-up are variable, different stoma types are grouped together, and often only large, symptomatic, or operated hernias are noted. Only Grier et al.[16] and Balslev[24] performed physical examination on end colostomy patients, with mean follow-up exceeding 5 years. They found parastomal hernias in 58% and 56% of their patients, respectively. Williams et al.[39] did the same for end ileostomy patients. Twenty-eight percent were found to have hernias. These series most accurately assess the magnitude of the problem.

TYPES OF HERNIA

Four distinct types of hernia or pseudohernia can develop near a stoma. The most common is the "true parastomal" hernia (Fig. 15-1), which has a peritoneal sac that emanates from an enlarged fascial opening. The sac may be found in a subcutaneous or interstitial position. A second type of hernia, designated "intrastomal" (Fig. 15-2), occurs when an intraperitoneal structure insinuates into the space between the serosal surfaces of a spout ileostomy or

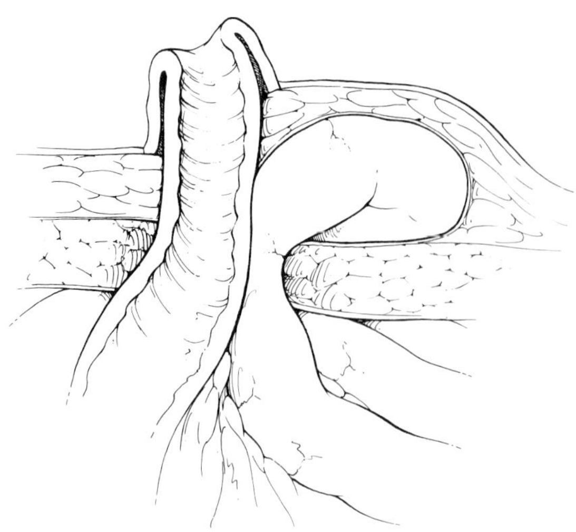

Fig. 15-1. True parastomal hernia.

the extension of the peritoneal cavity created whenever stoma prolapse occurs. The fascial defect is enlarged, if only slightly, but the sac may be composed only of the visceral peritoneum of the prestomal bowel. Both variants have been described but are rare.[10,11] The third and fourth hernia types are actually pseudohernias, but they are included here because they may cause symptoms similar to those of hernia, may be mistaken for hernia, and may require treatment similar to that for hernia. Fig. 15-3 depicts "subcutaneous prolapse." As with frank prolapse, redundancy and other factors may lead to

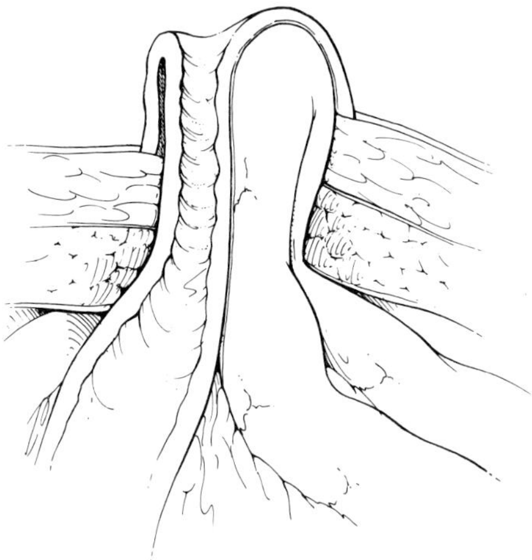

Fig. 15-2. Intrastomal hernia (may be associated with prolapse).

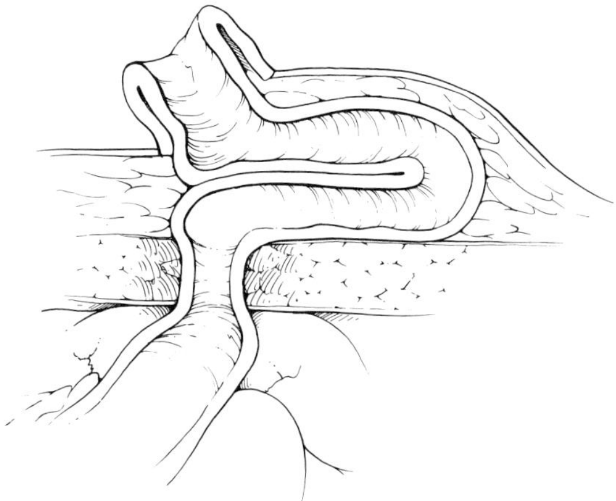

Fig. 15-3. Subcutaneous prolapse (pseudohernia) with intact fascial ring.

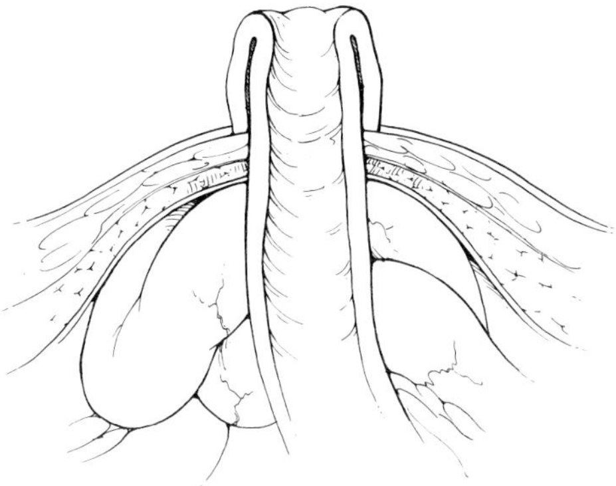

Fig. 15-4. Pseudohernia due to weakness of abdominal wall without fascial defect.

advancement of the prestomal intestine from the peritoneal cavity proper. The result is a subcutaneous redundant loop that creates a bulge when distended. Identification of this variant is important because there may be little or no fascial defect and local revision may suffice (if symptoms warrant repair). The final type (Fig. 15-4) is the classic "pseudohernia." Seen less and less frequently because it is peculiar to laterally placed stomas, the pseudohernia is a diffuse bulge without enlarged fascial defect or herniated structure in the subcutaneous space that develops over time because of the relatively weak or denervated muscles lateral to the rectus muscle.

More than 90% of the parastomal hernias seen today are of the true parastomal variety. The fascial defect is often relatively small, although it can be large, especially when the stoma trephine is close to the fascial closure of another incision. Small bowel and omentum commonly occupy the hernia sac, but virtually any intraperitoneal organ may enter it. Parastomal hernias seem to occur most commonly at either the mesenteric aspect of the stoma or laterally. Knowing the difference between prolapse and herniation is important. Prolapse results largely from intestinal redundancy and lack of fixation, whereas hernia implies excessive size of the fascial ring. Prolonged or repeated prolapse may lead to widening of the trephine and development of hernia, and patients with hernias may coincidentally develop prolapse.

EVALUATION AND MANAGEMENT OPTIONS

The evaluation of the patient with an ostomy who may have a hernia begins with a directed history eliciting the abdominal or stoma-related complaint, its duration, and its relationship to body position and physical activities. Local pain is common. A bulge may occur with straining, standing, or after a large meal. Intermittent difficulty with the appliance also may indicate occult hernia. It is important to inquire about signs and symptoms of intestinal obstruction (which may be very mild) and difficulty with irrigation of the stoma. Stool size and consistency and presence of prolapse also should be elicited.

Parastomal hernia may be relatively obvious or extremely difficult to diagnose. Examination requires that the patient be unclothed with the ostomy management system removed. The region of the stoma is examined. Palpation is done first with the patient recumbent and then standing. The patient is asked to relax and perform the Valsalva maneuver repeatedly. Perhaps the most valuable and often omitted technique in evaluation of patients with stoma problems is digital examination of the stoma during these maneuvers. Such examination allows palpation of the fascial aperture and the most direct evaluation of the subcutaneous parastomal region. The site of the stoma, presence of scars, degree of obesity, evidence of abdominal muscle denervation, quality of the skin locally, and potential alternative stoma sites should be noted during the examination.

In the patient whose symptoms suggest parastomal hernia but no hernia can be detected, CT scanning may be of value. In a population of patients with ileostomy, Williams et al.[39] found that 20% of parastomal hernias were detectable only by CT scan. Such detection allowed two symptomatic patients to undergo repair.

Not all hernias require repair. Central to the decision between operative and nonoperative treatment is the surgeon's accurate assessment of the nature of the hernia, its current or potential seriousness, and how adversely it affects the patient. The indications and contraindications for repair of parastomal hernia are listed in the box on p. 254. Most contraindications are relative because life-threatening complications require repair in all but the terminal patient.

Virtually all authors agree that for ostomy patients with an asymptomatic or mildly symptomatic hernia nonoperative management should be attempted. Most hernias are well tolerated. Serious complications are uncommon, and operative repair may be difficult, produce morbidity, and have a significant rate of recurrence.

Nonoperative management centers around the use of a binder or a belt that incorporates a plastic disk atop the flange of the ostomy device to maintain the hernia in a reduced state. Such an approach may allow the symptomatic, poor-risk patient to live comfortably with a hernia.

It has been suggested that only 10% to 20% of parastomal hernias ever will require repair.[5] This figure appears to be reasonable for paracolostomy her-

INDICATIONS AND CONTRAINDICATIONS TO PARASTOMAL HERNIA REPAIR

Indications

Absolute
- Incarceration
- Strangulation
- Obstruction
- Fistulization
- Perforation (related to incarceration or irrigation)
- Stoma ischemia

Relative
- History of incarceration
- Symptoms suggestive of obstruction
- Difficulty maintaining appliance fit
- Patient unable to see or manage stoma
- Irrigation difficulty
- Pain related to hernia
- Ulceration of overlying skin
- Cosmetic unacceptability
- Tight neck of hernia that is difficult to reduce
- Concomitant prolapse, stricture, or other indication for revision

Contraindications

Absolute
- End-stage malignancy

Relative
- Recurrent, metastatic, or inoperable malignancy
- Severe comorbid disease
- Temporary stoma

nias. In Balslev's study,[24] which included meticulous long-term follow-up, 9 of 62 (15%) patients with hernias required repair. There is some evidence that the necessity for repair is greater when the hernia is associated with an ileostomy. Williams et al.[39] found that 9 of 13 (69%) paraileostomy hernias had needed repair when he examined a group of long-term survivors. Of Fleshman and Lewis's series of paraileostomy hernias,[40] 50% required repair, although some may have had other reasons for revision besides hernia. The liquid, somewhat caustic effluent may make ileostomy hernia more difficult to manage nonoperatively. For similar reasons paraurostomy hernias also seem to require repair frequently. Schmidt et al.[22] report 6 of 8 of their series underwent repair, as did all 18 in a series by Marshall et al.[27] Unfortunately, both of these chart review studies suffer from identifying only patients who returned for examination because of particularly symptomatic hernias. By underestimating the total number of hernias, such studies may exaggerate the frequency with which repair is required. Nonetheless, it is probable that paraileostomy and paraurostomy hernias are more likely to require repair than paracolostomy hernias.

OPERATIVE REPAIR

The patient who fails nonoperative management or has an absolute indication for repair has several options. They include simple local repair, relocation of the stoma, and local repair with prosthetic mesh. Preparation for surgery requires thoughtful evaluation of the need for repair and identification of comorbid disease such as recurrent malignancy or inflammatory bowel disease. Potential risk factors for recurrence, such as obesity and pulmonary or urinary dysfunction, should be treated preoperatively whenever possible. The surgeon must consider factors such as hernia size, stoma location, and sites of associated scars that might influence repair type. In the perioperative period we use a standard mechanical and antibiotic bowel preparation for paracolostomy repair and restrict ileostomy patients to clear liquids. If prosthetic mesh will be used, both systemic and intraluminal antibiotics should be used. Our other management is similar to that for any clean-contaminated operation.

TECHNIQUES OF REPAIR

Local repair, as described by Thorlakson,[43] is the oldest and, until recently, the most widely practiced form of repair. Thorlakson's technique involved making a semicircular or an L-shaped skin incision just outside the ostomy management system zone, exposing and reducing the sac, and clearing the anterior fascia for several centimeters around the stoma and the fascial defect. Interrupted nonabsorbable sutures were used to "snug" the fascia and close the defect around the stoma. Other authors describe similar repairs, using the original laparotomy incision and developing an extraperitoneal flap to expose the parastomal fascia or incising at the mucotaneous junction, performing the repair, and rematuring the stoma. Local repair also may be effected by laparotomy, with mass closure of the defect from within.

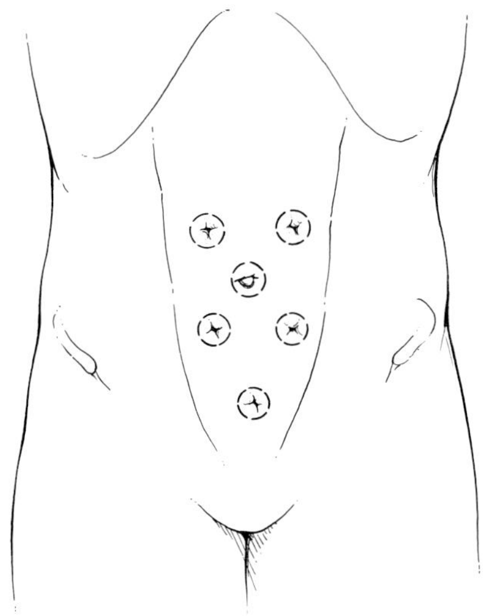

Fig. 15-5. Acceptable abdominal stoma sites.

Most authors consider relocation of the stoma to be the most reliable operative repair. Relocation usually requires laparotomy, lysis of adhesions, and fashioning a new stoma. Consequently morbidity is higher. The enterostomal therapist (ET) plays an important role in preoperative planning and the choice of alternative stoma sites. The patient is fitted with a sham ostomy management system at several potential sites and is observed in supine, sitting, standing, and various activity-related positions. The best and the second-best alternative sites are determined and marked. There are six generally acceptable stoma sites[6] (Fig. 15-5). In any given patient the number of sites available may be significantly less. Body habitus may be a restricting factor (obese patients may have difficulty seeing a stoma located at any of the three lowest sites) as may prior surgical scars and regions of denervation (proximity to them is believed to predispose to recurrence).[7]

There are two general techniques of stoma relocation. In 1967 Turnbull and Weakley[41] described a technique of relocating ileostomies without laparotomy, but we have no experience with their technique. Subsequently, Taylor et al.[44] and Kaufman[45] used this approach successfully to relocate two ileostomies and four urostomies. Although several surgeons have performed this operation safely, we have concerns about potential difficulties arising from the blind nature of the procedure. The inability to lyse adhesions safely, to ensure that no twisting has occurred, and to mobilize and assess the prestomal bowel make this operation riskier than is necessary.

We prefer the more classic resiting operation described by Devlin.[10] A circumstomal incision is made and the stoma is mobilized and closed. If the hernia is very large, the incision can be extended and used for laparotomy, but most often the previous incision is reopened. Reduction of the hernia and completion of the takedown of the stoma are accomplished through simultaneous intraperitoneal and extraperitoneal dissection. The new stoma site is created and the stomal intestine is delivered. The laparotomy incision is closed, and the old hernia is repaired with or without prosthetic material. After these incisions have been closed and draped outside the field, the new stoma is matured. If prosthetic material is used or if there is a large subcutaneous space, closed drainage is used.

The third general type of repair is local repair with prosthetic material. In the past 15 years development of well-tolerated synthetic mesh and its successful use in inguinal, ventral, and incisional hernia repair have fostered an increasing interest in this form of repair. Most such repairs avoid laparotomy and the need to fashion a new stoma. The recurrence rate is lower because repair with mesh circumvents reliance on the weakened musculofascial tissue in the region of the stoma. Many authors have described their favored technique of prosthetic local repair.[10,11,42,46-50] Various approaches have been used, including circumstomal, semicircular, or L-shaped incisions made just outside the appliance zone and prior vertical laparotomy incisions. Mesh has been placed in the extrafascial, properitoneal, or intraperitoneal plane, and bowel has been brought through the center of or beside the mesh.

In 1977 Rosin and Bonardi[42] first described prosthetic local repair. Their method uses a large elliptical circumstomal incision to dissect out the prestomal intestine, the hernia sac, and a rim of good fascia around the hernia. The sac is opened, its contents are reduced, and the peritoneum and fascia are closed in layers around the exiting bowel. A piece of Marlex mesh with a central orifice sized to fit snugly around the prestomal intestine is passed over the stoma and sutured to the fascia with interrupted nonabsorbable sutures. The subcutaneous tissues are irrigated and drained with closed suction. The skin defect is closed linearly, the former stoma is excised, and a new stoma is primarily matured in the center of the incision. Only one of the seven patients had a local infectious complication, and none developed recurrence or required removal of the mesh. Although these results were excellent (Table 15-3), the technique has some theoretical drawbacks. Having the mesh in the same field with the stoma and leaving the matured stoma in the incision may increase the chances of infectious complications. The proximity of the incision to the stoma also may interfere with the fit of the ostomy management system.

Table 15-3. Published results of parastomal hernia repair

Author	Year	Years of Follow-up*	Local Repair Success/Total	Relocation of Stoma Success/Total	Prosthetic Repair Success/Total
Marshall et al.[27]	1975	2.4	4/7	7/9	
Prian et al.[28]	1975	2.8	0/3	6/6	
Rosin & Bonardi[42]	1977	0-4			7/7
Taylor et al.[44]	1978	—		2/2	
Abdu[46]	1982	6.2			4/4
Hopkins & Trento[47]	1982	—			1/1
Kaufman[45]	1983	—		4/4	
Sugarbaker[52]	1985	5.1			7/7
Horgan & Hughes[53]	1986	0.8-5	0/2	1/1	
Williams et al.[39]	1990	—	0/2	3/9	1/1
Rubin[51]	In press	—	7/18	2/5	2/3
TOTAL			11/32	25/36	22/23

*Single numbers indicate mean follow-up; hyphenated numbers indicate range.

Four years later Leslie[48] described an alternative method that we favor (Figs. 15-6 and 15-7). An L-shaped incision is made outside the ostomy device zone. Whenever feasible, the former laparotomy or other incision is used as one limb of the L. The subcutaneous tissue is raised from the anterior rectus sheath as a flap until strong fascia is reached at the edges of the hernia defect. The stoma is not disturbed. The hernia is reduced, and, if possible, the fascia is repaired around the stoma with nonabsorbable sutures. A square sheet of prosthetic mesh (Leslie uses Mersilene) is then partially split and passed around the bowel and sutured atop the anterior sheath with nonabsorbable material. The split portion is overlapped, producing the correct degree of snugness. Leslie allows the redundant mesh to fold up along the bowel to reinforce the repair and prevent future prolapse and retraction. The flap is closed over a drain, and the ostomy management system is replaced.

Although this is essentially the repair we use today, we use several modifications. We drape the stoma from the surgical field to minimize the chance of contaminating the prosthetic material. Often we intubate the stoma with a large Foley catheter, a procedure that may assist in the often complex task of delineating the prestomal bowel from any herniated loops. We use Marlex mesh and affix it to the fascia with two concentric rows of interrupted 0-Prolene sutures, one near the outer edge of the mesh and one close to the reapproximated trephine to prevent lifting and subprosthetic insinuation of a hernia. Sutures are placed at 2 cm intervals, starting opposite the split side of the mesh and working toward the split around both sides of the stoma. In this

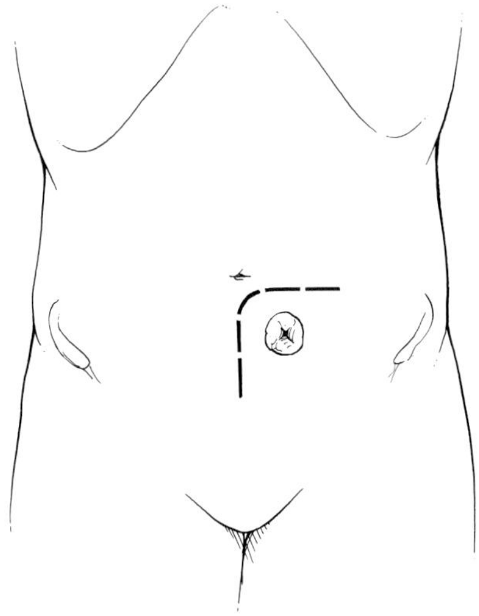

Fig. 15-6. L-shaped incision outside ostomy management system zone for extrafascial mesh repair.

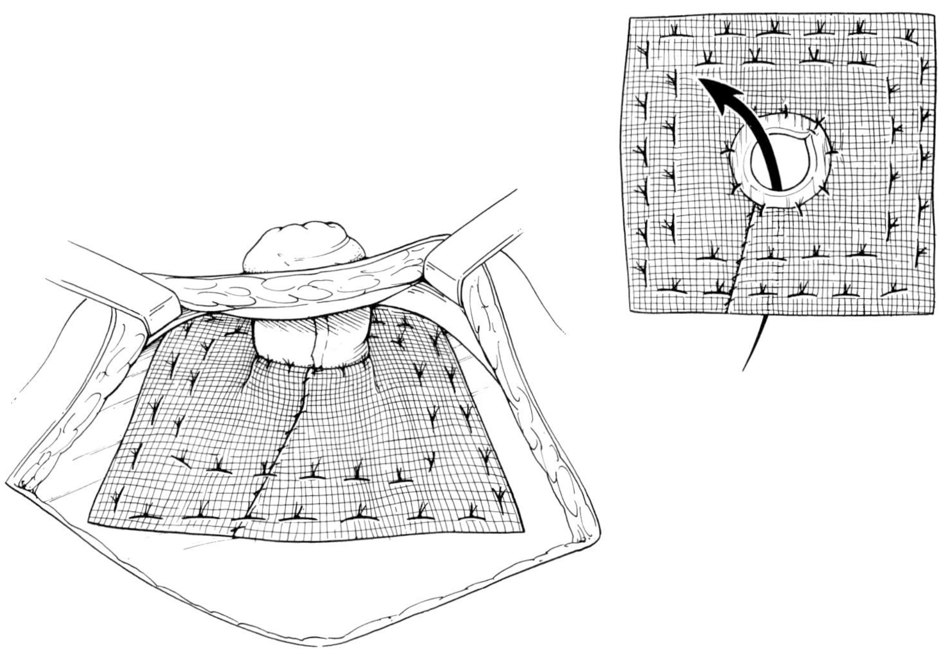

Fig. 15-7. Extrafascial mesh repair showing mesh sutured in place around stoma. Note collar sutured to stoma and concentric placement of anchoring sutures (inset). (Modified from Leslie D. The parastomal hernia. Aust N Z J Surg 51:485-486, 1981.)

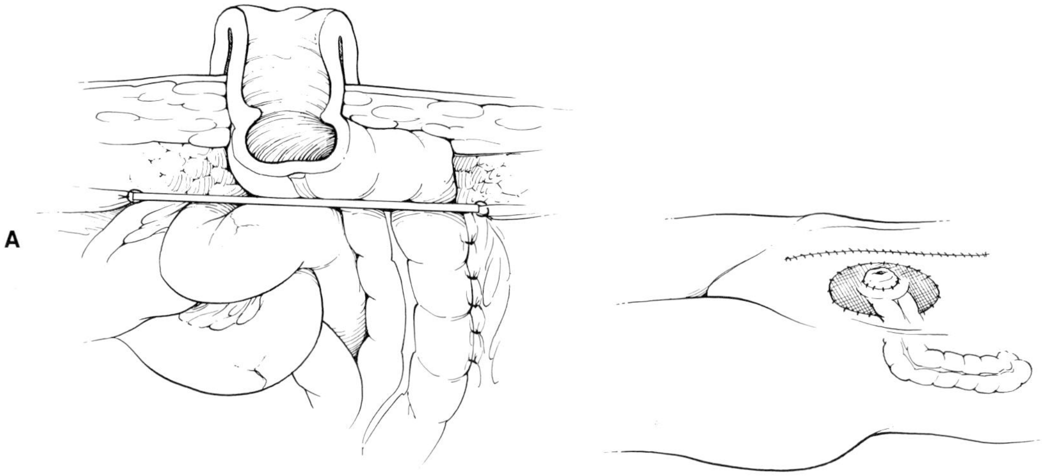

Fig. 15-8. A, Intraperitoneal mesh repair showing mesh in place and bowel entering from lateral edge. **B,** Note that bowel is also anchored to lateral abdominal wall peritoneum. (Modified from Sugarbaker PH. Prosthetic mesh repair of large hernias at the site of colonic stomas. Surg Gynecol Obstet 150:577-578, 1980.)

way the snugness of the repair can be adjusted gradually by increasing or decreasing the degree of overlap at the split in the mesh. A finger in the stoma helps in evaluating the size of the opening. Finally we use interrupted 3-0 silk seromuscular sutures (carefully avoiding the mucosa) to attach the mesh to the prestomal bowel. We believe that this attachment prevents insinuation of a small hernia sac inside the mesh repair and motion of the mesh against the bowel that might lead to perforation. We have not had adverse consequences because of the proximity of the mesh to the bowel.

Another useful technique, described by Sugarbaker,[49] is of particular value in patients with large hernias and patients whose anterior fascia is too attenuated for use in even a mesh repair (Figs. 15-8 and 15-9). In Sugarbaker's method the old laparotomy incision is reopened after intubating and draping the stoma. The hernia is reduced from within the peritoneal cavity, and a sheet of prosthetic material (Marlex mesh) is sutured in place to close the defect from the peritoneal side. Sugarbaker places all the sutures with deep bites in the peritoneum, posterior fascial sheath, and mesh at close intervals. He sutures the mesh circumferentially to the fascial ring except laterally, where the intestine is made to exit the peritoneal cavity, curving medially atop the mesh to become the stoma. Sugarbaker believes that his excellent long-term results have been derived in part from the oblique egress of the pre-

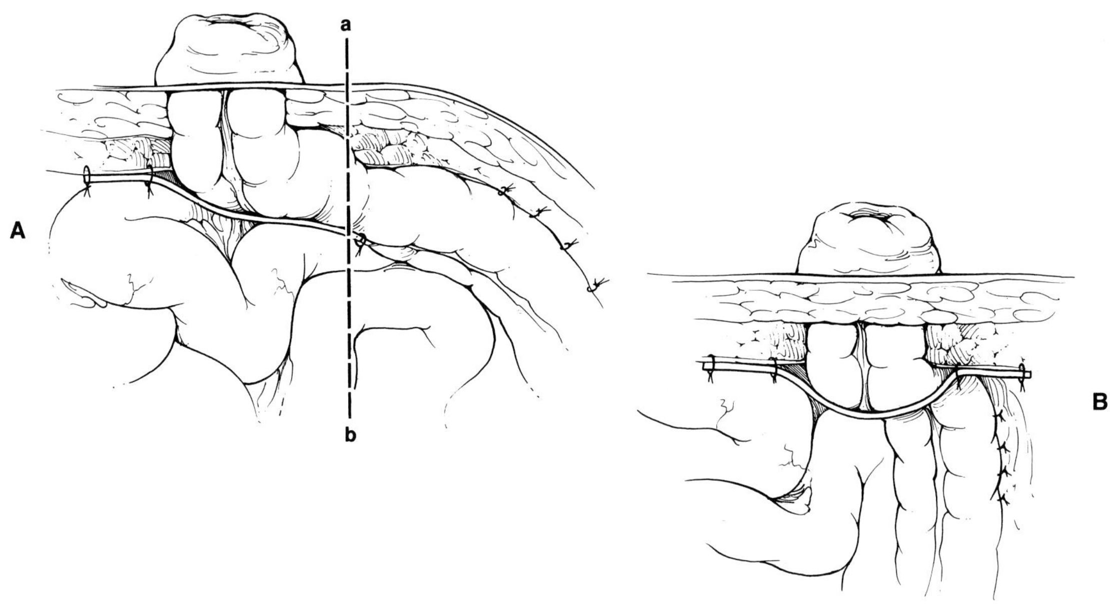

Fig. 15-9. A, Intraperitoneal mesh repair with detail of bowel entering tunnel below mesh. **B,** Cross-sectional view corresponds to *a-b* in **A.**

stomal bowel (essentially creating an extraperitoneal stoma). Increased intra-abdominal pressure is exerted on the mesh rather than on the fascial opening. An alternative form of this technique uses split mesh fixed circumferentially around the bowel. We also have used the latter technique with success and believe that we are better able to adjust the neofascial aperture in this way. Intraperitoneal mesh is particularly useful in a recurrent hernia in which there is a marked fascial defect or in which extraperitoneal mesh has been used previously. Devlin[10] has described a variant in which the mesh is placed in the properitoneal plane, theoretically avoiding a difficult intraperitoneal dissection.

Certain principles are applicable to all types of mesh repair. Perioperative antibiotics should be used. All incisions should be made outside the ostomy management system zone. Whenever possible, the stoma should be draped outside the operative field. The fascial defect beneath the mesh may be sutured, but this step is not essential. The mesh must, however, be sutured securely to strong fascia at least 3 cm from the hernia defect. Finally, when mesh is placed subcutaneously, the space should be drained by closed suction.

RESULTS

The techniques of local repair are described largely for historical interest because most reports since that of Thorlakson[43] have noted poor results. Table 15-3 lists the articles reporting follow-up of parastomal hernia repairs. Results of local repair are uniformly bad, with 65% of repairs resulting in recurrence. In the two series that report some long-term successes with simple local repair, the authors comment that the herniorrhaphies of this type that remained intact were in patients with small or incidental hernias and that many other small hernias did recur.[27,51]

Many experienced authors believe relocation of the stoma is the best method of repair for parastomal hernia.[1,4,10] Some consider resiting the only choice for large or recurrent hernias. In the series in which this technique was used, the long-term success rate was almost 70%.* Several of these authors noted that the patients undergoing resiting had the most difficult hernias.

The reported results of prosthetic local repair are very good, in fact, probably as good or better than those with resiting. Infections and other complications have not been a problem. The concern expressed by several authors that mesh infection with prolonged adverse sequelae would be a common complication with this technique has not been supported by the literature. Of 27 patients reported in several series, only four local infections occurred, only one was considered serious, and no patient required removal of the mesh.† In our experience infection involving the mesh often can be controlled without removal of the mesh.

SELECTION OF REPAIR TYPE

Once the indication for operative repair has been established, the surgeon must decide which type of hernia repair is best. This decision must be individualized. As a rule we do not recommend simple local repair, except for small asymptomatic hernias incidentally found at laparotomy. The choice between local prosthetic repair and resiting depends on the condition of the stoma and abdomen locally, the general condition of the patient, and, ultimately, the surgeon's preference. Both Goligher[1] and Corman[11] consider resiting preferable, although Goligher's data antedates much of the recent literature on mesh repairs. Table 15-3 suggests that the efficacy of these approaches is similar. Recurrence and complication rates are not significantly different. Our approach is to use whichever type of repair seems most appropriate for

*References 27, 28, 39, 44, 45, 51, 53.
†References 10, 39, 42, 46, 47, 51, 52.

the given patient. If a stoma is poorly situated, it should be resited if possible. A hernia around a stoma that is not transrectus is best repaired by relocation. Similarly a stoma that is out of sight in an obese patient should be resited. On the other hand, a mesh repair may be chosen for a patient who likes the current site and who has had no prior difficulties. In a patient with severe comorbid disease, performing an extraparietal mesh repair or a translocation without laparotomy may avoid the complications associated with a major abdominal operation. A patient with multiple scars across the other potential stoma sites may be best treated with local mesh repair. We have placed stomas in previous incision sites, but we prefer to avoid doing so if possible because we believe there is an increased recurrence rate and difficulty with the fit of the ostomy management system.

POSTOPERATIVE MANAGEMENT AND COMPLICATIONS

Except for the avoidance of heavy lifting and vigorous activity for at least 2 months, the postoperative management of these patients is the same as that for any patient with a new stoma. Winkler[3] believes that use of a corset or binder is essential in the short- and long-term management of these patients. We do not agree and believe that there is insufficient evidence at this time to justify this recommendation for all patients. However, the patient with a high risk of recurrence may benefit from a prophylactic corset or binder.

Serious complications other than recurrence are uncommon with parastomal hernia repair. Seroma, the most common complication, occurs to some degree in almost all patients. Most patients should be treated expectantly, although aspiration may be indicated for those who are significantly symptomatic. To prevent contamination, aspiration should be avoided, if possible, when prosthetic material has been used. Infectious wound complications are unusual; when present, they are usually minor. Few such complications are noted in the literature. Even when mesh is used, local infection occurs in less than 15% of patients and is serious in less than 5%. Recurrence is a problem, occurring in roughly 70% who undergo simple repair. Even prosthetic and resiting-type repairs have significant recurrence rates (5% to 35% range), and most studies have relatively short follow-up. Finally, there is always the risk that manipulating, moving, or dissecting near the stoma will cause a complication, such as an injury to the bowel or its blood supply, that will have adverse consequences in the early or late postoperative period.

PREVENTION

It is undeniable that parastomal hernia is a common problem in individuals with an ostomy and that it may cause serious complications or management problems. Repair, when required, may be difficult, and the condition is prone to recurrence. As with many other surgical complications, prevention is the most efficacious way to deal with the problem. Goligher[1] "knows of no certain preventive of this complication," but by adhering to a few principles, the risk of herniation can be minimized.

Preoperatively all possible efforts should be made to improve the risk factors for hernia. Preoperative planning and marking of the stoma site (preferably with the advice of the ET) are essential and have been covered in detail in the chapter on preoperative considerations (Chapter 3). Meticulous attention must be paid to the construction of the initial stoma as described in the chapters on the end sigmoid colostomy (Chapter 6) and the end ileostomy (Chapter 9). The choice of incision is important. One of us (M.S.R.) prefers to use a contralateral paramedian incision, believing that its use avoids proximity to the stoma and narrowing of the fascial bridge between stoma and incision. The other (H.R.B.) prefers a midline approach and avoids paramedian incisions altogether because such incisions may preclude using that side of the abdomen for future stomas. Neither of us would use a right paramedian incision in a patient with inflammatory bowel disease. In locating the stoma, the transrectus position is superior to the lateral one. An umbilical

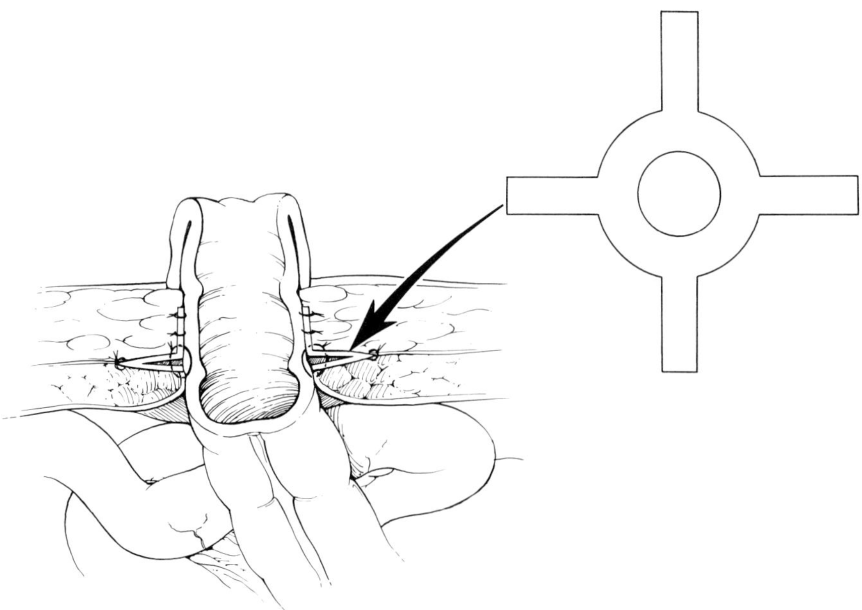

Fig. 15-10. Paracolostomy mesh reinforcement showing collar of mesh (inset) around stoma and anchored to anterior fascia. (Modified from Bayer I, Kyzer S, Chaimoff C. A new approach to primary strengthening of colostomy with Marlex mesh to prevent paracolostomy hernia. Surg Gynecol Obstet 163:579-580, 1986.)

stoma also will have a lower rate of hernia formation.[30] Trephine size should be only large enough to admit the bowel itself.[12] Points of controversy include the value of circumferential tacking of the bowel to the fascia[37,54] and the benefit of creating an extraperitoneal stoma. No studies have been done on the risks or values of tacking, and we do not believe that this practice is useful in preventing herniation. An interesting report by Bayer et al.[55] investigated the benefits and risks of placing a ring of Marlex mesh around all colostomies to prevent hernias (Fig. 15-10). Forty-three patients were followed for up to 4 years. None developed a hernia, and only seven had complications attributable to the mesh. We have no experience with this technique and will await a randomized prospective study of this method against conventional techniques before recommending it for routine use. It may be appropriate to use prophylactic mesh in the high-risk patient. Although some studies have supported the use of the extraperitoneal stoma[26,29] as described by Goligher,[56] the authors disagree on its use. Although of theoretic advantage, such a stoma may be technically difficult to construct and present problems in irrigation.

• • •

The surgeon must remember that for the long-term survivor the single most important part of the operation is the creation of the stoma. Even minor malfunctioning of the stoma may seriously hamper the patient's daily activities and life. The construction of the stoma should be meticulous, and it should be performed by, or be done under the guidance of, an experienced attending surgeon.

REFERENCES

1. Goligher JC. Surgery of the Anus, Rectum and Colon, 5th ed. London: Baillière Tindall, 1985, pp 703-705.
2. Goligher JC, DeDombal FT, Watts JM, Watkinson G. Ulcerative Colitis. Baltimore: Williams & Wilkins, 1968, p 312.
3. Winkler R. Stoma Therapy: An Atlas and Guide for Intestinal Stomas. Stuttgart: Georg Thieme Verlag, 1986, pp 53-57, 69-71.
4. Leslie D. The parastomal hernia. Surg Clin North Am 64:407-415, 1984.
5. Pearl RK. Parastomal hernias. World J Surg 13:569-572, 1989.
6. Nyhus LM, Condon RE. Hernia, 3rd ed. Philadelphia: JB Lippincott, 1989, pp 333-337, 567-570.
7. Ferrari BT, Ray JE, Gathright JB. Complications of Colon and Rectal Surgery: Prevention and Management. Philadelphia: WB Saunders, 1985, pp 236-246.
8. Todd IP. Intestinal Stomas. London: William Heinemann Medical Books, 1978, pp 12-15.
9. Ponka JL. Hernias of the Abdominal Wall. Philadelphia: WB Saunders, 1980, pp 389-390.

10. Devlin HB. Management of Abdominal Hernias. London: Butterworth, 1988, pp 177-186.
11. Corman ML. Colon and Rectal Surgery, 2nd ed. Philadelphia: JB Lippincott, 1989, pp 894-903.
12. Todd IP. The resolution of stoma problems. In Allan RN, Keighley MRB, Alexander-Williams J, Hawkins C. Inflammatory Bowel Disease. Edinburgh: Churchill Livingstone, 1983, pp 256-261.
13. Gabriel WB, Lloyd-Davies OV. Colostomy. Br J Surg 22:520, 530-532, 1935.
14. Sjodahl R, Anderberg B, Bolin T. Parastomal hernia in relation to site of the abdominal stoma. Br J Surg 75:339-341, 1988.
15. Birnbaum W, Ferrier P. Complications of abdominal colostomy. Am J Surg 83:64-67, 1952.
16. Grier WRN, Postel AH, Syarse A, Localio SA. An evaluation of colonic stoma management without irrigations. Surg Gynecol Obstet 119:1234-1242, 1964.
17. Green EW. Colostomies and their complications. Surg Gynecol Obstet 122:1230-1232, 1966.
18. Watts JM, DeDombal FT, Goligher JC. Long-term complications and prognosis following major surgery for ulcerative colitis. Br J Surg 53:1014-1023, 1966.
19. Roy PH, Saver WG, Beahrs OH, Farrow GM. Experience with ileostomies: Evaluation of long-term rehabilitation in 497 patients. Am J Surg 119:77-86, 1970.
20. Burns FJ. Complications of colostomy. Dis Colon Rectum 13:448-450, 1970.
21. Harbach LB, Hall RL, Cockett ATK, et al. Ileal loop cutaneous urinary diversion: A critical review. J Urol 105:511-515, 1971.
22. Schmidt JD, Hawtrey CE, Flocks RH, Culp DA. Complications, results and problems of ileal conduit diversions. J Urol 109:210-216, 1973.
23. Saha SP, Rao N, Stephenson SE. Complications of colostomy. Dis Colon Rectum 16:515-516, 1973.
24. Balslev AI. Parakolostomihernier. Ugeskr Laeger 135:2799-2804, 1973.
25. Kronborg O, Kramhoft J, Backer O, Sprechler M. Late complications following operations for cancer of the rectum and anus. Dis Colon Rectum 17:750-753, 1974.
26. Harshaw DH, Gardner B, Vives A, Sandaram KN. The effect of technical factors upon complications from abdominal perineal resections. Surg Gynecol Obstet 139:756-758, 1974.
27. Marshall FF, Leadbetter WF, Dretler SP. Ileal conduit parastomal hernias. J Urol 114:40-42, 1975.
28. Prian GW, Sawyer RB, Sawyer KC. Repair of peristomal colostomy hernias. Am J Surg 130:694-696, 1975.
29. Marks CG, Ritchie JK. The complications of synchronous combined excision for adenocarcinoma of the rectum at St. Mark's Hospital. Br J Surg 62:901-905, 1975.
30. Raza SD, Portin BA, Bernhoft WH. Umbilical colostomy: A better intestinal stoma. Dis Colon Rectum 20:223-230, 1977.
31. Abrams BL, Alsikafi FH, Waterman NG. Colostomy: A new look at morbidity and mortality. Am J Surg 45:462-464, 1979.
32. Wara P, Sorenson K, Berg V. Proximal fecal diversion: Review of ten years' experience. Dis Colon Rectum 24:114-119, 1981.
33. Stothert JC Jr, Brubacher L, Siminowitz DA. Complications of emergency stoma formation. Arch Surg 117:307-309, 1982.

34. Eldrup J, Weid U, Bischoff N, Peterson VM. Parakolostomihernier. Ugeskr Laeger 144:3742-3743, 1982.
35. Burgess P, Matthew VV, Devlin HB. A review of terminal colostomy complications following abdominoperineal resection for carcinoma [abstract]. Br J Surg 71:1004, 1984.
36. Phillips R, Pringle W, Evans C, Keighley MRB. Analysis of a hospital-based stoma-therapy service. Ann R Coll Surg Engl 67:37-40, 1985.
37. Pearl RK, Prasad ML, Orsay CP, et al. Early local complications from intestinal stomas. Arch Surg 120:1145-1147, 1985.
38. Phillips RKS, Ritchie JK, Hawley PR. Proctectomy and ileostomy for ulcerative colitis: The longer-term story. J R Soc Med 82:386-387, 1989.
39. Williams JG, Etherington R, Hayward MWJ, Hughes LE. Paraileostomy hernia: A clinical and radiological study. Br J Surg 77:1355-1357, 1990.
40. Fleshman JW, Lewis MG. Complications and quality of life after stoma surgery: A review of 16,470 patients in the UOA Data Registry. Semin Colon Rectal Surg 2:66-72, 1991.
41. Turnbull RB, Weakley FL. Atlas of Intestinal Stomas. St. Louis: CV Mosby, 1967, pp 1-5, 78-91, 131-143.
42. Rosin JD, Bonardi RA. Paracolostomy hernia repair with Marlex mesh: A new technique. Dis Colon Rectum 20:299-302, 1977.
43. Thorlakson RH. Technique of repair of herniations associated with colonic stomas. Surg Gynecol Obstet 120:347-350, 1965.
44. Taylor RL, Rombeau JL, Turnbull RB Jr. Transperitoneal relocation of the ileal stoma without formal laparotomy. Surg Gynecol Obstet 146:953-958, 1978.
45. Kaufman JJ. Repair of parastomal hernia by translocation of the stoma without laparotomy. J Urol 129:278-279, 1983.
46. Abdu RA. Repair of paracolostomy hernia with Marlex mesh. Dis Colon Rectum 25:529-531, 1982.
47. Hopkins TB, Trento A. Parastomal ileal loop hernia repair with Marlex mesh. J Urol 128:811-812, 1982.
48. Leslie D. The parastomal hernia. Aust N Z J Surg 51:485-486, 1981.
49. Sugarbaker PH. Prosthetic mesh repair of large hernias at the site of colonic stomas. Surg Gynecol Obstet 150:577-578, 1980.
50. Garnjobst W, Sullivan ES. Repair of paraileostomy hernia with polypropylene mesh reinforcement. Dis Colon Rectum 27:268-269, 1984.
51. Rubin MS. Personal communication, 1992.
52. Sugarbaker PH. Peritoneal approach to prosthetic mesh repair of paraostomy hernias. Ann Surg 201:344-346, 1985.
53. Horgan K, Hughes LE. Para-ileostomy hernia: Failure of a local repair technique. Br J Surg 73:439-440, 1986.
54. Lyons AS, Turell R. Operative correction of intestinal stoma difficulties. Am J Surg 101:55-60, 1961.
55. Bayer I, Kyzer S, Chaimoff C. A new approach to primary strengthening of colostomy with Marlex mesh to prevent paracolostomy hernia. Surg Gynecol Obstet 163:579-580, 1986.
56. Goligher JC. Extraperitoneal colostomy or ileostomy. Br J Surg 46:97-103, 1958.

16 STOMA PROLAPSE

Juan J. Nogueras and Steven D. Wexner

Many challenges await patients with a newly formed stoma. Some of these challenges include the need to meet the physical and psychologic challenges unique to their new body architecture. Any deviation from optimal conditions can impair stoma management and thus hinder patient acceptance of the stoma. The ideal stoma combines optimal cosmetic and functional results so that both patient and physician are pleased with the outcome. Stoma prolapse is one of many potential complications. In this condition the full thickness of the intestine protrudes through the stoma. This condition is not unique to any one type of stoma. Prolapse has occurred in both end and loop stomas, colostomies and ileostomies, and even in urostomies and continent ileostomies. Some authors have attempted to classify stoma prolapse into fixed and sliding categories.[1] The fixed variety of prolapse occurs most commonly as a result of improper stoma construction that involves excessive protrusion of the stoma beyond the abdominal wall. The sliding variety of prolapse, however, is not static in length. This type of prolapse is more prone to incarcerate and therefore is associated with higher risk for ischemia.

INCIDENCE

The incidence of stoma prolapse is variable. It is dependent on the type and the location of the stoma. In general, properly constructed end stomas have a lower incidence of prolapse than do loop stomas. Fleshman and Lewis[2] reported the incidence of stoma-related complications based on a review of 16,740 entries in the United Ostomy Association Registry. The incidence of prolapse for ileostomy, colostomy, and urostomy was 3%, 2%, and <1%, respectively. Other authors have reported the incidence of end-colostomy prolapse to range from 1% to 13%.[3,4] The reported incidences of prolapse for end ileostomies are similar, ranging from 2.6% to 16%.[5,6] This wide discrepancy in incidence among various series may reflect the differences in technique in stoma construction among institutions. Turnbull and Weakley[7] expressed their opinion that ". . . prolapse of the distal limb of the loop cannot yet be prevented. . . ."

Loop colostomies generally prolapse more often than do end colostomies. When loop stomas do prolapse, the prolapse occurs more often through the distal limb than through the proximal one (Fig. 16-1). The reported incidence of loop colostomy prolapse is 5% to 10%.[8]

A commonly associated finding with colostomy prolapse is a parastomal hernia (Fig. 16-2). It may result because the fascial and skin apertures for colostomies are larger than for ileostomies. This situation is especially true

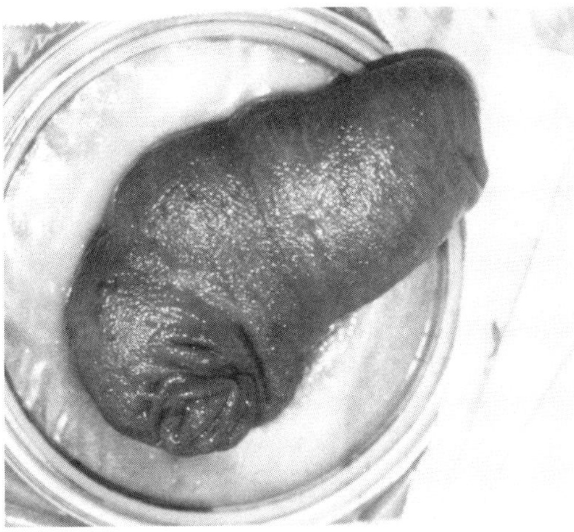

Fig. 16-1. Loop colostomy with prolapse of defunctionalized distal limb.

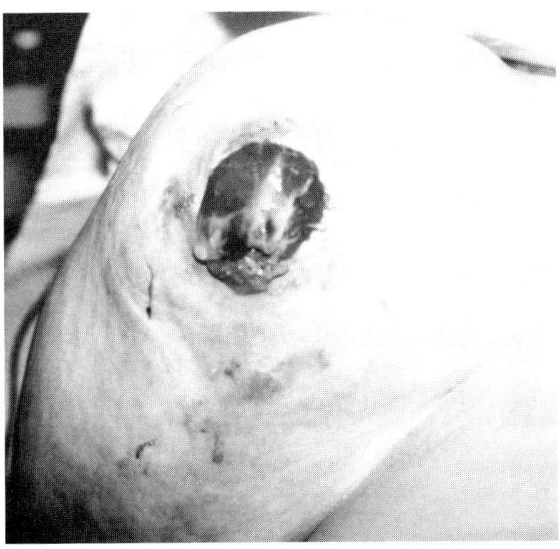

Fig. 16-2. Large parastomal hernia associated with ileostomy prolapse.

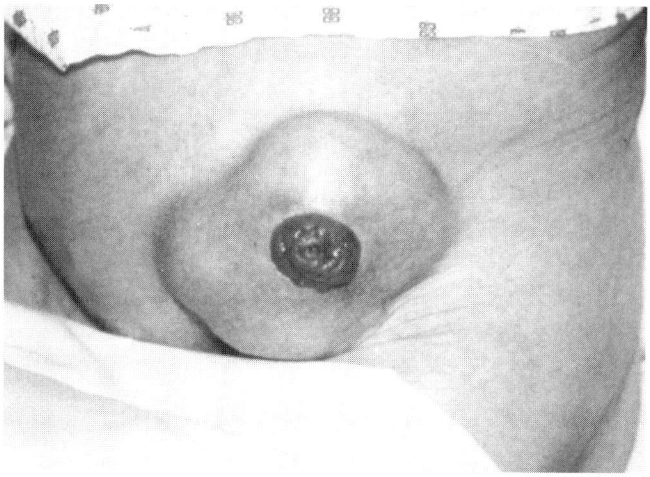

Fig. 16-3. End sigmoid colostomy with parastomal hernia. (From Bubrick MP, Rolstad BS. Intestinal stomas. In Gordon PH, Nivatvongs S, eds. Principles and Practice of Surgery for the Colon, Rectum, and Anus. St. Louis: Quality Medical Publishing, 1992, p 886.)

for end sigmoid colostomies because they are often created in obstructed colonic segments, mandating overly large fascial and skin openings. Parastomal hernias also can occur with end or loop ileostomies and with loop colostomies. The most common association, however, is with end colostomies (Fig. 16-3). In the series by Allen-Mersh and Thomson,[4] 50% of the patients with colostomy prolapse also had a parastomal hernia.

SYMPTOMS

Prolapse can cause unsightly bulging of the stoma, which can adversely affect how the ostomy patient accepts the stoma (Fig. 16-4). The presence of this bulge, especially if associated with a parastomal hernia, commonly results in difficulties with proper fitting of the ostomy management system. As a result of an improperly fitted appliance, leakage and parastomal skin irritation can ensue. Thus pain or bleeding from skin excoriation and poor ostomy management system fitting may be a symptom of prolapse. Even if the system is properly fitted, the prolapsed stoma is prone to injury from local trauma, and ulceration may develop. Ultimately obstruction from incarceration or even strangulation leading to possible peritonitis can occur. Fortunately, these complications are relatively rare but do require immediate recognition and treatment.

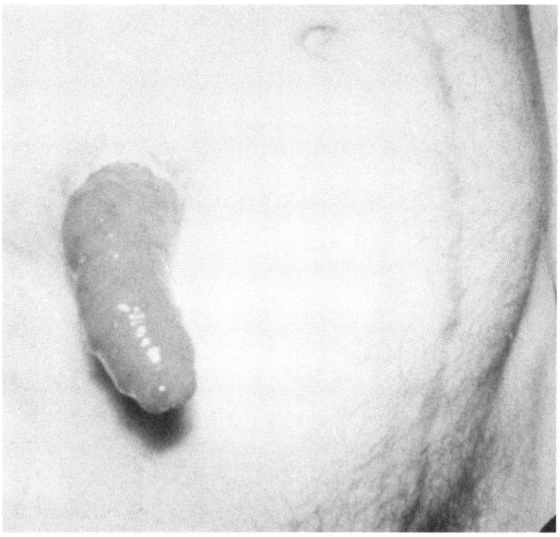

Fig. 16-4. End ileostomy with significant prolapse. (Courtesy Bonnie Sue Rolstad, R.N., C.E.T.N.)

PREDISPOSING FACTORS FOR STOMA PROLAPSE

Patient related	Surgeon related
Obesity	Improper site placement outside rectus abdominis muscle
Increased intra-abdominal pressure and chronic obstructive pulmonary disease	Oversized aperture
Bowel redundancy	Failure of mesenteric fixation (?)
Poor, weak fascia	Bowel redundancy

PREDISPOSING FACTORS

The development of stoma prolapse is usually insidious rather than sudden or acute. Certain circumstances do predispose to development of prolapse. These factors generally can be categorized into patient-related factors and surgeon-related factors (see box).

The obese patient is at higher risk for developing a variety of stoma complications, including prolapse, parastomal hernia, and retraction. Conditions that increase intra-abdominal pressure also predispose the stoma to prolapse.

It is not uncommon for a pregnant woman to notice increased projection of the stoma during the last trimester of pregnancy. Surgery should be avoided at this time because after childbirth the stoma usually returns to its normal position along with a resumption of normal intra-abdominal pressure. Chronic coughing or straining is another condition that results in increased intra-abdominal pressure and therefore predisposes to stoma prolapse. Technical factors associated with stoma prolapse include improper placement, creation of an oversized opening, exteriorization of excess bowel, and failure to resect redundant intra-abdominal bowel (especially colon).

During the construction of a stoma strict attention to technical details is imperative. A common causative factor in the development of prolapse is improper location of the stoma site. If the stoma is located outside the rectus abdominis muscle, it is more prone to prolapse and herniation. In the series by Weaver et al.[6] parastomal hernia and prolapse were associated with an improperly sited stoma in 10 of 17 patients. Fleshman and Lewis[2] reported malpositioning of the stoma in 12% of patients with stoma prolapse.

Another technical factor that may encourage stoma prolapse is an oversized abdominal wall aperture. In most situations the aperture should admit the breadth of two fingers, generally corresponding to an opening 2 to 2.5 cm in diameter. An abdominal wall opening that is too large, especially in the presence of other predisposing factors, will lead to the development of prolapse. Extra care must be taken when forming an end-sigmoid colostomy for an obstructing distal lesion because the colon proximal to the obstruction will be very dilated. Although dilation and bowel wall edema rapidly resolve after diversion, the aperture usually is created larger than necessary to permit exteriorization of the divided colon. The tendency to create an oversized stoma must be avoided because it is both unnecessary and inadvisable.

The failure of fixation of the bowel mesentery at the level of the internal opening has been cited as a cause for prolapse. The rationale for this belief stems from the notion that inadequate fixation of the seromuscular coat of the bowel to the abdominal wall fascia will result in a predisposition to prolapse. This theory remains a debatable point, however, and is not universally accepted.[9,10] Although the stoma can be secured to the posterior rectus sheath and peritoneum or to the anterior rectus sheath, neither of these adjunctive maneuvers obviates stoma prolapse. Moreover, the use of seromuscular sutures for fascial fixation encourages subsequent fistula formation. Furthermore, the cut mesenteric edge can be secured to the lateral peritoneum. Although this measure might prevent internal hernia formation, it has never been proven to affect the incidence of stoma prolapse. To reiterate, it is not the number of levels through which the sutures are placed but the size and location of the aperture that influence the incidence of stoma prolapse.

Patients with spinal cord injuries sometimes require the creation of a colostomy. Arun et al.[11] reviewed the experience of ostomy prolapse in paraplegic patients in an acute spinal cord injury unit. They concluded that prolapse is more likely to occur in paraplegic patients with an injury at or above the T-10 level. The exact reason for this association is unknown.

PREVENTION

The single most important factor in the prevention of stoma prolapse is adherence to sound surgical technique. Technical aspects have a direct effect on the ultimate outcome of the stoma, its function, and its propensity for complications. Factors that directly affect the predilection for prolapse include the selection of the stoma site, the creation of the abdominal wall aperture, and the technique of exteriorization.

The ideal location for a stoma is a site away from bony prominences, skin creases, old scars, the umbilicus, the belt line, and future incision sites. The stoma should be brought out through the rectus abdominis muscle. Preoperative marking of the stoma site by an ET therapist allows for proper site selection.

Creation of an abdominal wall aperture that is too large is likely to lead to prolapse and herniation. This technical error can be obviated by following the "two-finger" rule. If the aperture accepts two fingers placed through the internal opening so that both interphalangeal joints are at the level of the skin defect, an adequate opening has been achieved.

For exteriorization of the bowel through the stoma site, attention should be directed toward creating a well-vascularized stoma. Bowel redundancy proximal to the stoma should be resected to lessen stoma prolapse. The spout should be of proper length after eversion and maturation: 2 cm for an ileostomy and $<$2 cm for a colostomy.

Whittaker and Goligher[12] favored the use of the extraperitoneal approach for the construction of the stoma. In their experience this technique was associated with a decreased incidence of complications, including prolapse, when compared to a standard intraperitoneal colostomy. However, despite the authors' enthusiasm, these differences were not statistically significant. Ein[13] reported his experience with the creation of a divided-loop colostomy in 13 infants by using a modification of the extraperitoneal approach. During the 3-year study period, no prolapse was observed. Galladay et al.[14] reported their experience with the use of a pursestring technique for the prevention of prolapse. They sutured the seromuscular layer of the stoma to the underlying fascia in a running pursestring fashion. No incidences of prolapse occurred in a series of 85 pediatric patients.

Clearly a variety of techniques are available for the creation of a stoma.

However, adherence to sound surgical judgment, proper selection of the site, creation of the aperture, exteriorization of the segment, and suture of the mucocutaneous junction will reduce the chances for stoma prolapse.

MANAGEMENT

The physician caring for the patient with stoma prolapse must decide which course of therapy to pursue. If the prolapse is minimal and asymptomatic, an expectant course is indicated. In addition, if the patient has significant comorbid diseases, the risks of surgery may outweigh the potential risks associated with ostomy prolapse. However, if the patient is a reasonable surgical candidate and nonoperative means fail, surgical options should be considered. There are two surgical approaches to the management of stoma prolapse: local parastomal procedures and intra-abdominal procedures. The choice of surgical procedure should be tailored to the individual patient and to the type of stoma.

Ileostomy

A variety of local techniques are available for the management of a prolapsed ileostomy. In the 1930s, before the popularization of the Brooke ileostomy technique, it was common practice to place a split-thickness skin graft on the exteriorized limb of bowel. Turnbull and Weakley[7] described the use of a split-thickness skin graft for the management of prolapse. This maneuver was based on the work of Dragstedt et al.,[15] who noticed that prolapse rarely occurred in those stomas that had been covered with a split-thickness skin graft. This procedure subsequently was abandoned after long-term follow-up revealed that stenosis was a common sequela. Sohn et al.[16] described a technique of bidirectional myotomy with meshed split-thickness skin grafts for ileostomy prolapse. The rationale for the myotomy was to reduce peristaltic activity in the stoma, thereby reducing motion and fixation and maximizing chances for skin graft. The authors described four patients in whom this technique was successfully used.

Local repair of the prolapse can be performed by dividing the mucocutaneous junction. Some advocate leaving a rim of mucosa on the skin of the mucocutaneous junction, thereby eliminating the need for further skin excision and further widening of the skin aperture. Others advocate excising only a small amount of parastomal skin with the mucocutaneous junction. Once mucocutaneous division is accomplished, the bowel is dissected and delivered through the skin aperture, thus eliminating any excess proximal redundancy. The redundant bowel is resected, and a new primarily everted stoma is created.

Nonabsorbable mesh can be secured around the stoma at the level of the posterior rectus sheath. However, this option is generally reserved for patients with concomitant parastomal hernias. Yet it is generally preferable to avoid mesh. Another possible surgical approach to the prolapsed ileostomy is laparotomy with relocation of the ileostomy. This option is usually reserved for patients with associated large parastomal hernias or patients for whom a local approach has already failed.

End Colostomy

Several options are available in the management of the prolapsed permanent end colostomy, including local revision and laparotomy with relocation. If the stoma is temporary, however, reestablishment of intestinal continuity may be preferable to surgical repair of the prolapse. If the stoma is permanent, local measures should be attempted whenever possible. Gauderer and Izant[17] described a technique of postreduction intraluminal bowel fixation. After reduction of the prolapsed segment, the reduced bowel is attached to the parietal peritoneum with the use of large U sutures several centimeters away from the stoma. These sutures are bolstered to the skin with latex tubing. The authors used this technique on four children with prolapsed colostomies.[17] An encirclement technique based on the Thiersch procedure was described by Krasna.[18] Krasna described the use of a pursestring suture technique to encircle the stoma; however, the results associated with this technique have been unimpressive.

Abulafi et al.[19] described a modification of the Delorme procedure for prolapsed colostomy. A mucosal dissection is performed, with a redundant seromuscular layer left behind. Several pleating sutures are placed in the muscular coat, precluding the need for resection. Abulafi et al. have performed this procedure on two patients with good results.

If there is a large parastomal hernia associated with the prolapse, local hernia repair should be performed at the time of prolapse repair. The fascial defect is identified, and a primary suture repair is performed. If the defect is too large for primary repair or if a previous local repair has failed, relocation of the stoma offers a superior alternative to mesh fixation or repeat primary fascial suture closure.

Loop Colostomy

As already mentioned, loop colostomies have a higher predilection for prolapse than do end colostomies. The prolapse usually occurs in the defunctionalized distal limb. The reason for this finding is unclear.

If there is a symptomatic prolapse of a temporary loop colostomy, the surgeon should evaluate the patient for stoma reversal. If deemed appropriate, reestablishment of intestinal continuity will correct the prolapse.

If stoma reversal is not appropriate or possible, correction of the prolapse is necessary. One option in the management of a prolapsed loop colostomy is to convert the loop to an end colostomy. After a parastomal incision has been made, the stoma is mobilized from the mucocutaneous junction. After the loop colostomy has been divided, the redundant colon is resected; an end colostomy is created. Several options are available for the management of the distal limb. A mucous fistula can be created either at the stoma site or at a separate site. Alternatively, the distal limb can be left as a long Hartmann's pouch either in the abdomen or in the subcutaneous parastomal space.

When a large parastomal hernia is associated with the prolapse, the same options apply as with the end colostomy. The surgeon must choose between a local direct fascial repair and stoma relocation.

Incarceration

A more difficult situation arises when the patient has an incarcerated prolapsed stoma. Attempts at reduction usually are fraught with failure because of the edema and patient anxiety. Myers and Rothenberger[20] have described a nonoperative approach for the management of this condition. By sprinkling sugar on the incarcerated segment, the amount of edema is decreased, thereby allowing reduction of the prolapsed limb.

If vascular compromise is associated with gangrene of the prolapsed limb, reduction should not be attempted, and an emergency laparotomy should be performed. The compromised bowel should be resected, and a new stoma should be created at a new location. When gangrenous changes are limited to the extracorporeal intestine and peritonitis is absent, a parastomal approach may be used if a well-vascularized stoma can be created.

SUMMARY

Ostomy prolapse is a common complication after colostomy or ileostomy construction. Presentation may range from asymptomatic protrusion to incarceration with vascular compromise. A variety of surgical options is available for the management of this condition. The physician caring for the ostomy patient with prolapse must be aware of all of these options.

The surgeon who creates stomas must adhere to the basic surgical principles of stoma construction. Prolapse is one of the stoma-associated complications that is directly related to the surgical technique. Prevention, therefore, is preferable to treatment of this often avoidable complication.

REFERENCES

1. Gordon PH, Nivatvongs S. Principles and Practice of Surgery for the Colon, Rectum, and Anus. St. Louis: Quality Medical Publishing, 1992, p 873.
2. Fleshman JW, Lewis MG. Complications and quality of life after stoma surgery: A review of 16,470 patients in the UOA Data Registry. Semin Colon Rectal Surg 2:2, 66-72, 1991.
3. Chandler JG, Evans BP. Colostomy prolapse. Surgery 4:84, 1978.
4. Allen-Mersh TG, Thomson JPS. Surgical treatment of colostomy complications. Br J Surg 5:75, 1988.
5. Watts JM, DeDombal FT, Goligher JC. Long-term complications and prognosis following major surgery for ulcerative colitis. Br J Surg 53:1014, 1966.
6. Weaver RM, Alexander-Williams J, Keighley MR. Indications and outcome of reoperation for ileostomy complications in inflammatory bowel disease. Int J Colorectal Dis 1:3, 1988.
7. Turnbull RB, Weakley FL. Atlas of Intestinal Stomas. St. Louis: CV Mosby, 1967, pp 131-199.
8. Pearl RK, Prasad ML, Tan AB. Loop stomas: Indications, techniques for construction, take-down, and management of complications. Semin Colon Rectal Surg 2:2, 1991.
9. Corman ML. Colon and Rectal Surgery. Philadelphia: JB Lippincott, 1989, p 894.
10. Fazio VW. Complications of intestinal stomas. In Ferrari BT, Ray JE, Gathright JB. Complications of Colon and Rectal Surgery: Prevention and Management. Philadelphia: WB Saunders, 1985, pp 227-250.
11. Arun H, Ledgerwood A, Lucas CE. Ostomy prolapse in paraplegic patients: Etiology, prevention, and treatment. J Am Paraplegia Soc 2:13, 1990.
12. Whittaker M, Goligher JC. A comparison of the results of extraperitoneal and intraperitoneal techniques for construction of terminal ileac colostomies. Dis Colon Rectum 3:19, 1976.
13. Ein SH. Divided loop colostomy that does not prolapse. Am J Surg 2:147, 1984.
14. Galladay ES, Bernay F, Wagner CW. Prevention of prolapse in pediatric enterostomas with purse string technique. J Pediatr Surg 9:25, 1990.
15. Dragstedt LR, Dack GM, Kirsner JB. Chronic ulcerative colitis: A summary of evidence implicating bacterium necrophorum as an etiologic agent. Ann Surg 114:653, 1941.
16. Sohn N, Sculman N, Weinstein MA, Robbins RD. Ileostomy prolapse repair utilizing bidirectional myotomy and a meshed split-thickness skin graft. Am J Surg 6:145, 1983.
17. Gauderer MW, Izant RJ Jr. A technique for temporary control of colostomy prolapse in children. J Pediatr Surg 6:20, 1985.
18. Krasna IH. A simple purse string suture technique for treatment of colostomy prolapse and intussusception. J Pediatr Surg 14:801-802, 1979.
19. Abulafi AM, Sherman IW, Fiddian RV. Delorme operation for prolapsed colostomy. Br J Surg 12:76, 1989.
20. Myers JO, Rothenberger DA. Sugar in the reduction of incarcerated prolapsed bowel: Report of two cases. Dis Colon Rectum 5:34, 1991.

17 MANAGEMENT OF INTESTINAL FISTULAS

W. Douglas Wong and W. Donald Buie

Few complications of gastrointestinal surgery are as disturbing to both surgeon and patient as a postoperative external intestinal fistula. For the surgeon it implies a possible failure in judgment or an aberration in surgical technique. It presents an immediate and often formidable challenge to (1) stabilize the patient by correcting the effects of sepsis, fluid and electrolyte or acid-base imbalance, and any nutritional problems, (2) gain control of the fistula, and (3) achieve eventual closure and integrity of the gastrointestinal tract. For the patient the grim prospect of a protracted, highly morbid illness with a long, costly hospitalization and the potential for mortality is compounded by the psychologic trauma and abhorrence of stool draining from the abdomen.

Such patients are best managed by a multidisciplinary team approach that includes the surgeon, the internist and/or gastroenterologist, the ET nurse, and a dedicated general nursing staff. This team must be cognizant of the metabolic, septic, nutritional, and wound care consequences of such a fistula. The team members must direct care aggressively in order to prevent mortality, which, in general, has declined in recent years to less than 20% because of improved multidisciplinary care.[1]

The focus of this chapter is the management of enterocutaneous fistulas, including those originating from the duodenum, jejunum, ileum, and colon, with emphasis given to those originating from the small intestine. A four-phase management plan is outlined to address both nonoperative and surgical management, including the rationale, indications, timing, and decision-making for definitive surgery.

CLASSIFICATION

External fistulas can be classified by several different methods. In addition to forming a rational basis for discussion, classification systems are useful in predicting the morbidity and mortality associated with a specific fistula and the probability of spontaneous closure. For purposes of this discussion, fistulas are classified on an anatomic basis as simple or complex (see box). Simple fistulas have a short tract that is in direct communication with the skin but has no septic focus and no other organ involvement (Fig. 17-1). Complex fistulas can be divided into two types. *Complex type 1 fistulas* are those that are associated with an abscess or that have multiorgan involve-

ANATOMIC CLASSIFICATION OF FISTULAS

Simple
- Short, direct tract
- No associated abscess
- No other organ involvement

Complex
- Type 1
  - Associated with abscess
  - Multiple organ involvement
- Type 2
  - Opens into base of disrupted wound

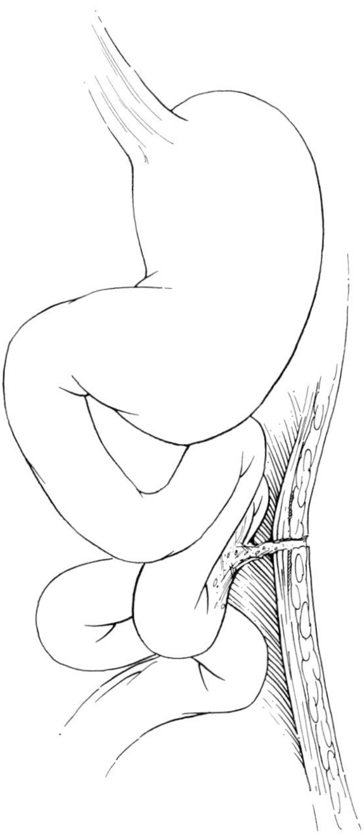

Fig. 17-1. Simple enterocutaneous fistula.

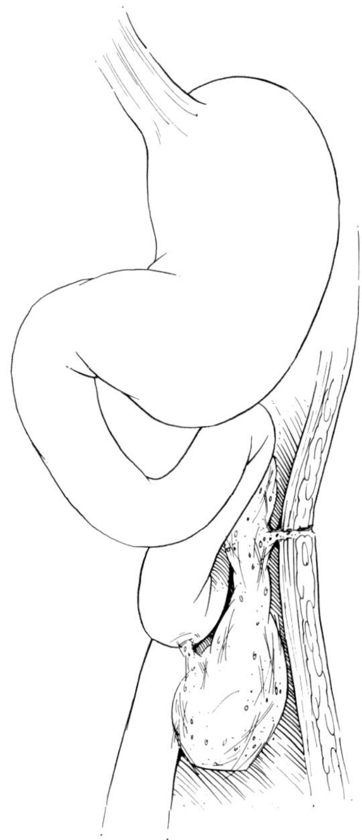

Fig. 17-2. Complex type 1 fistula with associated abscess.

ment (Fig. 17-2). *Complex type 2 fistulas* are those that open into the base of a disrupted wound (exposed fistula) (Fig. 17-3). By their nature, complex fistulas are associated with higher rates of morbidity and mortality as well as a lower rate of spontaneous closure.[1-4]

All fistulas, whether simple or complex, may be divided into two groups based on the site of intestinal origin. Fistulas that arise in the upper small bowel generally are associated with a higher morbidity and mortality and a lower rate of spontaneous closure when compared to those originating from the large intestine.[3]

Fistula output relates directly to the site of origin. Fistulas of the large bowel almost always have low output, whereas those of the small bowel can have either low or high output.[5] Most authors use 200 cc/24 hr as the distinction between high- and low-output fistulas.[1] However, not all authors agree with this distinction, and some use 500 cc/24 hr to define high- vs. low-output fistulas.[5]

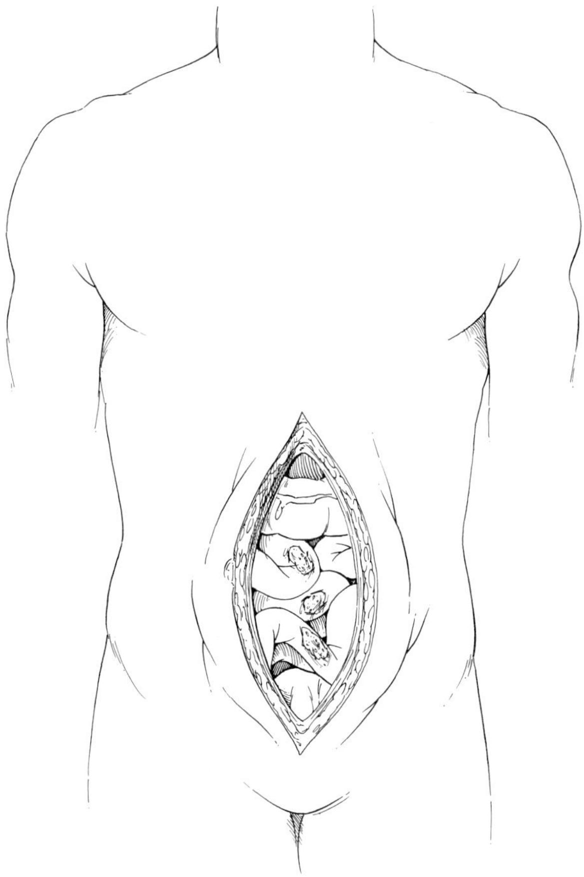

Fig. 17-3. Complex type 2 fistula with multiple fistulous openings associated with a large abdominal wall defect.

ETIOLOGY

Acquired enterocutaneous fistulas may occur either postoperatively or spontaneously (see box on p. 282). Postoperative fistulas are much more common, comprising well over 90% in some series.[6] They are primarily caused by anastomotic breakdown.[7] These fistulas are largely preventable if basic surgical principles of anastomotic construction are observed, including adequate blood supply, lack of tension, and good suture technique. Intrinsic intestinal disease and characteristics of individual patients also contribute to the occurrence of postoperative fistula. Incidental intestinal injury during lysis of adhesions figures prominently in several series.[1,6,8-10]

Less common are the spontaneous causes secondary to either intrinsic intestinal disease or external trauma. Inflammatory bowel disease is pres-

ETIOLOGY OF ACQUIRED ENTEROCUTANEOUS FISTULAS

- I. Postoperative occurrence
  - A. Anastomotic problems
    - 1. Technical factors
      - a. Tension
      - b. Blood supply
      - c. Technique
    - 2. Intestinal factors
      - a. Inflammation
      - b. Ischemia
      - c. Malignancy
      - d. Infection
    - 3. Systemic factors
      - a. Malnutrition
      - b. Steroids
      - c. Malignancy (including chemotherapy and x-ray therapy)
      - d. Systemic disease (diabetes, renal failure)
  - B. Incidental injury
    - 1. Lysis of adhesions
- II. Spontaneous occurrence
  - A. Intrinsic disease
    - 1. Inflammation (inflammatory bowel disease, diverticulosis)
    - 2. Malignancy
    - 3. Infection (tuberculosis, actinomycosis, amoebiasis)
    - 4. Ischemia (embolus, thrombosis, low flow)
    - 5. Foreign body
    - 6. Collagen vascular disease
    - 7. Radiation
  - B. Extrinsic disease
    - 1. Trauma
    - 2. Other organ

ently the most common cause of spontaneous enterocutaneous fistulas. These fistulas are difficult to treat and usually are very resistant to spontaneous closure.[7,8]

MORBIDITY AND MORTALITY

The morbidity and mortality associated with intestinal fistulas depend on the type of fistula, its etiology, and individual patient characteristics. These factors explain in part the differences in morbidity and mortality rates between selected series, which to a large degree reflect the caseloads and referral patterns of individual institutions.[11]

Morbidity from intestinal fistulas is difficult to quantitate. It arises primarily from fluid and electrolyte imbalance, sepsis, malnutrition, and the local effects of corrosive small bowel fluid on skin.[11] These physiologic derangements, which are all interrelated, are central to an understanding of the pathophysiology of fistulas. Large volume losses of electrolyte and protein-rich secretions combined with third-space losses secondary to surgical trauma and infection cause rapid fluid shifts, upsetting general homeostasis. Sepsis, which is commonly associated with enterocutaneous fistulas, may arise from either a localized abscess or continuous gastrointestinal contamination. Sepsis has far-reaching effects on all organ systems and contributes to poor wound healing, poor nutritional status, and multiple system organ failure. Malnutrition, in turn, contributes to fistula formation and poor wound healing and increases the patient's susceptibility to infection.

In addition, the physical and emotional effects of a serious complication requiring prolonged hospitalization and often additional surgical procedures cannot be overlooked. Iatrogenic morbidity occurs primarily from central venous catheters used for nutrition and includes complications of insertion, septicemia, phlebitis/thrombosis, and hyperglycemia from hypertonic glucose solutions.[6]

Mortality rates from intestinal fistulas have declined in recent years, but they remain relatively high, ranging from 6%[5,8] to 23% in some series.[1,4,7] As already mentioned, this disparity is caused largely by differences in patient populations. In a recent series Schein and Decker[12] reported a 37% mortality rate in high-output postoperative small bowel fistulas despite modern supportive therapy.

In a classic paper Edmunds et al.[13] noted that mortality was related to three factors: fluid and electrolyte imbalance, malnutrition, and sepsis. Fluid and electrolyte imbalance is primarily related to fistula output. Initially 35% to 40% of patients with fistulas have severe fluid and electrolyte disturbance and acid-base imbalance.[11] The effluent from high-output fistulas originating close to the ligament of Treitz is made up largely of pancreatic and biliary secretions, which contain high concentrations of sodium and bicarbonate. As a consequence, fistulas arising in the upper small bowel are associated with a higher morbidity and mortality and a lower rate of spontaneous closure than those originating from the large intestine.[3] In a series reported by Fazio et al.[4] the mortality rate for high-output fistulas was 31%, as opposed to 5% in low-output fistulas.

The importance of malnutrition was demonstrated in 1964 by Chapman et al.,[14] who found that patients who received <3000 cal/day had a 55% mortality rate, whereas those who received >3000 cal/day had a mortality rate of only 12%. The absence of food intake for several days (especially during the postoperative period), the hypercatabolism of sepsis with the breakdown of lean body mass, and the loss of hypertonic protein-rich secretions from the fistula all contribute to malnutrition. Under normal circumstances the intestinal secretions are digested and the amino acids are resorbed and resynthesized into protein. When a fistula is present, most of these secretions are lost.

Uncontrolled sepsis remains the most common cause of death in patients with enterocutaneous fistulas and contributes to a high rate of associated complications. In most series it accounts for approximately 70% of all deaths.[3,12,15,16] Altomare et al.[15] found that 54% of septic patients died, in contrast to 14% of nonseptic patients. Similarly Reber et al.[6] described mortality rates of 85% in patients in whom sepsis was uncontrolled vs. 8% in patients with controlled sepsis. Such patients are often postoperative and in a state of immunosuppression from surgery. If there has been an anastomotic disruption, devitalized tissue is present, forming a nidus for abscess formation with continued contamination from the gastrointestinal tract.

Fistula etiology is also predictive of mortality. Fistulas associated with malignancy and radiation have a high mortality rate.[16,17] Patients with fistulas arising from inflammatory bowel disease have a lower mortality rate,[18] yet this rate is higher than that for simple postoperative anastomotic fistulas (simple type 1), which have the lowest associated mortality.[3,4]

Many other factors contribute to the high mortality rate associated with fistulas. Advancing age often has been related to a higher mortality rate; however, this connection has not been consistently demonstrated.[15] Many significant risk factors are associated with increasing age, and the presence or absence of these risk factors may be more important than chronologic age in determining outcome. Patients with malignancy who develop an unrelated fistula have an increased mortality rate.[15,16] Anemia and hypoalbuminemia also have been implicated, with associated mortality rates of 31% and 42%, respectively.[15,17] Perhaps the greatest risk factor for increased mortality is the presence of an open fistula (complex type 2), which drains into the base of an incision. Mortality rates in this situation range from 50% to 60% and have not improved significantly, even with advances in supportive care.[3,12,17]

In 1989 Levy et al.[2] developed a risk score that correlated eight so-called severity factors: multiple fistulas, intra-abdominal abscess, septicemia, ileus, adult respiratory distress syndrome, upper gastrointestinal hemorrhage, renal or hepatic failure, and thromboembolic complications. They found that any patient with three or more of these factors has a mortality rate of 50%.

REASONS FOR NONCLOSURE

Many factors contribute to the persistence of an intestinal fistula. The most important of these are (1) undrained sepsis (Fig. 17-4), (2) distal obstruction (Fig. 17-5), and (3) underlying disease (e.g., Crohn's disease, radiation-induced bowel injury, and malignancy) (Fig. 17-6).

Other potential factors are separation of the bowel ends (Fig. 17-7), a short (<2 cm) fistula tract (Fig. 17-8), a foreign body, a bowel wall defect >1 cm in diameter, and epithelialization of the tract (Fig. 17-9).[19-22] Reber et al.[6] have

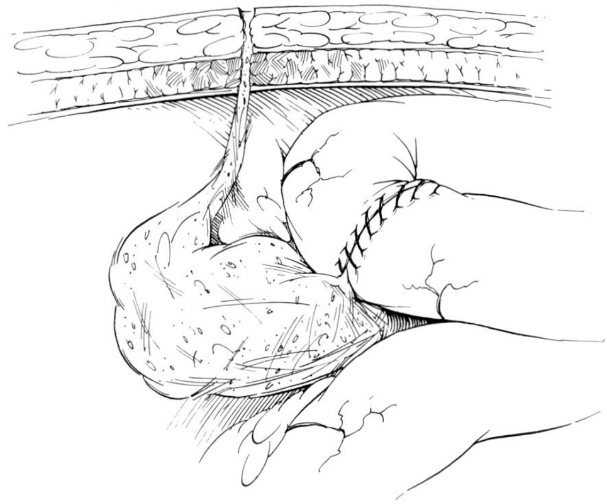

Fig. 17-4. Underlying sepsis can be a reason for nonclosure.

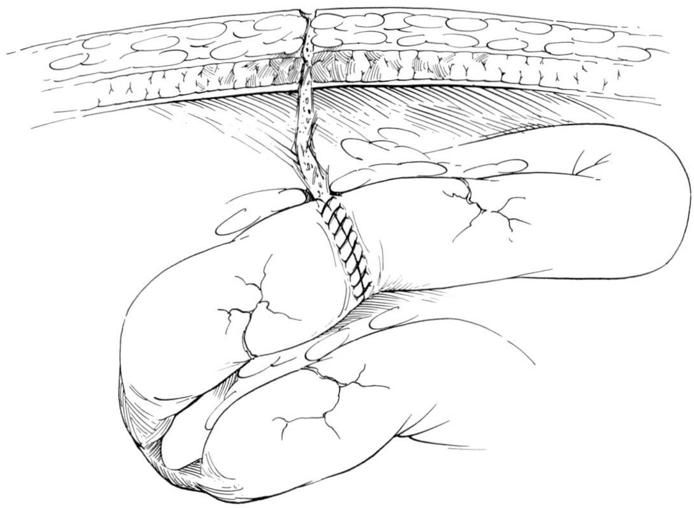

Fig. 17-5. Distal obstruction may inhibit closure of a fistula.

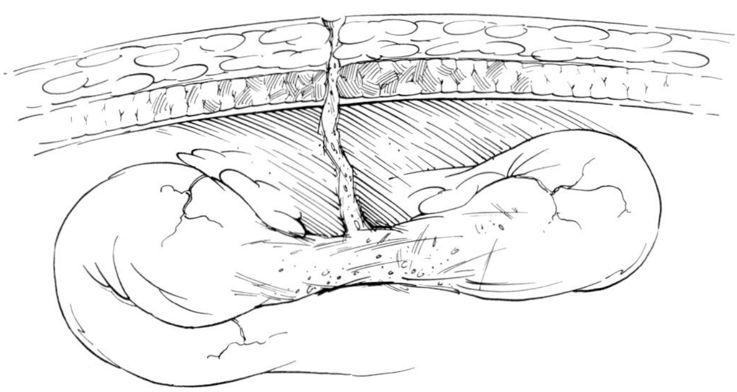

Fig. 17-6. Underlying bowel disease may be a reason for nonclosure.

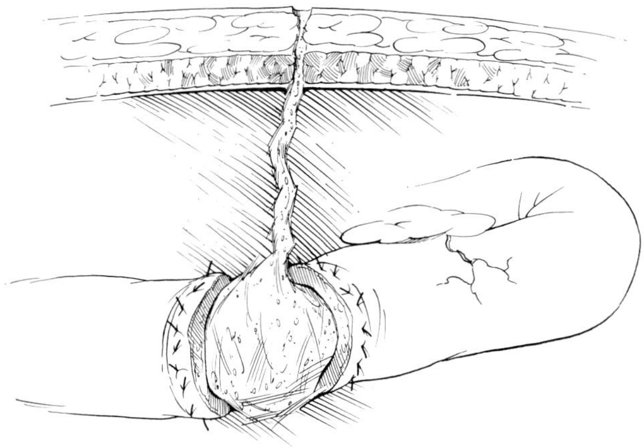

Fig. 17-7. A disrupted anastomosis as a reason for nonclosure.

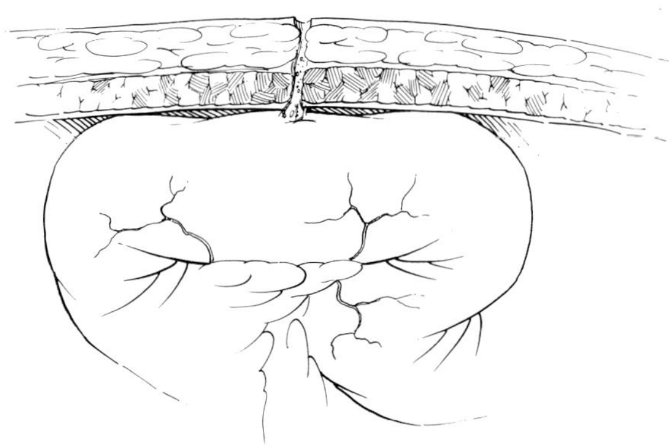

Fig. 17-8. A short tract may explain failure of a fistula to close spontaneously.

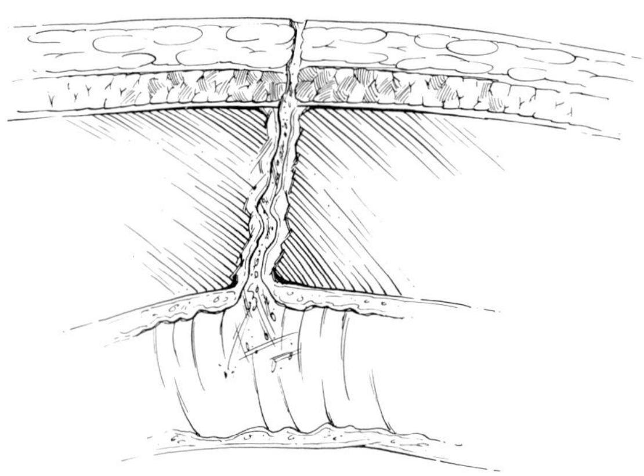

Fig. 17-9. Epithelialization of the tract may prohibit spontaneous closure.

reported that in the absence of mitigating factors, the spontaneous closure rate is 32%. They also stated that once sepsis has been controlled 90% of fistulas that close spontaneously do so within 1 month. Persistent sepsis, however, affected closure rate significantly. In those patients whose sepsis was controlled within 1 month, 48% of fistulas closed spontaneously with an 8% mortality, compared to a 6% closure rate and 85% mortality when sepsis was not controlled.

Hugh et al.[23] have stressed that distal obstruction with adhesions or abscess is a critical factor in fistula persistence. The fistula acts as a vent, and because the obstruction is usually partial, the diagnosis is often difficult to confirm. Of 93 patients with colovesical fistula reported on by Fazio et al.,[24] 38 (41%) had persistent distal obstruction as a contributing factor.

Persistence of underlying disease is responsible for nonclosure of many fistulas. In a study of enterocutaneous fistulas in patients who underwent surgery for Crohn's disease, 6 of 7 patients with no active disease had closure with conservative management, whereas only 1 of 20 patients with documented active disease had spontaneous closure.[18] In the series by Reber et al.,[6] when an enteric fistula was associated with Crohn's disease, only 8% of fistulas closed spontaneously. When abdominal irradiation was a factor, only 14% of fistulas healed with conservative treatment.

McIntyre et al.[5] have presented data suggesting that (1) a postoperative fistula is more likely to close than a spontaneously occurring one (26% vs. 17%), (2) a simple fistula is more likely to close than a complex one (37% vs. 15%), and (3) surprisingly, a high-volume fistula is just as likely to close as a low-volume fistula (25% vs. 28%).

MANAGEMENT

The management of patients with intestinal fistulas can be very challenging and requires a team approach. Treatment can be divided into four phases: stabilization, investigation, conservative treatment, and decision/definitive surgery.

Phase 1: Stabilization

At the time of fistula presentation, patients are often in the postoperative period and have been without adequate nutrition for several days. Prior to the discharge of intestinal contents from either a drain site or a surgical wound, clinical progress usually has been poor. The combination of third-space losses from inflammation and fistula discharge rapidly depletes the patient's intravascular volume. The first priority in this situation is the immediate restoration of intravascular volume with crystalloid, colloid, and blood (when appropriate) to establish tissue perfusion and adequate urine output.

The patient must be evaluated to determine whether immediate surgery is necessary. Emergency surgery carries a high mortality (55%)[2] and should be performed for only three reasons: a septic focus requiring surgical drainage, uncontrolled hemorrhage, or evisceration. If an abscess has been identified and is approachable through the abdominal wall, percutaneous drainage should be considered (Fig. 17-10). After localization through CT scanning or ultrasound, a needle is introduced into the cavity, the contents are aspirated, and a sample is sent for aerobic and anaerobic culture. Water-soluble contrast can be injected at this time to delineate the site of origin before draining the abscess.[25] The latter is accomplished with either a catheter introduced by the Seldinger technique or through a local procedure. In the septic patient every effort should be made to identify and drain all abscesses. Uncontrolled sepsis in a patient in whom an abscess is suspected but cannot be identified may require a formal laparotomy if the patient's condition continues to deteriorate. The importance of surgical intervention to control sepsis has been emphasized by Reber et al.,[6] who found that, in patients who required surgery to control sepsis, 90% eventually achieved spontaneous closure. When laparotomy is necessary for control of sepsis, no attempt should be made to definitively repair the fistula; instead, proximal diversion along with drainage of the abscess should be performed and definitive repair should be reserved for when the patient has been restored to health (Fig. 17-11).

Antibiotics should be reserved for patients who are septic. Patients who are not septic and who have a simple fistula tract (without associated abscess) do not require antimicrobial therapy. The administration of antibiotics in no way obviates the need for adequate surgical drainage. Initial use should be empiric, covering intestinal organisms such as coliforms, *Bacteroides,* and enterococci. Prior to initiation of treatment, fistula drainage should be Gram-stained and cultured to determine bacterial flora and sensitivities. The average number of antibiotics used in a series by Soeters et al.[1] over the course of fistula therapy was six to eight. Thus indiscriminate use of antibiotics will select out organisms with high levels of antibiotic resistance.

Early in this initial management phase, attempts should be made to diminish intestinal output. This approach not only decreases the fluid and electrolyte losses experienced by the patient but makes wound and skin care easier. All patients should have NPO designation, not only to decrease luminal contents but to decrease gastrointestinal stimulation and pancreaticobiliary secretion. In addition, all patients should be given H_2 antagonists to prevent stress erosions and to decrease gastric secretions. In 1978 Reber et al.[6] demonstrated a 60% decrease in fistula output with the addition of IV cimetidine.

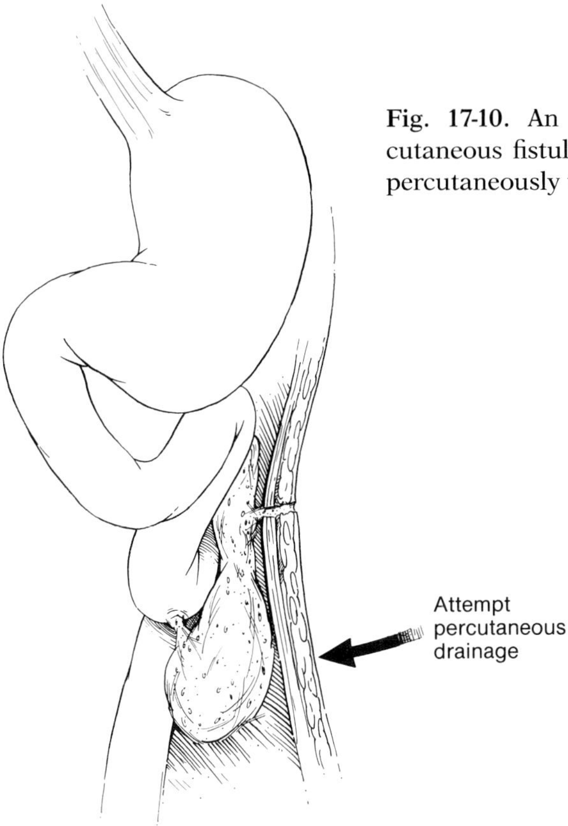

Fig. 17-10. An abscess associated with an enterocutaneous fistula (complex type 1) should be drained percutaneously whenever feasible.

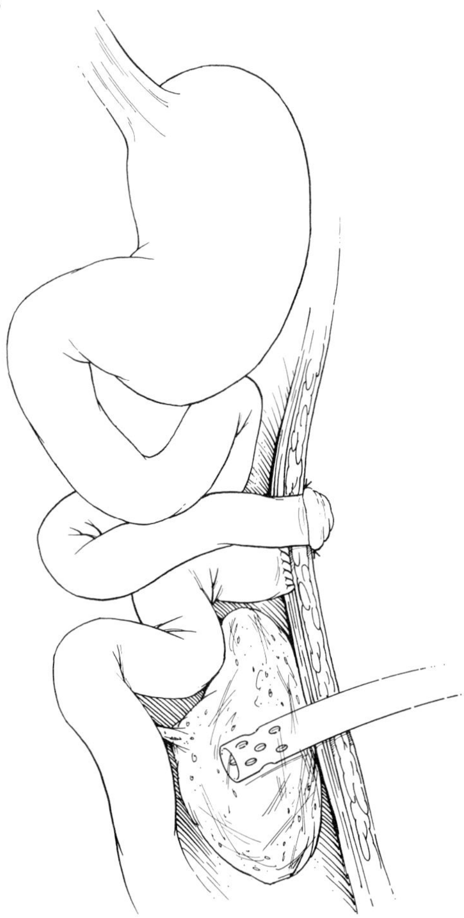

Fig. 17-11. When percutaneous drainage fails (or is not technically feasible) for complex type 1 fistulas, a laparotomy with drainage of abscess plus proximal diversion should be performed.

This method can be extremely helpful in decreasing drainage from high-output fistulas from the upper gastrointestinal tract.

Several studies have shown that nasogastric tubes do not increase the closure rate of fistulas.[1,8] The use of such tubes should be restricted to patients with partial small bowel obstruction. Long-term use can be detrimental, causing erosions, bleeding, and late strictures.[9] If a patient is expected to have prolonged postoperative ileus, consideration should be given to placing a gastric tube.

Wound and skin care. During the stabilization phase of fistula management, early attention must be directed at wound and skin care. Many of the complications of enteric contents eroding the abdominal wall can be minimized by early intervention. A skilled and knowledgeable ET nurse working with a dedicated general nursing team is invaluable. Efforts should be directed toward abdominal wall–fistula management, containment of the effluent, and patient support. For a comprehensive discussion of this aspect of management, the reader is referred to Chapter 18.

Phase 2: Investigation

Once the patient has been resuscitated and stabilized and the sepsis has been controlled, the fistula must be investigated to determine (1) the course and origin of the fistula tract, (2) the presence of a persistent abscess, (3) the condition of the adjacent bowel, and (4) the presence of distal obstruction or discontinuity. The best means of evaluating a fistula is a fistulogram. The fistulogram is done with the use of a soft-tip catheter (e.g., Foley) or a pediatric feeding tube (if the skin opening is small). Leakage of contrast material onto the skin is prevented by inflating the Foley balloon. A water-soluble contrast material is used, and it should be injected gently to prevent rupture. Once the origin of the fistula has been determined, either an upper gastrointestinal and small bowel follow-through or a barium enema should be performed to visualize the adjacent bowel and rule out distal obstruction. The choice of study depends on the level of fistula origin.[26]

The role of CT scanning in the initial evaluation of a fistula tract is limited to the identification of an associated abscess and, occasionally, to delineate three-dimensional anatomy. CT scanning also may help to define the extent, nature, and location of underlying disease.[27] CT is most useful for reevaluating patients who are not responding to conservative treatment when an inflammatory process is suspected.[26] Other examinations, such as cystoscopy and intravenous pyelography, are used as necessary if other organ systems are involved.

Phase 3: Conservative Treatment

Total parenteral nutrition. The development of total parenteral nutrition (TPN) has revolutionized the treatment of enterocutaneous fistulas.[28] In 1972 Wolfe et al.[29] demonstrated that TPN decreased the output of experimental enterocutaneous fistulas by 93%. Subsequent clinical studies have confirmed this figure.[8] However, the effect of TPN on spontaneous closure rate is less clear. Most authors claim slightly improved rates of spontaneous closure with TPN.[1,6,8] This association has led some authors to believe that spontaneous closure is primarily a function of fistula etiology, anatomy, and associated sepsis.[4] Disagreement also exists about the effect of TPN on mortality. Uncontrolled sepsis is still the most common cause of mortality, and TPN does not alleviate this problem.[1] The improvement in mortality rates over the past 20 years also may be attributed to the general improvement in other forms of supportive care. Undoubtedly, the greatest contribution TPN has made, as stated by Reber et al.,[6] is the simplification of nutritional management for patients with enterocutaneous fistulas. TPN has allowed better timing for operative intervention when required, improved the nutritional status of patients undergoing reoperation, and increased the rate of postoperative recovery.

TPN should be started early, after volume, electrolyte, and clotting deficits have been corrected and sepsis is under control. It is administered through a central venous catheter, most commonly placed in the subclavian vein. The nutritional goal is 30 to 40 kcal/kg/day with a calorie-nitrogen ratio of 150:1. Approximately 0.25 to 0.35 g of nitrogen/kg body weight/day is necessary to maintain a positive nitrogen balance. Lipid emulsion (250 ml of 20% solution) should be given 3 days a week to increase the caloric density and to prevent essential fatty acid deficiency. It may be given daily with a concomitant reduction in glucose solution in patients with diabetes, congestive heart failure, and chronic obstructive pulmonary disease to decrease the glucose load, the volume of administration, and carbon dioxide production. In addition, trace elements, multivitamins, and vitamin K must be given weekly.

Initially patients must be watched closely for fluid and electrolyte balance by monitoring daily weights, hydration status, and serum electrolyte levels. All electrolytes can be replaced through TPN, except for large amounts of calcium and phosphate, which may be limited by solubility. The potassium level may fluctuate markedly, and since replacement solutions are limited to 80 mEq/L, either use of a supplemental line or oral administration may be required. Magnesium, an important electrolyte for energy-requiring processes, is often overlooked.[25] Low levels of magnesium are associated with large gastrointestinal fluid losses and may make hypocalcemia resistant to treatment.

Enteral nutrition. TPN has become the mainstay of nutritional therapy for patients with enterocutaneous fistulas; however, enteral nutrition also may play a role. Complete nutritional support with enteral feeding is possible in selected patients. In most cases TPN is necessary initially to stabilize the patient and to establish positive nitrogen balance. Often TPN must be continued to maintain an anabolic state because only a portion of the necessary calories can be given enterally.

Enteral nutrition in the form of low-residue diets has been shown experimentally[29] and clinically[30] to significantly decrease fistula output, although to a lesser extent than TPN. Low-residue diets are relatively low in cost, simple to administer, and require very little special equipment or preparation. In addition, they help to preserve gut integrity.[31] Unfortunately, low-residue diets have limited application in gastroduodenal and upper small bowel fistulas unless the diet can be delivered to a point distal to the fistula. With distal small bowel or colonic fistulas, low-residue diets may be tolerated quite well because an adequate length of small bowel will affect complete absorption. At least 4 feet of functioning bowel must exist between the ligament of Treitz and the fistula or between the fistula and the ileocecal valve to allow adequate absorption.

Low-residue diets should not be used in patients with sepsis or peritonitis. Adynamic ileus, intra-abdominal abscess, and distal obstruction also must be ruled out prior to the initiation of enteral feeding. The diet can be administered through a nasogastric tube, a nasoduodenal tube, a feeding jejunostomy, or a needle-catheter jejunostomy (elemental diets only). Tube placement always should be checked either visually (at surgery) or radiographically before feeding is started.

Elemental or low-residue diets are hyperosmolar and should be administered by continuous infusion to minimize cramping and dumping. Initially the diet should be diluted to half-strength and administered at a rate of 50 cc/hr because the upper small bowel cannot tolerate hyperosmolar infusion. When the small bowel is being used, the rate should be increased before osmolarity. In some patients the small bowel may not tolerate more than half-strength enteral feed, and supplemental TPN will be required.[31]

Very few series have involved the use of enteral nutrition exclusively. Bury et al.[30] reported a 54% spontaneous closure rate and a 14% to 80% decrease in fistula output. Voitk et al.[32] reported a 75% spontaneous closure and a fistula-related mortality rate of 16%.

Somatostatin. Several studies have described the use of somatostatin in patients with enterocutaneous fistulas to decrease fistula output.[33-35] The proposed mechanism of action is a reduction in gastrointestinal secretions, primarily through the inhibition of gastrin, gastric acid, biliary flow, pancreatic output, and intestinal secretions. Somatostatin also is believed to inhibit gastrointestinal motility, thus increasing intestinal transit time.[34]

In a review of 175 patients treated with native somatostatin and TPN, the overall spontaneous closure rate was 78% with a mean closure time of 7 days.[34] However, side effects with native somatostatin are numerous; they include hyperglycemia and rebound phenomena upon discontinuation of the drug. Somatostatin analog has demonstrated neither of these side effects. Nubiola et al.[34] treated 27 patients with enterocutaneous fistulas by using somatostatin 201-995 analog. Within 24 hours of administration, fistula output was dramatically reduced (mean reduction of 55%). Of 27 patients, 21 experienced spontaneous closure at a mean of 6 days (3 to 10 days). All six failures involved high-output fistulas; one patient died of continued sepsis, and the remaining five had an anatomic reason for nonclosure demonstrated at surgery (three complete anastomotic disruptions and two distal obstructions). Mean spontaneous closure in a previous group of patients treated with TPN alone was 3 to 5 weeks. The most encouraging results occurred with high-output small bowel fistulas in which the addition of somatostatin increased the spontaneous closure rate from 50% to 90%.

Somatostatin analog seems to be most effective in postoperative, high-output fistulas. Its primary effect seems to be shortening of the time to closure. It has no effect on fistulas that are anatomically incapable of closure and does not appear to be effective in the treatment of fistulas related to intrinsic intestinal disease such as Crohn's disease and ulcerative colitis.[36]

Fibrin glue. Many different substances have been injected into fistula tracts to obliterate them. Cyanoacrylate glue, prolamine, and, most recently, fibrin glue all have been used.[37-39] The most successful agent to date appears to be fibrin glue. It is applied endoscopically if the internal origin can be visualized. The tract is irrigated clear, and the patient is given preoperative and postoperative antibiotics. Aprotinin, a fibrinolysis inhibitor, is added to the solution to reduce enzymatic breakdown. In 1990 Eleftheriadis et al.[39] reported on seven patients with high-volume postoperative enterocutaneous fistulas who were treated through endoscopic application of fibrin glue in the second postoperative week. There were no complications, and an average of 2.4 sessions were required to close the fistulas. The mechanism of action appears to center around the ability of fibrin to induce a cellular response to injury and to assist in neovascularization and fibroblast proliferation.

When the intestinal opening cannot be identified, the tract can be visualized percutaneously by using a flexible endoscope, as described by Lange et al.[38] in 1990. Eighty-three patients were prepared with systemic antibiotics, and the fistula tracts were irrigated with streptokinase and streptodornase. The endoscope or fistuloscope was advanced along the fistula tract, and fibrin glue was injected to obliterate it. Of 48 patients who underwent a gastroscopic or colonoscopic approach, 36 had successful occlusion of their fistulas. An additional 16 of 35 patients had successful closure after fistuloscopy and percutaneous obliteration. One patient died of air embolism, and another patient had pneumoperitoneum secondary to air insufflation. Air insufflation is not currently performed because the tracts usually are mature enough to remain open for visualization. Patients with an opening >2 cm in diameter or extensive necrotic masses were excluded from treatment. Treatment failure occurred in fistulas <1 cm long, fistulas arising in irradiated tissue, fistulas associated with active Crohn's disease, and fistulas that could not be completely obliterated with sealant.

Fistula obliteration with fibrin glue is a promising new option for the nonoperative treatment of fistulas. Whether it should be used in conjunction with other conservative therapy or reserved for high-risk patients who have failed conservative therapy remains to be determined.

Outcome of conservative therapy. Overall, spontaneous closure can be anticipated in 60% to 70% of fistulas,[3,6,7,16] depending on anatomy, etiology, and concurrent sepsis. Simple type 1 fistulas have the highest success rate, with reported closure rates approximating 90%.[3] In contrast, complex type 2 fistulas have the lowest rate of spontaneous closure, at less than 10%.[2,3] Fistulas arising secondary to intrinsic disease processes also have very low rates of spontaneous closure when compared to postoperative fistulas. Reber et al.[6] reported spontaneous closure rates of only 8%, 26%, and 14% in patients with Crohn's disease, cancer, and radiation, respectively. Similar results were reported by Rose et al.[16]

Fistulas occurring in patients with Crohn's disease can be subdivided into two types according to etiology.[18] Those fistulas secondary to spontaneous extension of active disease have a very low rate of spontaneous closure (10%), whereas those occurring secondary to leakage of an anastomosis usually close with conservative management (86%).

Phase 4: Decision/Definitive Surgery

Indications and timing of definitive surgery

Simple and complex type 1 fistulas. It cannot be overemphasized that control of sepsis must be the number one priority in the management of an enterocutaneous fistula. Control of sepsis must be undertaken as soon as it is recognized during the course of management and must be sought and treated in phase 1 and/or phase 2 of management. Definitive surgery for the fistula should not be attempted at this time. Once sepsis has been controlled, a persistently draining fistula in a sepsis-free environment for 6 to 8 weeks constitutes an indication for definitive surgical repair of simple and/or complex type 1 fistulas as long as the patient is both metabolically and nutritionally stable. Reber et al.[6] documented that 90% of fistulas that close spontaneously will do so within 1 month of control of sepsis but less than 10% will do so in the second and third months after sepsis control. Hence they concluded that there is no reason to delay definitive surgery beyond 3 months after control of sepsis. One possible exception is the low-volume distal fistula with progressively diminishing output in a patient who shows continuing clinical improvement. Therefore good clinical judgment is important, and definitive surgical therapy must be individualized for the patient's circumstances. On the other hand, early surgical intervention may be indicated in certain situations that make the fistula unlikely to close. The two most commonly cited reasons are discontinuity of the bowel ends and distal obstruction.[5,6] Active Crohn's disease, abdominal irradiation, malignancy, and a short tract (<2 cm) also constitute reasons for earlier surgery.[6,19]

Even when earlier surgical treatment is indicated, it is best to delay surgery for a minimum of 6 weeks because it has been well documented that obliterative peritonitis follows many major procedures, particularly those associated with fistulization. This process is most likely to occur from 10 to 21 days after surgery and persists for 6 to 8 weeks.[22] The dense, woody adhesions make dissection extremely hazardous, and multiple enterotomies frequently occur, which may compound the patient's problem. Fazio et al.[4] have reported that although the fistula cure rate did not change whether the surgery was done in less than 10 days, 10 to 42 days, or more than 6 weeks, the mortality was significantly higher in the middle period (21%). This rate was compared to a 13% mortality when surgery was done before 10 days and an 11% mortality when 6 weeks were allowed to pass. Therefore definitive surgery should be delayed for at least 6 weeks. However, there are instances in which very early surgical intervention (less than 10 days) is indicated when the abdomen can be reentered before sepsis becomes established and before the obliterative adhesive process develops.[4]

The timing of surgical intervention also may be influenced by the status of the abdominal wall. It is preferable to delay elective surgery until the abdominal wall is soft, supple, and not inflamed. This situation generally can be appreciated by palpation and inspection.

The site may have some bearing on spontaneous closure and the indication and timing of the definitive surgery. MacFadyen et al.[8] reported spontaneous closure in 100% of duodenal fistulas, 88% of jejunal fistulas, 79% of colonic fistulas, but only 40% of fistulas arising from the ileum.

Complex type 2 fistulas. Guidelines to the indications for and the timing of surgical treatment for simple or complex type 1 enterocutaneous fistulas, as outlined earlier, should not be applied to the more complex fistulas, in which mortality rates of 25% to 50% are commonly reported.[4,40] Complex type 2 fistulas (those associated with large abdominal wall defects) constitute a major challenge to the surgeon and the management team. The indications for and the timing of definitive surgical intervention differ from those associated with simple enterocutaneous fistula because of the complexity in this seriously ill group. Whereas 30% to 80% of simple and complex type 1 fistulas can be expected to heal spontaneously within 6 weeks, a complex type 2 fistula almost invariably requires definitive surgery at some juncture.

Conter et al.[41] reported on a series of 51 patients with complex enterocutaneous fistulas managed by delayed reconstructive surgery; they noted a mortality of 4% and overall restoration of gastrointestinal continuity in 94%. Conter et al. stressed that in their opinion "the single most important factor is delaying of definitive surgery for an extended period of time." In this report the mean time from fistula recognition to definitive operation was 4.2 months (range of 10 weeks to 13 months).

Guidelines for the timing of surgery for complex fistulas are not well defined because few papers address this important question. Nutritional and metabolic status and immunocompetence should be restored, and adequate time should be allowed for the obliterative peritonitis to resolve. Since the majority of patients with complex fistulas have had considerable peritoneal contamination and inflammation, a longer time is generally required for this reaction to resolve. The abdominal wall should be soft and pliable to palpation in contrast to the woody induration suggestive of an ongoing inflammatory process. Conter et al.[41] suggested digitalizing any existing stoma if it is available in order to further clarify abdominal status. By judicious individualized timing of appropriate surgery, successful reconstruction with acceptable morbidity and mortality in these complex fistulas can be achieved.

Definitive surgery. This discussion deals with definitive surgery and treatment in patients who have persistent fistulas despite adequate conservative measures. The optimum timing of such surgery has already been addressed.

Simple fistulas

SMALL BOWEL (JEJUNUM AND ILEUM). Small bowel resection of the fistula segment with primary anastomosis is the treatment of choice[6,22] (Fig. 17-12). Success rates of 90% can be achieved.[6] Any temptation to try direct suture repair should be avoided because Reber et al.[6] have reported that this method failed in 41% of 32 patients in whom this was tried. In some instances dissection of the entire length of the small bowel and resection of the diseased segment is not safe, and a bypass or exclusion procedure should be considered (see discussion of special considerations).

After induction of anesthesia, a Foley catheter is inserted and the abdomen is prepared. Every attempt should be made to exclude the draining fistula site from the main operative wound. This exclusion can be accomplished by suture closure of the skin or by an exclusion barrier (e.g., Opsite or

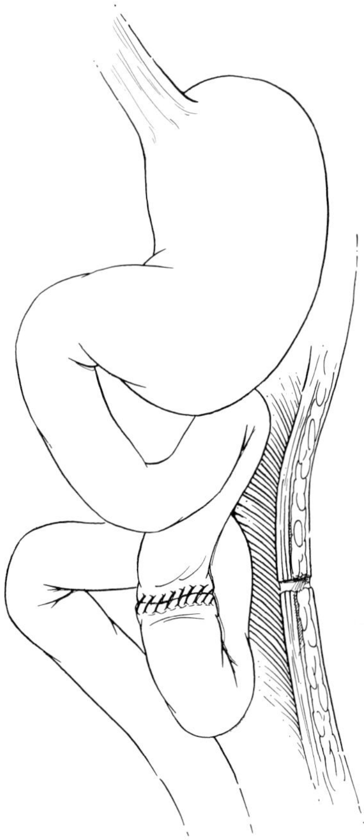

Fig. 17-12. The operation of choice for a simple fistula is resection and primary end-to-end anastomosis.

Vidrape) or another similar method. The abdomen should be opened through the old scar, but first it should be entered through an uninvolved area in longitudinal continuity with the original scar. This area often is located in the upper midline. Such entry minimizes the chances of small bowel injury to the potentially densely adherent loops that are expected to be present under the old scar. Once entry has been accomplished, Metzanbaum scissors are used to dissect the small bowel from under the old incision, which is extended as the bowel is cleared. The intent should be to divide all the adhesions and to free the small bowel in its entirety. This process may be tedious and time-consuming, and extreme care should be taken to avoid further injury to the small bowel.

Once the fistula site has been encountered, it is cut across at the level of the abdominal wall. Spillage from the opening in the small bowel should be controlled by temporary direct suture. A loop of small bowel is sought for beginning the dissection to separate the loops and free the small bowel through its entire length. Resection of the segment of small bowel is then performed back to soft, pliable intestine on either side of the fistula. At this point distal obstruction should be ruled out. In many cases such obstruction can be reasonably determined through inspection and palpation of the small bowel. However, in some instances doubt may exist and a Baker tube can be used to aid in identification of an occult obstruction. Once the tube has been passed distally, the balloon is inflated and the tube is gradually withdrawn, with any sites of narrowing noted. If found, the obstruction should be relieved by either strictureplasty or resection. In some instances enteroscopy with a colonoscope passed transanally and cannulation of the ileocecal valve and examination of the small bowel directly may be of value. This procedure necessitates that the patient be placed in modified lithotomy position with legs in the Allen stirrups at the outset. Once distal obstruction has been ruled out, primary anastomosis of the small bowel can be accomplished. We prefer a one-layer 4-0 silk handsewn anastomosis. Alternatively, a functional end-to-end stapled anastomosis can be used.

In most cases an extensive dissection has been necessary, and prolonged postoperative ileus occurs. Consideration should be given to performing a Stamm gastrostomy to avoid prolonged nasogastric intubation and patient discomfort. The abdominal cavity is irrigated with saline, and hemostasis is checked and secured. The abdominal wall fistula tract is debrided and usually is left open. Alternatively, the internal aspect at the peritoneal level can be sutured closed with 2-0 polyglycolic acid suture. The abdominal wall is then closed in the usual manner.

TPN is continued during the postoperative period. Suction is maintained on the gastrostomy until flatus or stool is passed. At this point the gastrostomy tube can be clamped and intermittently irrigated for patency. Oral fluids can be started, and the patient's diet can be advanced as tolerated. When sufficient oral nutrition can be maintained, TPN is discontinued. It is best to retain the gastrostomy tube for at least 2 weeks after discharge or until the patient is thriving without complication.

DUODENAL FISTULAS. Duodenal fistulas present a different management problem. Anatomic considerations make simple resection and anastomosis infeasible in most cases. Spontaneous closure rates vary from 37% to 100%.[6,8,42] Overall mortality occurs in 18% to 35% of patients.[6,42] Two types of fistulas occur: (1) end duodenal fistulas, which are almost invariably a complication of duodenal stump leakage after Billroth II anastomosis; or (2) lateral duodenal fistulas of the second, third, or fourth part of the duodenum. End duodenal fistulas usually have low output, and with adequate drainage they should heal spontaneously.[19] Rarely, such fistulas may require a serosal patch or Roux-en-Y duodenal jejunostomy. Lateral duodenal fistulas of the second portion usually have high output and rarely close spontaneously. They are associated with increased mortality and most require operative management.[19] The operative treatment of choice is the application of a serosal patch.[22] If one half to two thirds of the duodenal circumference is intact, a Roux-en-Y jejunal patch is preferred by Malangoni et al.[43] and Wolffman et al.[44] If, however, less than one half of the circumference is present, a Roux-en-Y jejunal end-to-end or end-to-side anastomosis is performed to avoid stenosis.[44] When a fistula arises from the third or fourth portion of the duodenum, the segment usually can be mobilized and resected and an end-to-end anastomosis in front of the superior mesenteric artery can be achieved.[22] Very rarely a Whipple pancreaticoduodenectomy is needed for a complicated duodenal fistula.[42]

Complex type 1 fistulas. The general approach to definitive surgery for a complex type 1 fistula (initially associated with intra-abdominal abscess) is identical in most respects to that of a simple fistula. In fact, many complex type 1 fistulas have been converted to simple fistulas by earlier control of sepsis either by percutaneous drainage or by laparotomy drainage of abscess and proximal diversion. The goal of surgical treatment should be to resect the small bowel segment with primary reanastomosis and closure of the proximal stoma when present. The same technique and principles as previously outlined are followed. Dense adhesions of small bowel loops are likely to be present at the site of the previously drained abscess. If the timing of the surgery has been appropriate, these adhesions usually can be separated with preservation of small bowel. Occasionally small bowel is so adherent and indurated that an additional adjacent segment may require resection. Once distal obstruction has been ruled out, the anastomosis can be performed. If all aspects of the procedure have been uneventful, the proximal stoma, if present, can be safely closed at this time. If, however, the circumstances of the primary anastomosis have been less than ideal, the stoma can be left standing and can be closed at a later date, once healing has been ensured.

Complex type 2 fistulas. Complex fistulas, particularly those associated with a large abdominal wall defect, rarely close spontaneously (7% to 10%).[3,41] They carry a mortality of 50% to 60%.[3,12] In a series by Schein and Decker,[12] the mortality was almost threefold that of the other forms of fistulas. Sitges-Serra et al.[3] defined these more serious fistulas as being associated with an abdominal wall defect >20 cm^2. These complex fistulas occur as a result of (1) major wound dehiscence secondary to underlying intra-abdominal wall sepsis and intestinal leakage, or (2) a laparostomy as a planned procedure in order to control massive intraperitoneal sepsis. Of 45 patients with fistulas associated with a major abdominal wall defect, Schein and Decker[12] reported that 25 fistulas were caused by spontaneous dehiscence, whereas 20 were the result of an open wound management policy.

A common pathophysiologic mechanism is illustrated by the following example. A patient sustains an anastomotic leak with massive peritoneal contamination and then undergoes repeated laparotomies in an attempt to control sepsis. The obliterative peritonitis is compounded by the repeat laparotomies, and further small bowel injury often ensues. The abdominal wall becomes edematous and often infected, and attempts at closure under tension result in wall necrosis. Increased intra-abdominal pressure secondary to ileus and fluid accumulation further compounds the process. Draining intestinal juices digest the anterior bowel wall. Eventually dehiscence occurs, leaving the fistula and multiple loops of small bowel exposed. This situation is the mark of a true surgical disaster. It is often the result of injudicious management of intra-abdominal infection at the initial insult.

Those patients who have undergone a planned laparostomy usually benefit from adequate control of sepsis, but the open method contributes to the development of a type 2 fistula. Nevertheless, such patients may well have been salvaged by this treatment method.

Patients with a complex type 2 fistula present a demanding therapeutic challenge to the surgeon and management team. Surgical management is described here through a two-phase plan—initial control and late reconstruction.

INITIAL CONTROL. Proximal gastrointestinal diversion in an area remote from the abdominal wall defect is the ideal initial surgical therapy, but such diversion may be very difficult to achieve. Some authors have advocated exteriorization of the ends of the fistulized bowel or exclusion bypass. Although these approaches may be ideal if they can be achieved, often they are not possible because the bowel is edematous and distended and the mesentery is commonly foreshortened. Schein and Decker[12] have emphasized that multiple fistulas at the base of the defect may be better left undisturbed rather than risking resection of an undefined mass. They have stated that a proximal jejunostomy, even if done at a point just distal to the ligament of Treitz, is tolerated reasonably well and that the surgeon should not rule out high proximal jejunal diversion for fear of unknown consequences. If a fistula associated with a large abdominal wall defect is close to the surface and properly walled off from the remainder of the peritoneal cavity and if sepsis is under control, such situations may not need proximal diversion; a creative draining collection system (see Chapter 18) may suffice to control output until definitive restorative surgery can be performed safely.

When a large open wound defect is present, some authors advocate initially covering the defect with mesh and later with a split-thickness skin graft for definitive coverage[12]; others have advocated the use of pedicle flaps.[45] In our experience neither coverage method is routinely necessary; most such wounds can be allowed to granulate and contract.

LATE RECONSTRUCTION. Once initial control of a fistula in association with a dehisced or open wound has been achieved, definitive reconstructive surgery should be delayed for several months and sometimes for as long as 1 year. This delay allows for adequate resolution of the extensive inflammatory process and improves the likelihood of successful reconstruction. The 6-week guideline for simple or even complex type 1 fistulas is not appropriate for the more difficult problems posed by complex type 2 fistulas.

Conter et al.[41] reported on a series of 51 patients with complex fistulas (15 patients, or 29%, had large abdominal wall defects; 36 patients, or 71%, had either multiple or recurrent fistulas) managed by a policy of delayed reconstructive surgery. The mean time to definitive surgery was 4.2 months. The spontaneous closure occurred in 5 of the 51 patients (10%). Forty-six patients, therefore, underwent reconstructive surgery, 38 by resection and anastomosis (three recurrences, two of the three closed spontaneously), five by simple diversion, and three by fistula takedown and repair (two of three recurred). Morbidity was 57%. Fistula-related mortality was 4%. Gastrointestinal continuity was restored in 94%. The authors attribute their excellent results to this delayed approach. Fazio et al.[4] reported on four patients with multiple fistulas and severe sepsis who were treated by urgent surgery and proximal diversion with wide-open drainage and delayed reconstructive surgery. All four patients were successfully managed and eventually had gastrointestinal continuity restored.

Complex type 2 fistulas, while presenting a formidable challenge, can be managed successfully by initial aggressive therapy, including adequate control of intra-abdominal sepsis, and control of fistula output, in conjunction with nutritional and adjunctive metabolic support followed by judiciously timed delayed reconstructive surgery.

Special considerations

CROHN'S DISEASE AND EXTERNAL FISTULAS. One of the features of Crohn's disease is propensity to fistulization. Spontaneous closure with active Crohn's disease is unlikely. Driscoll and Rosenberg[46] noted that 10 of 11 patients with active Crohn's disease who had enterocutaneous fistulas required surgical treatment. In an initial report by the Birmingham group,[18] who reported on 39 Crohn's external fistulas, nine postoperative fistulas involving no active disease closed spontaneously with medical treatment. In contrast, all 30 patients with active Crohn's disease required surgical resection. In a subsequent report this group found that only seven of 24 postoperative fistulas closed spontaneously, and they concluded that surgical resection and anastomosis is the best option when surgery is required.[21] Attempts at simple closure of the fistula in four patients resulted in abscesses in three. Of three patients treated with strictureplasty, two developed leaks. Of 20 patients with Crohn's disease and spontaneously occurring fistulas, spontaneous closure occurred in only one. Therefore surgical resection is almost always advised for fistulas associated with active Crohn's disease. In most situations anastomosis can be done primarily, although in some patients with extensive concomitant intra-abdominal sepsis, the creation of a proximal stoma may be prudent. Results of strictureplasty in active Crohn's disease with enterocutaneous fistulas were poor (only one of three was successful).

RADIATION-INJURED BOWEL. When an enterocutaneous fistula arises from irradiated bowel, the ordinary guidelines for definitive surgery do not apply. The irradiated bowel usually is encased in dense adhesions with a frozen pelvis. In such instances resection with primary anastomosis is either not feasible or not safe. Therefore the most distal portion of nonirradiated small bowel should be divided, leaving the distal end closed and the proximal end anastomosed to the transverse colon as a bypass procedure (Fig. 17-13). Lui et al.[47] have reported on the successful use of vascularized muscle flaps from a distant nonirradiated field to achieve safe repair of bowel defects in three refractory enterocutaneous fistulas associated with radiation injury. The role of this adjunctive procedure has not yet been established. Bypass for most

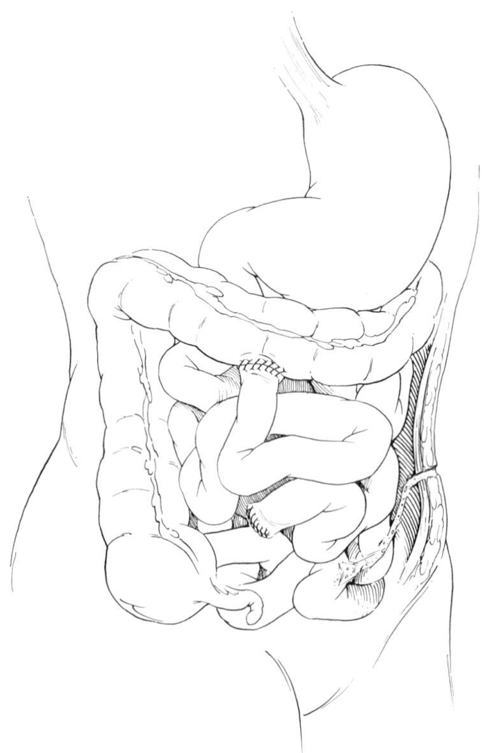

Fig. 17-13. A radiation-induced fistula is often best managed with a bypass procedure.

enterocutaneous fistulas arising from irradiated small bowel is the treatment of choice.[22]

MALIGNANCY. When an underlying malignancy exists with an enterocutaneous fistula, there is no hope of spontaneous closure and operative therapy is required. If possible, a standard cancer operation should be performed with wide en bloc excision of the fistula tract and any adjacent organ structures in continuity with it. It is not possible to tell whether such adherence is secondary to neoplastic invasion or solely inflammatory. If widespread metastatic disease is evident, palliative resection or bypass may be all that is possible. Soeters et al.,[1] in a review of 100 enterocutaneous fistulas at the Massachusetts General Hospital between 1960 to 1970, found that 26 fistulas (26%) were associated with cancer, 12 occurring spontaneously and 14 postoperatively.

COLOCUTANEOUS FISTULAS. In general, colocutaneous fistulas are low-output fistulas associated with fewer nutritional and metabolic consequences to the patient than other types and therefore usually are tolerated reasonably well. There is some discrepancy in the literature about the rates of spontaneous closure and hence the timing of surgical intervention. Sitges-Serra et al.[3] reported spontaneous closure in 11 of 12 colocutaneous fistulas with 0% mortality. They noted, however, that 20% to 25% required some form of surgical intervention to achieve adequate drainage of the abscess or fistula site. In contrast, Schein and Decker[12] reported on 15 patients with colocutaneous fistulas in whom surgical intervention (usually in the form of dismantling of the disrupted anastomosis) was necessary in 60%. Mortality in this series was 20%. However, it may not be valid to compare these two series because it is likely that they involve two different presentations of colocutaneous fistulas. Sitges-Serra et al.[3] stated that colocutaneous fistulas generally occur late, suggesting that in their series most fistulas were likely initially confined leaks that found their way to the wound after being initially walled off. In a series by Schein and Decker,[12] the patients had diffuse fecal peritonitis; hence the differing results, both in mortality and spontaneous closure rates.

For established colocutaneous fistulas, some authors have reported high spontaneous closure rates, ranging from 75% to 79%.[8,13] In contrast, however, Zera et al.[48] reported only a 20% spontaneous closure rate and therefore advised early surgery. Doglietto et al.[49] also reported that in their experience only 25% of colocutaneous fistulas closed spontaneously in contrast to a 73% closure rate for upper gastrointestinal and small bowel fistulas. They also favored an early surgical approach for large bowel fistulas. Fazio et al.[24] reported on 93 colocutaneous fistulas associated with diverticular disease. Eighty-eight fistulas developed postoperatively, whereas five were spontaneous. Ninety-two patients were treated surgically, 80% by one-stage or two-stage resection and anastomosis. Morbidity was 48% with one mortality.

Surgery was successful in achieving closure in 77% of patients. Crohn's disease was diagnosed in 10 of the patients with complicated and persistent fistulas.

Although there is no unanimity in the literature about the likelihood of spontaneous closure, it is generally agreed that a contained colocutaneous fistula is well tolerated by the patient and a reasonable period of time should be given to allow closure. If closure has not occurred by 6 weeks after control of sepsis and fistula has been achieved, surgical intervention should be considered. The goal of surgery is one-stage resection and primary anastomosis after complete mechanical and antibiotic bowel preparation.

SUMMARY

External fistulas, whether simple or complex, present a significant challenge to the gastrointestinal surgeon. A team approach is essential. With careful attention given to basic surgical principles and good judgment on the part of the surgeon, most patients can be restored to health and gastrointestinal continuity can be reestablished.

REFERENCES

1. Soeters PB, Ebeid AM, Fischer JE. Review of 404 patients with gastrointestinal fistulas. Ann Surg 190:189-202, 1979.
2. Levy E, Frileux P, Cugnenc PH, Honiger JH, Olivier JM, Par R. High-output external fistulae of the small bowel: Management with continuous enteral nutrition. Br J Surg 76:676-679, 1989.
3. Sitges-Serra A, Jaurrieta E, Sitges-Creus A. Management of postoperative enterocutaneous fistulas: The roles of parenteral nutrition and surgery. Br J Surg 69:147-150, 1982.
4. Fazio VW, Coutsoftides T, Steiger E. Factors influencing the outcome of treatment of small bowel cutaneous fistula. World J Surg 7:481-488, 1983.
5. McIntyre PB, Ritchie JK, Hawley PR, Bartram CI, Lennard-Jones JE. Management of enterocutaneous fistulas: A review of 132 cases. Br J Surg 71:293-296, 1984.
6. Reber HA, Roberts C, Way LW, Dunphy JE. Management of external gastrointestinal fistulas. Ann Surg 188:460-467, 1978.
7. Sansoni B, Irving M. Small bowel fistulas. World J Surg 9:897-903, 1985.
8. MacFadyen BV, Dudrick SJ, Ruberg RL. Management of gastrointestinal fistulas with parenteral hyperalimentation. Surgery 74:100-105, 1973.
9. Fischer JE. The management of high-output intestinal fistulas. Adv Surg 9:139-176, 1975.
10. Aguirre A, Fischer JE, Welch CE. The role of surgery and hyperalimentation in the therapy of gastrointestinal-cutaneous fistulae. Ann Surg 180:393-401, 1974.
11. Fischer JE. The pathophysiology of enterocutaneous fistulas. World J Surg 7:446-450, 1983.
12. Schein M, Decker GAG. Postoperative external alimentary tract fistulas. Am J Surg 161:435-438, 1991.

13. Edmunds LH Jr, Williams GM, Welch CE. External fistulas arising from the gastrointestinal tract. Ann Surg 152:445-471, 1960.
14. Chapman R, Foran R, Dunphy JE. Management of intestinal fistulas. Am J Surg 108:157-164, 1964.
15. Altomare DF, Serior G, Pannarale OC, Lupo L, Palasciano N, Memeo V, Rubino M. Prediction of mortality by logistic regression analysis in patients with postoperative enterocutaneous fistulae. Br J Surg 77:450-453, 1990.
16. Rose D, Yarborough MF, Canizaro PC, Lowry SF. One hundred and fourteen fistulas of the gastrointestinal tract treated with total parenteral nutrition. Surg Gynecol Obstet 163:345-350, 1986.
17. Coutsoftides T, Fazio VW. Small intestine cutaneous fistulas. Surg Gynecol Obstet 149:333-336, 1979.
18. Hawker PC, Givel JC, Keighley MRB, Alexander-Williams J, Allan RN. Management of enterocutaneous fistulae in Crohn's disease. Gut 24:284-287, 1983.
19. Bergamini TM, Richardson JD. External gastrointestinal fistulas. Principles of management and treatment. J Ky Med Assoc 85:186-190, 1987.
20. Rubelowsky J, Machiedo GW. Reoperative versus conservative management for gastrointestinal fistulas. Surg Clin North Am 71:147-157, 1991.
21. Keighley MRB, Heyen F, Winslet MC. Entero-cutaneous fistulas and Crohn's disease. Acta Gastroenterol Belg 50:580-600, 1987.
22. Hill GL. Operative strategy in the treatment of enterocutaneous fistulas. World J Surg 7:495-501, 1983.
23. Hugh TB, Coleman MJ, Cohen A. Persistent postoperative enterocutaneous fistula: Pathophysiology and treatment. Aust N Z J Surg 56:901-906, 1986.
24. Fazio VW, Church JM, Jagelman DG, Weakley FL, Lavery IC, Tarazi R, VanHillo M. Colocutaneous fistulas complicating diverticulitis. Dis Colon Rectum 30:89-94, 1987.
25. Fischer JE. Enterocutaneous fistulas. In Najarian JS, Delaney JP, eds. Progress in Gastrointestinal Surgery. Chicago: Year Book Medical, 1989, pp 377-387.
26. Alexander ES, Weinberg S, Clark RA, Belkin RD. Fistulas and sinus tracts: Radiographic evaluation, management, and outcome. Gastrointest Radiol 7:135-140, 1982.
27. Frick MP, Feinberg SB, Stenlund RR, Gedgaudas E. Evaluation of abdominal fistulas with computed body tomography (CT). Comput Radiol 6:17-25, 1982.
28. Dudrick SJ, Wilmore DW, Vars HM, Rhoads JE. Long-term total parenteral nutrition with growth, development, and positive nitrogen balance. Surgery 64:134-142, 1968.
29. Wolfe BM, Keltner RM, Willman VL. Intestinal fistula output in regular, elemental, and intravenous alimentation. Am J Surg 124:803-806, 1972.
30. Bury KD, Stephens RV, Randall HT. Use of a chemically defined, liquid, elemental diet for nutritional management of fistulas of the alimentary tract. Am J Surg 121:174-183, 1971.
31. Deitel M. Elemental diet and enterocutaneous fistula. World J Surg 7:451-454, 1983.
32. Voitk AJ, Echave V, Brown A, McArdle AH, Gurd FN. Elemental diet in the treatment of fistulas of the alimentary tract. Surg Gynecol Obstet 137:68-72, 1973.
33. diConstanzo J, Camo N, Martin J. Somatostatin in persistent gastrointestinal fistula treated by total parenteral nutrition. Lancet 2:338-339, 1982.
34. Nubiola P, Badia JM, Martinez-Rodenas F, Gil MJ, Segura M, Sancho J, Sitges-Serra A. Treatment of 27 postoperative enterocutaneous fistulas with the long half-life somatostatin analogue SMS 201-995. Ann Surg 210:56-58, 1989.
35. Geerdsen JP, Pedersen VM, Kjaergard HK. Small bowel fistulas treated with somatostatin: Preliminary results. Surgery 100:811-814, 1986.

36. Hild P, Dobroschke J, Henneking K, Rieck B. Treatment of enterocutaneous fistulas with somatostatin. Lancet 2:626, 1986.
37. Bianchi A, Solduga C, Ubach M. Percutaneous obliteration of a chronic duodenal fistula. Br J Surg 75:572, 1988.
38. Lange V, Meyer G, Wenk H, Schildberg FW. Fistuloscopy—An adjuvant technique for sealing gastrointestinal fistulae. Surg Endosc 4:212-216, 1990.
39. Eleftheriadis E, Tzartinoglou E, Kotzampassi K, Aletras H. Early endoscopic fibrin sealing of high-output postoperative enterocutaneous fistulas. Acta Chir Scand 156:625-628, 1990.
40. Hollender LF, Meyer C, Avet D, Zeyer B. Postoperative fistulas of the small intestine: Therapeutic principles. World J Surg 7:474-480, 1983.
41. Conter RL, Root L, Roslyn JJ. Delayed reconstructive surgery for complex enterocutaneous fistulae. Am Surgeon 54:589-593, 1988.
42. Tarazi R, Coutsoftides T, Steiger E, Fazio VW. Gastric and duodenal cutaneous fistulas. World J Surg 7:463-473, 1983.
43. Malangoni MA, Madura JA, Jesseph JE. Management of lateral duodenal fistulas: A study of fourteen cases. Surgery 90:645-651, 1981.
44. Wolffman EF Jr, Trevino G, Heaps DK, et al. An operative technique for the management of acute and chronic lateral duodenal fistulas. Ann Surg 159:563-569, 1964.
45. Levy E, Palmer DL, Frileux P, et al. Septic necrosis of the midline wound in postoperative peritonitis. Ann Surg 207:470-479, 1988.
46. Driscoll RH, Rosenberg IH. Total parenteral nutrition in inflammatory bowel disease. Med Clin North Am 62:185-201, 1978.
47. Lui RC, Friedman R, Fleischer A. Management of postirradiation recurrent enterocutaneous fistula by muscle flaps. Am Surgeon 55:403-407, 1989.
48. Zera RT, Bubrick MP, Sternquist JC, Hitchcock CR. Enterocutaneous fistulas. Effects of total parenteral nutrition and surgery. Dis Colon Rectum 26:109-112, 1983.
49. Doglietto GB, Bellantone R, Pacelli F, Bossola M, Negro F, Crucitti F. Enterocutaneous fistulas: Effect of nutritional management and surgery. Ital J Surg Sci 19:375-380, 1989.

18 NURSING CONSIDERATIONS WITH INTESTINAL FISTULAS

Bonnie Sue Rolstad and W. Douglas Wong

Nursing management of the patient with an intestinal fistula, whether short-term or long-term, is complex and dynamic. Critical resourcefulness, flexibility, and collaboration are essential elements for successful management. The occurrence of a fistula is unplanned and may be viewed by the patient as catastrophic. A fistula represents a breech in integrity of the body over which the patient has little control.

The enterocutaneous fistula may occur in a patient who has recently had surgery or radiation therapy and may be malnourished, having diminished physical and emotional resources. The clinical course ahead offers little hope of immediate relief because hyperalimentation, additional surgery, and prolonged or numerous hospitalizations may be required. Normal patient responses include feelings of helplessness, frustration, anxiety, and shame.[1,2]

Within this complex of clinical issues, an organized approach to care needs to be established. Effective management of intestinal fistulas requires expert technical knowledge and skills, thorough patient and family education, and ongoing emotional support for both patient and caregivers.

CLINICAL GOALS

During the stabilization phase of fistula management, early attention to skin care, output monitoring, and patient support are essential. Complications can be prevented (or limited) by early intervention. The five primary goals in the nursing management of patients with an enterocutaneous fistula are (1) perifistular skin management, (2) containment of effluent, (3) odor control, (4) patient support, and (5) cost containment.[3,4] Achieving all these goals at the same time may not be possible, and prioritization may be necessary. For example, containment of effluent may be achieved without meeting the cost-containment goal.

ASSESSMENT OF CLINICAL FEATURES

In order to develop an effective plan of care, specific clinical features require assessment. These features include the fistula source, the characteristics of the effluent, the duration of the problem, the cutaneous location and abdominal topography around the opening, the condition of perifistular skin, and the patient's effectiveness in coping.[5]

Knowledge of the source of the fistula affects management interventions related to odor control, skin protection, and volume of output. Potentially, an ileocutaneous fistula may require aggressive skin protection and adequate pouch capacity for high output. In contrast, a colocutaneous fistula often requires minimal skin protection with a pouching system intended primarily for odor control (Fig. 18-1). If diagnostic studies are pending when fistula care is initiated, the fistula source may be approximated based on odor, pattern of output, volume, color, corrosive characteristics, and consistency of effluent. For example, a fistula with low-volume, gassy, infrequent output; brownish color; and malodorous, noncorrosive effluent is probably of left-sided colonic origin.

Fistulas may be of recent onset, or they may represent a long-standing problem. Determination of the time since presentation provides information for making predictions about the possibility of spontaneous closure. If a fistula, even when properly treated, has been present for months and the fistula tract is epithelialized, the fistula usually will not close spontaneously.

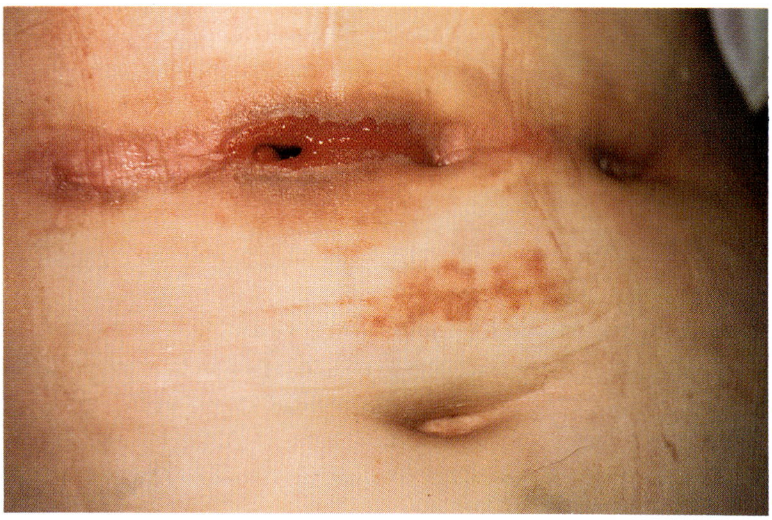

Fig. 18-1. Colocutaneous fistula with intact skin. (Courtesy Bonnie Sue Rolstad, R.N., C.E.T.N.)

In this situation fistula care is maintained until surgery. When surgery is not an option, supportive care becomes the focus. Knowledge of duration of the fistula also is helpful in planning patient education and psychologic support. The newly diagnosed patient has a knowledge deficit about the problem, initial fears, and anxiety—all of which are important clinical issues. For long-term conditions, both patient and family may need assistance with nursing care at home and often with the management of anxiety or depression.

Cutaneous locations of enterocutaneous fistulas are rarely ideal for management. These fistulas commonly appear at incisions or drain sites and within fat folds. Other problem locations include the umbilicus, stomas, and bony prominences (Fig. 18-2). In order to provide technical solutions to these often complex clinical problems, the principles and techniques used in ostomy and chronic wound care must be adapted to the management of intestinal fistulas.

Perifistular skin assessment frequently reveals compromised tissue, such as maceration caused by continuously moist dressings around the site, erosion secondary to the composition of the effluent, or erythema resulting from products used to treat compromised areas. Recent presentation of the fistula with intact skin requires early interventions aimed at protection. If the skin is compromised, reassessment of the current approach with plans for aggressive skin protection are indicated.

Beyond the technical issues, individuals with fistulas and their significant others have informational and emotional needs.[2,6] Assessment of knowledge

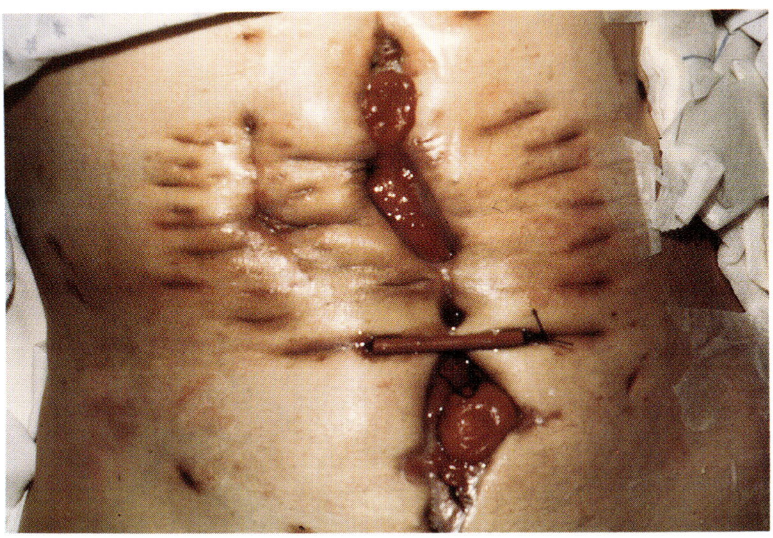

Fig. 18-2. Enterocutaneous fistulas shown here are located within a midline incision in association with an ileostomy and a mucous fistula. (Courtesy Bonnie Sue Rolstad, R.N., C.E.T.N.)

may be as simple as determining whether the patient understands the terminology, anatomy, medications, and rationale for perifistular wound care. Effective coping approaches may be evident by patients seeking answers, expressing concern, and participating in problem-solving.

PERIFISTULAR SKIN MANAGEMENT

Because fistulas are flush to the skin, they discharge effluent directly onto the epidermis. Prevention of denudation, inflammation, maceration, infection, or pain is not always possible (Fig. 18-3). However, effective perifistular skin management is usually possible. Prevention and early treatment represent the keys. Initial recognition of patients with enterocutaneous fistulas who are at higher risk of compromised skin integrity includes assessment of the patient's general condition, disease processes, age, immunosuppression, and antibiotic therapy.

The most common causes of compromised skin integrity with enterocutaneous fistulas are contact dermatitis and candidiasis infection.[7]

Irritant Contact Dermatitis

Irritant contact dermatitis, the most common skin irritation, results from mechanical and chemical injury. Mechanical injury occurs because of forceful and/or frequent removal of tape or other adhesives associated with

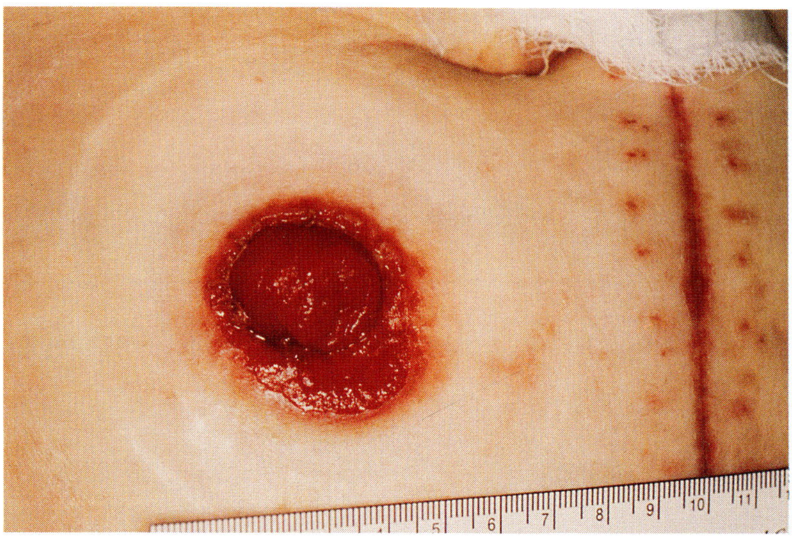

Fig. 18-3. Perifistular skin denudation associated with a mucocutaneous fistula. (Courtesy Bonnie Sue Rolstad, R.N., C.E.T.N.)

pouches. It is also caused by the pressure and sliding of unstabilized tubes or drains. Clinical presentation may involve erythema or patchy denudation in areas where adhesives have been placed. Preventive approaches include the use of skin sealants (e.g., copolymers in liquid film form), porous tapes, Montgomery straps, and solid-form skin barriers as platforms for frequently taped areas as well as gentle adhesive removal. Frequency of removal and adhesive tack also affect the potential for mechanical injury. If possible, pouching systems should be removed every 3 to 4 days since daily removal predisposes the patient to mechanical injury.[3]

Another form of irritant contact dermatitis results from contact with chemical irritants. Cutaneous assessment reveals areas of erythema or denudation of skin where the skin has come in contact with an irritant. Effluent with a high or low pH value or active proteolytic enzymes is particularly irritating to the epidermis. Other chemical irritants include solvents, soaps, hypochlorite (Dakin's) solution, acetic acid, and tincture of benzoin.[8-12] Prevention and treatment focus on protection from these agents or removal of irritants from the treatment protocol. Approaches to management may include the use of skin sealants (on intact skin only), petrolatum-based or zinc-based ointments (e.g., petrolatum or zinc oxide paste), and skin protectors with hydrophobic characteristics (e.g., solid-form skin barriers or transparent film dressings).[13,14]

Ointments and pastes are applied around the cutaneous fistula site. (If the site is occluded, drainage is trapped under the skin protector, resulting in compromised skin.) A secondary absorbent dressing is then applied over the skin protector and changed as needed. Commonly used absorbent dressings are gauze, polyurethane foams, and calcium alginates.

Ointments and copolymer skin sealants usually need to be applied two to three times per day, whereas adhesive protectants can be left in place up to 7 days or changed when the seal shows signs of erosion. Absorbent secondary gauze dressings are changed as needed.

Allergic Contact Dermatitis

Allergic contact dermatitis is a sensitivity reaction to substances used on the skin. Cutaneous reactions are manifest by intense erythema, itching, vesiculation, and denudation. Treatment includes identification of the offending product and removal of that product from use. True allergic reactions are documented through the use of patch tests. Clinicians are cautioned about arbitrarily removing a suspected product from use without patch testing.[15] Products used in perifistular skin care have universal components that would rule out the use of entire subgroups of equipment, thus significantly limiting treatment options.

Candidiasis Infection

Candidiasis is a common cutaneous infection that occurs in patients with fistulas because of the moist, warm cutaneous areas that are present. The proliferation of *Candida albicans* leads to erythematous, patchy, papular, pruritic, and, frequently, vesicular lesions. Prevention is best achieved by maintaining a dry epidermis. When gauze is being used, frequent dressing changes are recommended to avoid moisture on the skin. Water-insoluble skin sealants and solid-form skin barriers are useful for skin protection. Treatment involves exposing the skin to air or applying an antifungal agent.

ABDOMINAL WOUND CARE

Fistulas may occur adjacent to or within an open abdominal wound. However, wound management differs according to the circumstances. When the fistula is not located within the open abdominal wound, measures must be taken to prevent further contamination to the open wound. (An open wound is considered contaminated.) The risk of wound infection depends on the type and amount of bacterial contaminants in the wound, the condition of the wound at the end of the surgical procedure, the host's body defenses, and the specific antimicrobial agents in the tissue.[16] Fecal spillage into the open wound base increases the bacterial burden of the wound and delays wound healing. Therefore one component of topical wound management is isolation of the effluent from the fistula. In the contaminated wound, clean (rather than sterile) technique is used. If the wound requires pouching, the use of clean equipment is recommended because it offers an effective and less expensive intervention.

Once the fistula effluent has been isolated, routine protocols for moist wound healing are recommended for the open abdominal wound. Principles of wound care include maintenance of a moist wound bed, packing of tunnels and undermined areas, avoidance of the use of antiseptics, debridement as necessary, and protection of the periwound skin. Traditional approaches to open wound care include packing the wound with gauze and normal saline three to four times a day. Although this procedure is uncomplicated, it does not ensure a moist wound bed and it is expensive. Gauze may become embedded in the desiccating wound and result in tissue trauma and nonselective debridement during removal. In addition, gauze and saline represent an expensive, time-consuming approach to wound care.

More physiologic approaches to wound care include gentle irrigation and packing of wounds. Wounds may be irrigated with noncytotoxic solutions such as saline or Pluronic F68.[12] If avascular tissue is to be removed from the wound, irrigation with a 35 ml syringe and a 19-gauge needle provides maximum pressure with the least amount of trauma to the tissue. Wound packing may include the use of hydrogel sheets or hydrogel-saturated gauze once or twice a day. The material is loosely packed in the wound and placed in areas that tunnel or are undermined in order to fill dead space. Other wound dressing materials include copolymer absorption dressings or calcium alginate dressings that absorb exudate and provide an interface for moist wound dressings. A secondary cover dressing is then used and secured with tape or Montgomery straps. Depending on the size and condition of the wound, a transparent film dressing may be used as the secondary dressing and changed once a day. This approach is particularly practical and cost-effective for patients at home who are ambulatory.[8]

If the wound is infected or if there is concern about infection, 0.25% acetic acid, 1% povidone-iodine, 3% hydrogen peroxide, or 0.5% sodium hypochlorite solution has been recommended. However, research in tissue repair has yielded information about the toxicity of these antiseptics.[10,12,17-19] Lineaweaver et al.[11] compared the bactericidal and cytotoxic effects of serial dilutions of hydrogen peroxide and acetic acid in cultured human fibroblasts. Results indicated that cellular toxicity exceeded bactericidal potency. The outcome of Lineaweaver's research indicated that 0.25% acetic acid, 1% povidone-iodine, 3% hydrogen peroxide, and 0.5% sodium hypochlorite solution are "unsuitable for wound care."

When the fistula is located within or close to an open wound, packing is rarely indicated. The wound and the fistula usually are managed together (Figs. 18-4 through 18-7). The exception is the large undermining wound that

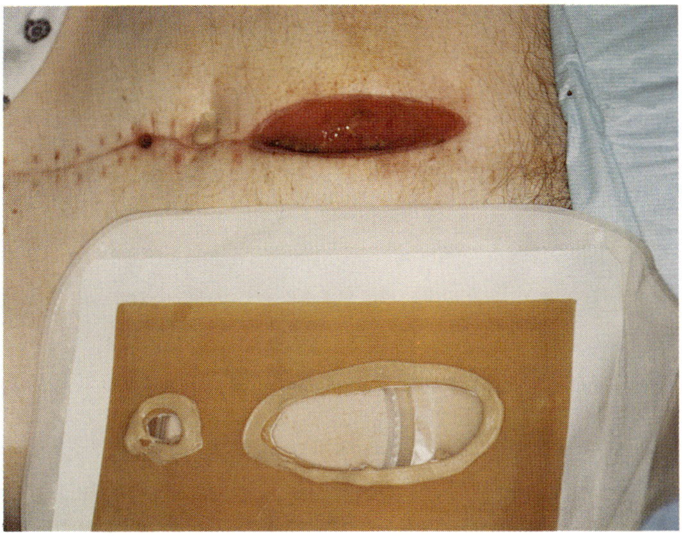

Fig. 18-4. An enterocutaneous fistula within an open abdominal wound and a second fistula located superiorly within the incision are "pouched" together. Skin barrier paste is applied to the wound-drainage collection system. (Courtesy Bonnie Sue Rolstad, R.N., C.E.T.N.)

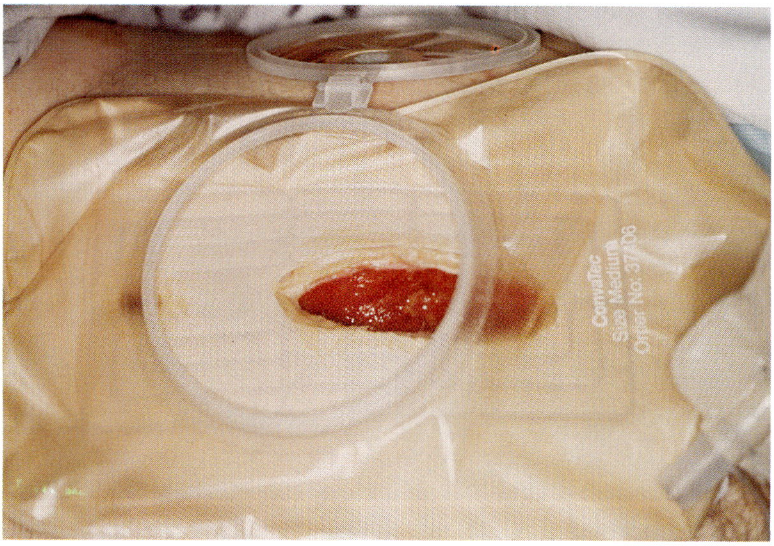

Fig. 18-5. Pouching method used for patient in Fig. 18-4. (Courtesy Bonnie Sue Rolstad, R.N., C.E.T.N.)

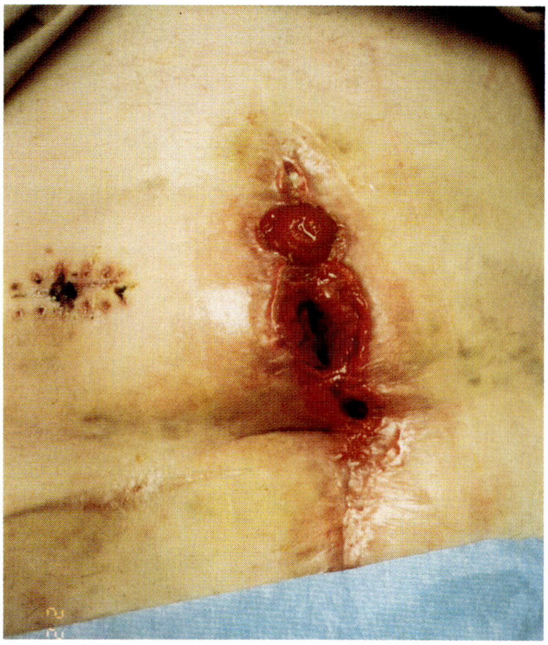

Fig. 18-6. Combined pouching is required for enterocutaneous fistulas within an abdominal incision and an ileostomy that is located superiorly. (Courtesy Bonnie Sue Rolstad, R.N., C.E.T.N.)

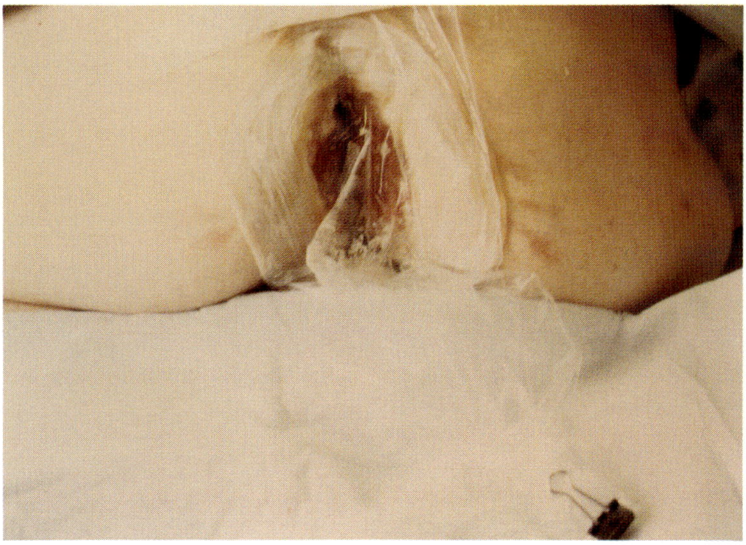

Fig. 18-7. Pouching of the wound and the fistula without packing. (Courtesy Bonnie Sue Rolstad, R.N., C.E.T.N.)

may need additional packing. In this situation a normal saline and gauze packing may be used to protect dead space from pooling of effluent.

CONTAINMENT OF EFFLUENT

Containment of effluent with gauze, foams, and alginates is effective for fistulas with no odor, minimal output, and noncorrosive drainage (Fig. 18-8). However, when the volume of effluent exceeds 10 to 100 ml in 24 hours, pouching and, occasionally, suction are indicated.[1,4,5,20] The advantages of pouching fistulas include accurate measurement of volume, increased patient comfort, avoidance of contamination of incisions and other wounds, decreased contact with potentially infectious materials for caregivers and others in contact with the patient, protection of perifistular skin, odor control, increased patient mobilization, and cost-effectiveness.

Selection of Equipment

Management of complex fistulas involves the most technically difficult pouching situations. Selection of a pouching system requires knowledge of available equipment and indications for its use. However, the technique used in application is frequently as important as the selection of the pouching system. Flexibility in adaptation and ongoing reevaluation are essential components in refinement of an effective system.

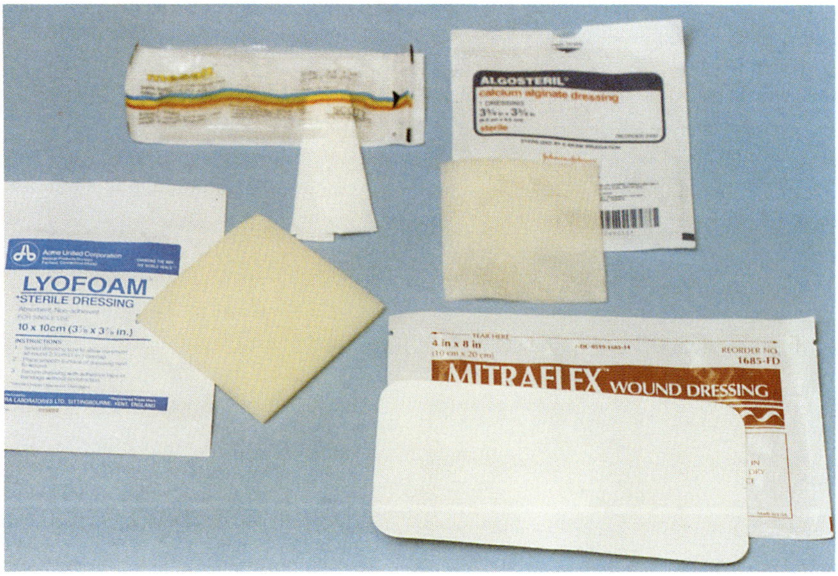

Fig. 18-8. Wound dressings shown are composed of polyurethane or calcium alginate and impregnated gauze. (Courtesy Bonnie Sue Rolstad, R.N., C.E.T.N.)

Clinical decision-making in pouch selection is based on specific criteria. Primary criteria include characteristics of the effluent, topography of the abdomen, and inspection of the wound. When the patient's technical needs have been met, attention is directed to secondary issues, such as patient mobility, aesthetics, ease of management, and cost-effectiveness.

Characteristics of effluent. Volume, consistency, odor, and composition of effluent are important variables to consider when selecting a pouching system. Pouches used in the management of low-volume enterocutaneous fistulas (<500/ml/24 hr) are fecal pouches, nondrainable or drainable with wide spouts. Nondrainable pouches are indicated when volume is such that the pouch requires removal once every 1 to 2 days. Drainable pouches are emptied every 3 to 4 hours (or when one third full) by the nurse or the patient and changed every 3 to 4 days.

When output increases to higher volumes (>1000 ml/24 hr), the seal may become detached because of overfilling. If the pouch is emptied every 2 to 4 hours, a drainable pouch with a wide outlet may continue to be used. However, when overfilling and leakage occur because of the inability to empty the pouch frequently enough, urinary drainage pouches that connect to a bedside bag may be used. Examples of situations warranting consideration of straight drainage include overfilling of the pouch at night; a confused, medicated, or exhausted patient who cannot alert the nursing staff about the need to empty the pouch; and high-volume "dumping" fistulas. The consistency of effluent affects the success of this decision since particulate matter may clog the

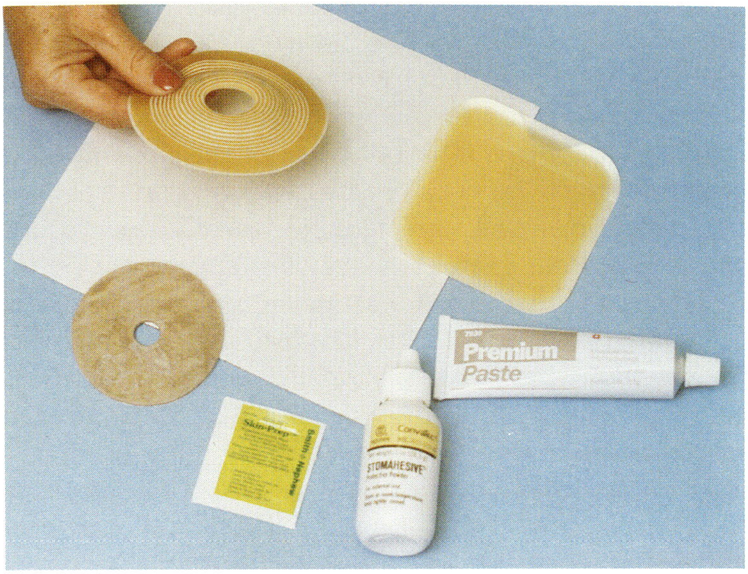

Fig. 18-9. Skin barriers include liquid skin sealant, skin barrier powder, solid-form barriers, and paste. (Courtesy Bonnie Sue Rolstad, R.N., C.E.T.N.)

drain. When patients are taking solid food by mouth, straight outlet valves are ineffective unless the lumen of the tubing is large (Greensmith device).[21] The odor barrier film of urinary pouches and straight drainage systems is not as effective as that of fecal pouches. Therefore deodorants and more frequent changes may be necessary when urinary pouches are used.

When the system requires changes more frequently than every 24 hours, there is greater risk of mechanical injury to the skin, increased expense, and increased patient frustration. In these situations the use of suction may be instituted. Effluent must be predominantly liquid since the catheter can become clogged with particulate matter. A suction catheter can be placed in the wound bed with intermittent or continuous drainage. A gauze dressing then can be placed over the catheter with a transparent film dressing covering the entire system.[22] Suction is a temporary intervention that limits patient mobility, provides limited odor control, and is costly.

The composition of the effluent raises questions about infection control and perifistular skin protection. Pouching a fistula is a clean procedure that requires the use of gloves but not sterile technique. Therefore sterile pouching systems, which are somewhat expensive, are not necessary. When the composition of the effluent is corrosive, skin barriers with hydrophobic characteristics are warranted. Karaya is not recommended in these situations because it erodes, leaving the skin exposed to effluent and decreased wear time. Solid-form skin barriers containing NaCMC (sodium carboxymethylcellulose) and polyisobutylene (e.g., Stomahesive, Premium Barrier) are preferred (Fig.

18-9). They are available with one-piece or two-piece pouching systems or in individual pieces that can be custom fit. Protection of skin edges surrounding a fistula opening with a skin barrier paste or a topically applied adhesive cement is recommended with high-volume, corrosive output (see Fig. 18-4).

Topography of abdomen. Determination of the abdominal topography includes location of the cutaneous opening, size and number of sites, tissue type (whether flaccid or firm), retracted and scarred areas, and presence of drains. Some fistulas occur in areas that can be managed easily. These fistulas are located away from creases and bony prominences with approximately 3 inches of circumferentially flat skin unobstructed by retention sutures, drains, stomas, or open incisions. Such fistula wound sites, when <3 inches in diameter, are managed with little need for adaptive equipment. Ostomy pouching systems can be used in these situations (Fig. 18-10). One-piece or two-piece systems are used with skin barriers already attached. Transparent or opaque pouches are available. The pouching system is changed every 3 to 4 days, and the pouch is emptied when it is one third full (see box).

CHANGING A FISTULA POUCH

The pouching system needs to be changed (1) when leakage occurs or (2) on a scheduled basis (e.g., every 3 to 7 days). Impending leakage is signaled by a skin barrier that appears to be waterlogged or by patient complaints about burning or excessive itching. For scheduled pouch changes, a time of the day when function is minimal should be selected. If necessary, suction should be kept on hand to control output. Otherwise, wicking drainage away with 4 × 4–inch sterile pads is effective. If the protocol is expected to be painful, arrangements should be made for analgesia. The analgesic agent should be administered 1 hour before the procedure, or topical lidocaine should be available. The patient is placed in a supine position to smooth out abdominal contours and to create flat surfaces.

The procedure for changing a fistula pouch is as follows:

1. Gather equipment and assemble supplies before removing the pouch.
   a. Pouching system and skin barrier
   b. Paste
   c. Measuring guide and pattern
   d. Closure clip
   e. Scissors
   f. Wicks and/or suction
   g. Water and basin
   h. Clean gloves
   i. Disposal bag
2. Prepare the pouching system.
   a. If a drainage spout is in use, close the spout with a closure clip.
   b. If the pouching system has been changed before, use the pattern and follow directions for changing at the bedside. If the system is being refitted, proceed to the next step.

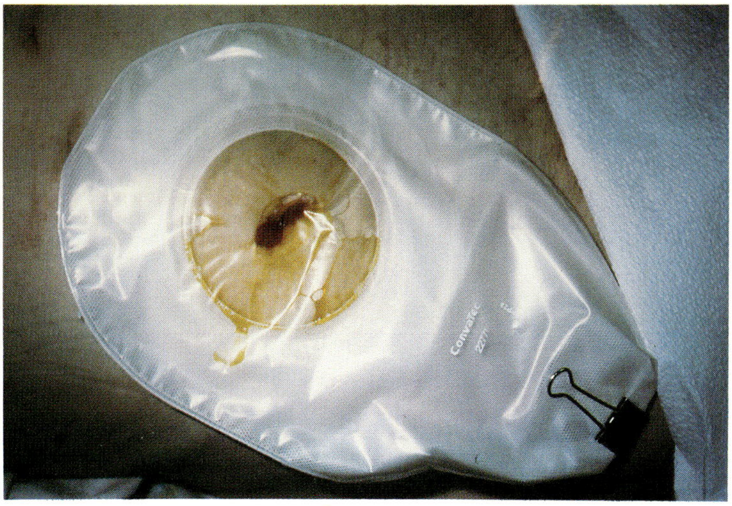

Fig. 18-10. Effluent containment is achieved with this type of one-piece ostomy pouching system. (Courtesy Bonnie Sue Rolstad, R.N., C.E.T.N.)

3. Remove the pouch.
   a. Wear clean gloves to moisten the adhesive with 4 × 4–inch sterile pads or cottonballs. Support the skin while the adhesive is being detached.
   b. Discard the used system and save the closure clip.
   c. If the clip is soiled, wash it in soap and water before reusing it.
4. Fit the pouching system.
   a. Measure the opening from its farthest points and fashion a pattern on a piece of firm paper or plastic. This pattern will be dated and used again. Trace the pattern onto the skin barrier and cut the skin barrier so that it is slightly larger than the pattern. If a separate pouch is in use, cut the pouch ⅛ inch larger than the skin barrier.
   b. When a one-piece pouching system is in use, simply remove the paper backing that covers the adhesive surface. When a two-piece system is being used, remove the paper backings on the pouch and attach the skin barrier to the pouch. Remove the paper backing on the skin barrier.
5. Apply the pouch.
   a. Rinse the skin with clear water and dry. Continue to control output so that the skin is dry when the pouching system is applied.
   b. Apply additional skin barriers, adhesives, etc., as determined at this point, to provide a flat skin surface.
   c. Apply the pouching system and hold it in place for a few minutes. Holding it steady will allow the pectin skin barrier and other adhesives to conform and attach well to the abdomen.
   d. Instruct the patient to lie flat for 5 to 30 minutes, depending on the complexity of the situation. This step allows additional setup time before the patient does any bending.

Fistulas associated with complicated topography require adaptive, less aesthetically acceptable equipment. Large pouches, multiple pieces of equipment, suction, and casting are included in this category. Such fistulas are characterized by poor abdominal location (e.g., creases, bony prominences, umbilicus, costal margins) and topographic obstacles proximal to the opening (e.g., retention sutures, drains, stomas, open wounds). Often cutaneous openings are large (e.g., >3 inches), located within a deep wound, and have multiple sites.

The main objective in the management of fistulas is to develop a system that provides a mirror image of the abdomen in proximity to the fistula. Equipment selection is designed to fill irregular contours, to provide support for soft or flaccid tissue while allowing flexibility for the firm abdomen, and to bypass topographic obstacles. Wound drainage collection systems, ostomy products, and chronic wound care products are used in fistula care. These pouching systems involve single or multiple pieces, are transparent, may/may not have access windows, and are adjustable in size; they may or may not have skin barriers already attached (Fig. 18-11).

Preparation of the skin when irregular contours are present involves assessment of the condition of the tissue and product selection. The skin is first cleaned with tap water and a soft tissue. If tissue is macerated or denuded, a skin barrier powder that is hydrophilic and binds fluid to create a sticky surface is used. When the skin is intact but has a high risk of denudation, a

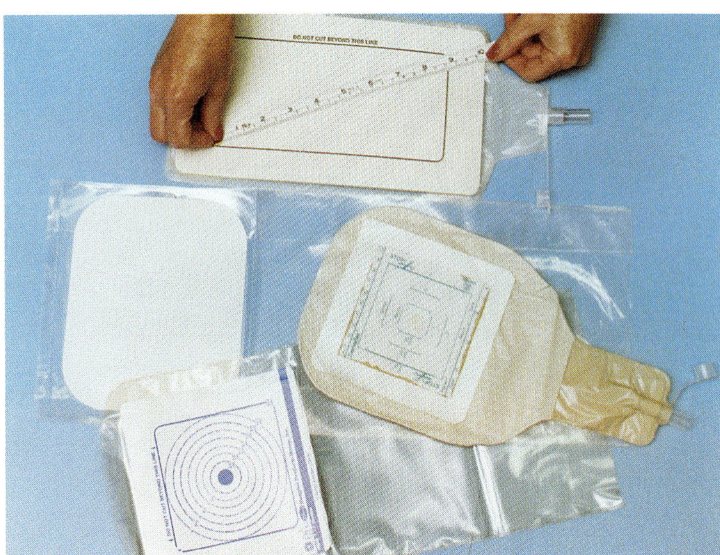

Fig. 18-11. Wound-drainage collection systems, with (or without) skin barriers, outlet valves, and open spouts shown. (Courtesy Bonnie Sue Rolstad, R.N., C.E.T.N.)

water-insoluble skin sealant may be used for protection. Defects in the skin are filled or leveled with a skin barrier paste or a solid-form skin barrier. Skin barrier sheets or pieces may be cut and layered into deep areas in order to provide a flat surface for pouching. If the retracted area is slight, a solid-form skin barrier wafer may be used without further adaptation. Occasionally, a Silastic molding of the skin may be necessary to fill irregular contours[23] (Figs. 18-12 and 18-13). However, this approach is costly and requires frequent re-

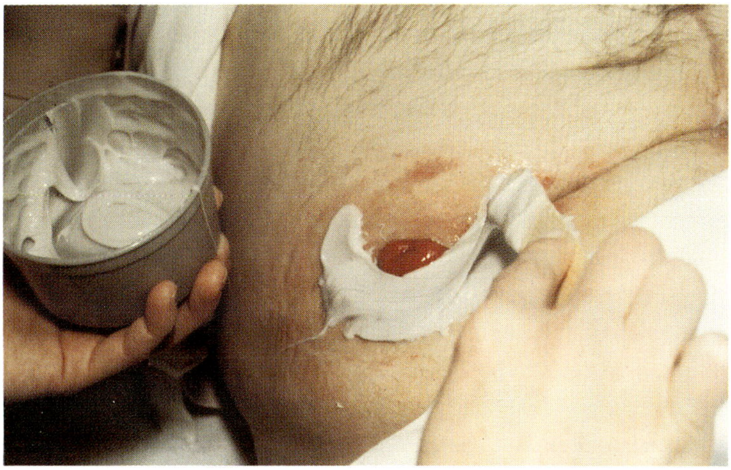

Fig. 18-12. Silastic casting: application of the molding to the skin. (Courtesy Bonnie Sue Rolstad, R.N., C.E.T.N.)

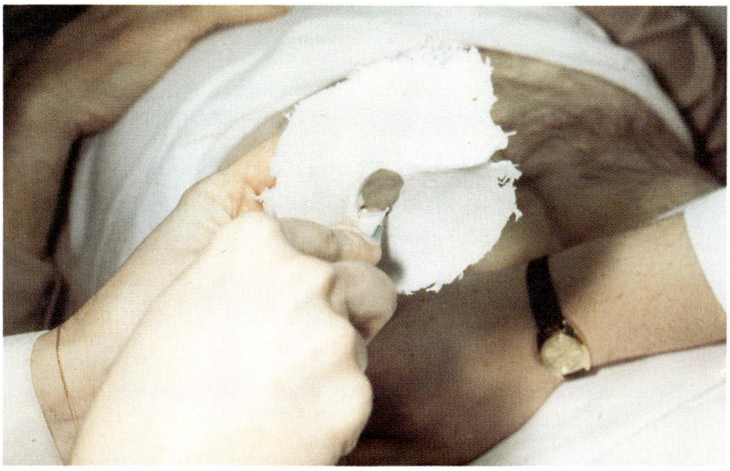

Fig. 18-13. Silastic casting: preparation of a setup mold before application to the abdomen. (Courtesy Bonnie Sue Rolstad, R.N., C.E.T.N.)

casting as abdominal contours change. A latex or silicone cement may be needed to provide additional adhesive. However, it is important to remember that additional adhesive is not a substitute for a properly fitted pouching system. Using more adhesive does not ensure greater security from leakage.

A solid-form skin barrier is also necessary in fistula care to provide increased skin protection and conformability. These barriers have an adhesive surface. They may already be attached to a pouch, or they may be individually fashioned to the fistula size and then attached to the pouch adhesive.

Pouches available are clean or sterile, nondrainable or drainable, transparent or opaque, and come in adult and pediatric sizes. They are available in single or multiple pieces, with or without skin barriers attached, with or without access windows, and may have presized or size-adjustable adhesive surfaces. Ostomy pouching systems and wound drainage collection systems are initial options to consider since they involve little assembly and they are available, cost-effective, and generally understood by nursing staff. Wound drainage collection systems are pouches with access windows and large surface areas of skin barriers attached for custom fitting. These systems have large lumen drainage outlets but are adaptable for straight drainage. Even when observation and treatment of the wound is not required, a wound drainage collection system may be indicated because of its ease in use and the size of the adhesive surface.[24-26]

When the cutaneous opening of the fistula requires a small, flexible pouching system or one with a larger adhesive surface than wound drainage collection systems can accommodate, a pouching system can be custom fit. Pediatric pouches or custom-made pouches with condom catheters can be fashioned for small, difficult-to-access areas[27] (Figs. 18-14 and 18-15). Large drain pouches and separate skin barriers with size-adjustable adhesive surfaces are indicated for cutaneous openings with large, irregular shape openings. Occasionally two large drain pouches, both having 8 x 8–inch adhesive surfaces, are overlapped and placed on the skin to increase the adhesive surface available. This technique is referred to as "saddlebagging." When a midline incision requires pouching but is too large for the methods described here, a trough procedure can be done. A solid-form skin barrier wafer is pieced around the wound and transparent film dressings are applied to cover the top two thirds of the site. A traditional pouching system is then used at the bottom of the wound. This procedure directs effluent down toward the pouch and allows the use of a smaller opening pouching system.[28]

When a tube or a drain is inserted into the fistula site or is located near the area to be pouched (e.g., sump), it may be necessary to pouch the tube with the fistula. A catheter access port may be used to deliver the tube through the

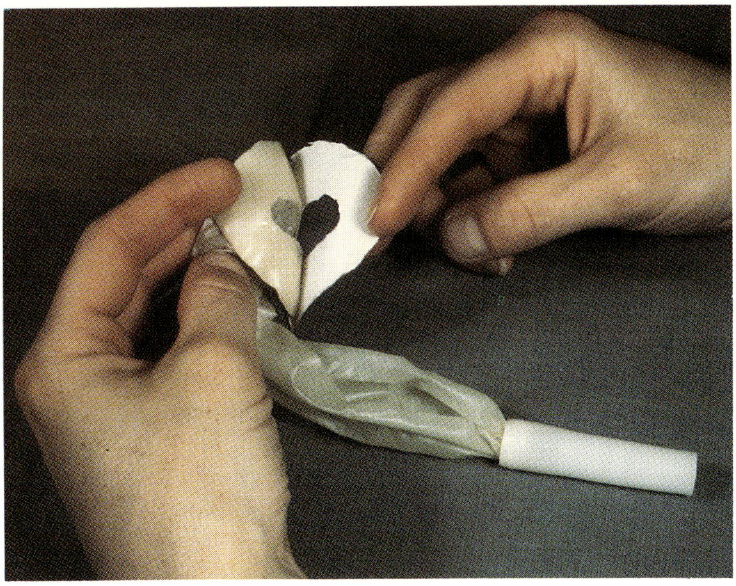

Fig. 18-14. Preparation of a condom catheter with skin barrier and cement. (Courtesy Bonnie Sue Rolstad, R.N., C.E.T.N.)

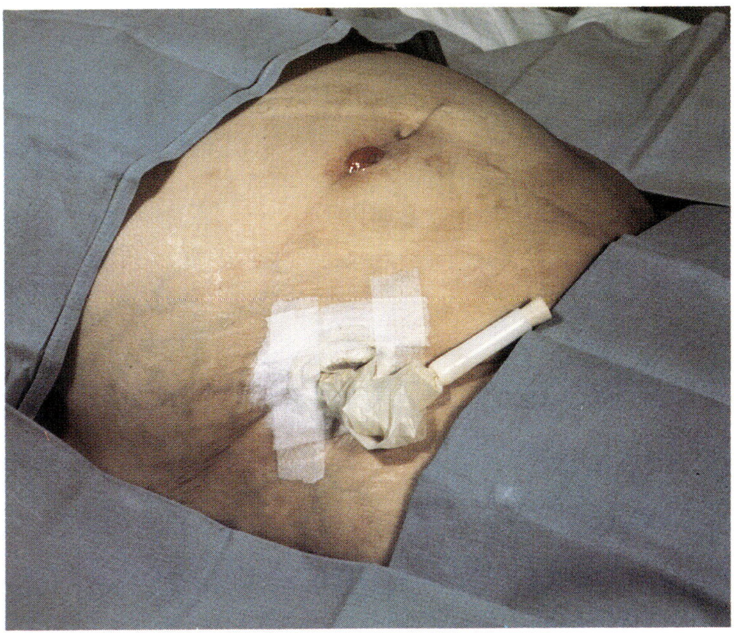

Fig. 18-15. Condom catheter pouching system shown in place. (Courtesy Bonnie Sue Rolstad, R.N., C.E.T.N.)

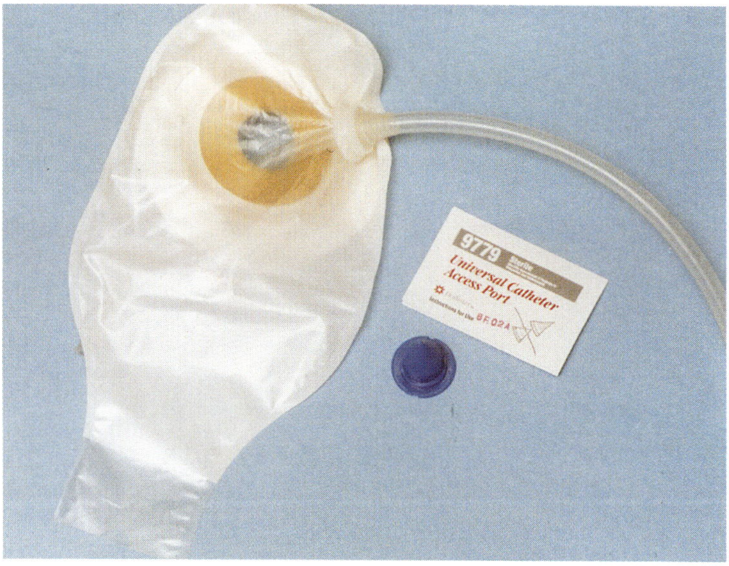

Fig. 18-16. Access port for a drainage catheter can be seen attached to straight drainage or suction. (Courtesy Bonnie Sue Rolstad, R.N., C.E.T.N.)

front of the plastic pouch. The device also seals off potential leakage sources from the opening made in the plastic (Fig. 18-16).

Inspection of wound. Often, access to the wound is needed when the pouch is in place. Advancement or removal of drains, inspection of the wound, or diagnostic procedures may require pouch removal if an access window is not available. Some wound drainage collection systems are equipped with access windows that are convenient and cost-effective.

ODOR CONTROL

Odor control is a concern with patients who have fecal fistulas. It is routinely the most common patient complaint because the odor is pungent and tends to linger. When a dressing is being used to contain effluent, there is no odor barrier. A charcoal-impregnated dressing may be placed over the gauze dressings to control odor (Fig. 18-17). However, charcoal dressings are inactivated when they come in contact with moisture. Charcoal-impregnated dressings are indicated with low-volume fistulas when this specialty dressing is changed every 24 to 48 hours.

A distinction must be made between pouches with odorproofing vs. odor-resistant characteristics. Most pouches are odorproof. However, urinary pouches and some large fistula drain pouches are odor-resistant. In either

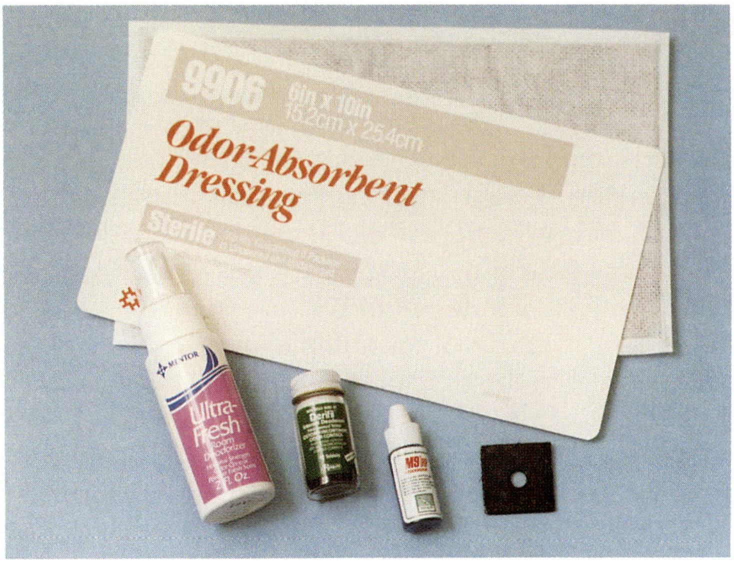

Fig. 18-17. Products used to deodorize effluent include polyurethane foam impregnated with carbon, carbon dressing, charcoal filter for pouch, liquid or tablet deodorizer to be inserted into the pouch, and room spray. (Courtesy Bonnie Sue Rolstad, R.N., C.E.T.N.)

case offensive odors require attention. Deodorants may be taken orally (e.g., bismuth subgallate, chlorophyllin), placed in the pouch (e.g., liquids, powders), or sprayed in the room. The preferred methods are pouch deodorization and room sprays, which avoid the risk of potential systemic interactions. Deodorants used in the pouch must be instilled after every pouch emptying in order to be effective. Room deodorizers should neutralize rather than mask odors.

Simple, often-overlooked methods of odor control are to check pouch spouts to be sure that they are clean, to dispose of soiled materials used in the pouch change or emptying, to check the pouch to be certain that it is not leaking, and to replace a pouch or a tube that has been in use too long. Patients can be instructed to assist with these checkpoints in order to eliminate odor problems.

PATIENT SUPPORT

Patients with an enterocutaneous fistula are faced with numerous psychosocial issues, but three important ones are independence, control, and concerns about the future.[2] Coping strategies used by these patients are varied. Intellectualization, denial, confrontation, isolation, and rationalization are only a few. Supportive counseling is a useful intervention for helping the patient to cope because it decreases the patient's anxiety and the sense of isolation.

Effective technical management of the fistula is primary to patient adaptation. Patients who have leakage and odor associated with their pouching system are anxious and insecure. Therefore securing the pouching system is the initial step toward patient support. Once the containment system has been made secure, mobility and aesthetic issues can be addressed. Mobility is restricted when some pouching systems are used. An example of this restriction is a patient using suction for collection of exudate. Immobilization may lead to the secondary problems of pneumonia or pressure ulcers. Attention to respiratory activity and pressure reduction on the bed are critical in preventing these problems. Suction or straight drainage can be disconnected during ambulation. However, the ongoing need for suction should be reevaluated frequently in order to respond to the concerns of patient dignity and mobility. When pouching systems are used for fistulas over long periods of time, opaque pouches or fabric pouch covers may be used. This intervention decreases the perspiration associated with plastic and removes the soiled pouch from view.

Restricted mobility and ongoing treatment threaten the patient's independence and lead to concerns about the future. All patients worry about their ability to function normally. In addition, they are concerned about their freedom to interact in relationships with others. Loss of love and approval from significant others is another important issue. The employed person may be worried about loss of a position and future income. Prolonged or numerous hospitalizations threaten the person's independence, finances, and emotional stability. In response to these needs, supportive counseling with consistent caregivers is most helpful. The collaborative approach also aids the caregivers because the primary physicians and the ET nurse become primary support resources as they help one another. In addition, a mental health professional is a useful support to patients, whether they need short-term or long-term care.

Issues of control are common concerns for patients with a fistula. In order to respond to these needs, patients and significant others are included in teaching sessions from the beginning. Understanding the rationale for interventions and encouraging participation with procedures reinstates a measure of control for the patient.[29] Initially patients are encouraged to inform the nurse when the pouch requires emptying. Later they are asked to participate in skin care and dressing changes or pouch assembly. When such physical participation is not possible, the patient may take on the role of overseer and supervisor of care. At discharge, the caregiver, whether patient or significant other, provides a return demonstration of skills for the nurse. Follow-up appointments for ongoing evaluation are scheduled with the ET nurse.

COST CONTAINMENT

As expected, clinical efficacy takes priority over cost. When access to the wound or large adhesive surfaces are required, few alternatives exist that are appropriate, regardless of cost. However, knowledge of equipment costs is important. Fistula pouching systems vary in regard to both expense and nursing time required. Costing is based on the numbers of procedures and amount of equipment needed to maintain the fistula weekly. The most expensive method of managing a fistula is the use of gauze dressings. Somewhat less expensive is a wound drainage collection system or a custom-made system with multiple components. Ostomy pouches used for fistula management involve one fifth the expense of a wound drainage collection system.[5]

REFERENCES

1. Alexander-Williams J, Irving M. Intestinal Fistulas. Bristol: John Wright & Sons, Ltd./ Stonebridge Press, 1982, pp 84-102.
2. Rolstad BS. Facilitating psychosocial adaptation. J Enterostom Ther 14:28-34, 1987.
3. Boarini JH, Bryant RA, Irrgang SJ. Fistula management. Semin Oncol Nursing 2(4): 287-292, 1986.
4. Irrgang S, Bryant RA. Management of enterocutaneous fistula. J Enterostom Ther 11:211-225, 1984.
5. Bryant RA. Management of drain sites and fistulas. In Bryant RA. Acute and Chronic Wounds: Nursing Management. St. Louis: Mosby–Year Book, 1992, pp 248-287.
6. Watson PG. Meeting the needs of patients undergoing ostomy surgery. J Enterostom Ther 12:121-124, 1985.
7. Bubrick MP, Rolstad BS. Intestinal stomas. In Gordon PH, Nivatvongs S. Principles and Practice of Surgery for the Colon, Rectum, and Anus. St. Louis: Quality Medical Publishing, 1992, pp 893-895.
8. Doughty DB. Principles of wound healing and wound management. In Bryant RA. Acute and Chronic Wounds: Nursing Management. St. Louis: Mosby–Year Book, 1992, pp 31-68.
9. Watt RC. Pathophysiology of peristomal skin. In Broadwell DC, Jackson BS. Principles of Ostomy Care. St. Louis: CV Mosby, 1982, p 244.
10. Johnson A, White A, McAnalley B. Comparison of common topical agents for wound treatment: Cytotoxicity for human fibroblasts in culture. Wounds 1(3):186-192, 1989.
11. Lineaweaver W, Howard R, Soucy D, et al. Topical antimicrobial toxicity. Arch Surg 120:267-270, 1985.
12. Rodeheaver G. Controversies in topical wound management. Wounds 1:19-34, 1989.
13. Wroblewski JJ. Ointments, creams, gels: Wounding with topical skin care preparations. Ostomy/Wound Management 15 (Summer):46-54, 1987.
14. Felice P. Wound management and the dermal ulcer. Ostomy/Wound Management 8 (Summer):20-24, 1985.
15. Hampton BG. Peristomal and stomal complications. In Hampton BG, Bryant RA. Ostomies and Continent Diversions: Nursing Management. St. Louis: Mosby–Year Book, 1992, pp 105-125.

16. Polk HC Jr, Simpson CJ, Simmons BP, Alexander JW. Guidelines for prevention of surgical wound infection. Arch Surg 118:1213-1217, 1983.
17. Alvarez O, Rozint J, Meeham M. Principles of moist wound healing: Indications for chronic wounds. In Krasner D. Chronic Wound Care: A Clinical Source Book for Healthcare Professionals. King of Prussia, Pa.: Health Management Publications, 1990, pp 266-289.
18. Brennen SS, Leaper DJ. The effect of antiseptics on the healing wound: A study using the rabbit ear chamber. Br J Surg 72:780-782, 1985.
19. Branemark PI, Ekholm R. Tissue injury caused by wound disinfectant. J Bone Surg 49A:48-62, 1967.
20. Felice MM. Draining wound management: Techniques for skin preservation. In Krasner D. Chronic Wound Care: A Clinical Source Book for Healthcare Professionals. King of Prussia, Pa.: Health Management Publications, 1990, pp 247-252.
21. Scott NA, Irving MH. Gastrointestinal Fistulae [monograph]. Basel, Switzerland: Sandoz Pharma Ltd., 1989, pp 1-20.
22. Jeter KF, Tinele TE, Chariker M. Managing draining wounds and fistulae: New and established methods. In Krasner D. Chronic Wound Care: A Clinical Source Book for Healthcare Professionals. King of Prussia, Pa.: Health Management Publications, 1990, pp 240-246.
23. Laing BJ. Making silicone casts for enterocutaneous fistulas. ET J Fall:11, 1977.
24. Tonn J. Management of fistula care with a wound drainage collector. J Enterostom Ther 15:87-90, 1988.
25. Jackson BS, Powers ML, Rush-Martin C, et al. A case control clinical trial of two wound drainage collection systems. J Enterostom Ther 15:191-195, 1988.
26. Wessel L. Management of a wound with multiple drains. J Enterostom Ther 16:26-28, 1989.
27. Wilson V, Roback SA, Leonard AS. A new appliance for the premature or newborn baby with an intestinal stoma. Surgery 77:715, 1975.
28. Pettengill C. Treatment of extraordinary wounds: Ingenuity and cooperation. J Enterostom Ther 16:29-33, 1989.
29. Watterworth B, Podrasky DL. Meeting the learning needs of the person discharged home with an open wound. J Enterostom Ther 16:12-15, 1989.

19 SKIN PROBLEMS IN STOMA MANAGEMENT

Robert D. Fry and Mary Ellen Swatske

The integrity of the skin adjacent to an abdominal stoma is jeopardized by a number of factors: the erosive effects of proteolytic enzymes in the effluent of an ileostomy; the irritating and crystal-forming properties of alkaline urine from an ileal conduit; the high bacterial concentration in feces from a colostomy; allergies to various components of enterostomal equipment, including agents used to remove adhesives and to prepare the skin for placement of an ostomy management system; and mechanical trauma caused by stripping adhesives from the skin or by pressure from an improperly fitted ostomy device. These hazards exist in the best of circumstances, even when the stoma has been properly fashioned and satisfactorily positioned on the abdominal wall, with precise approximation of the intestinal mucosa to the skin. Peristomal skin problems are magnified manyfold by failure to establish an adequate everting spigot for an ileostomy or by placement of a stoma in a skin crease or scar, which hampers efforts to establish a seal between the skin and the ostomy management system.

Patient education is essential to the prevention of peristomal skin problems. Much time is required to teach a patient the proper management of an ostomy, the importance of meticulous and gentle skin care, the correct method to fit and place an ostomy device, and the necessity of prompt recognition of inflammation of the peristomal skin. Unfortunately, even when the basic principles are followed, problems may arise. The cause of most common peristomal skin problems can be divided into four categories: chemical irritation, infection, allergy, and trauma.

CHEMICAL IRRITATION

Dermatitis caused by the leakage of stool or urine onto the peristomal skin is the most common dermatologic problem associated with an intestinal stoma. Leakage of the effluent may be the result of several factors already noted: a poorly located stoma, an ileostomy fashioned without an adequate everting nipple, an ill-fitting ostomy management system, or the inappropriate use of skin barriers. Ileostomy drainage that comes in contact with the skin can cause erythema within an hour, and ulceration of the skin surface can occur within a few hours.[1] Leakage also can cause skin erosion and its associated problems (Figs. 19-1 and 19-2). Regardless of the stoma type, chyme, urine, or feces that stays in prolonged contact with the skin will result in inflammation

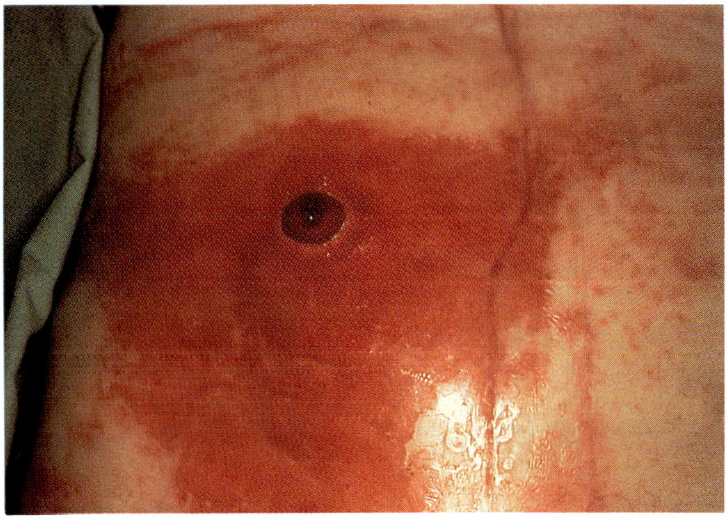

Fig. 19-1. Ileostomy with extensive skin erosion caused by leakage of ostomy management system.

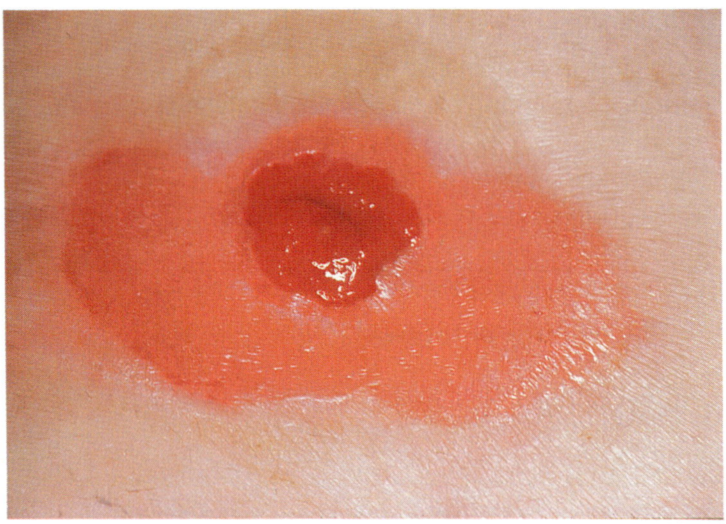

Fig. 19-2. With a flush ileostomy stoma, failure to maintain a seal has resulted in erosion of the skin adjacent to the stoma.

manifested by erythema and subsequent ulceration. Leakage may occur because of scars adjacent to the stoma that have been concealed by a faceplate. Such "hidden leaks" may be difficult to recognize because seepage does not occur at the outer margin of the faceplate.[2] The resulting irritant dermatitis is characterized by marked pruritus and scratching, which perpetuate the inflammation and further compromise adherence of the ostomy device.

Prolonged skin contact with urine may result in encrustation consisting of verrucous plaques of triple phosphate (calcium, magnesium, and ammonium phosphate) or uric acid crystals.[3] This crystal formation is associated with alkaline urine and may cause tears at the mucocutaneous margin or on the mucosa of the stoma.

Exposure of the peristomal skin to chyme or, more commonly, urine may cause pseudoepitheliomatous hyperplasia[4] (Figs. 19-3 and 19-4). This benign cutaneous proliferative disorder, which is the result of chronic inflammation, is characterized by reddish-brown nodules that may become confluent at the mucocutaneous border. Histologic examination will reveal irregular acanthosis with downward proliferation of the epidermis accompanied by acute and chronic inflammation.

Cutaneous inflammation also can be caused by inappropriate use of soaps, detergents, glues, and solvents. Soaps and detergents may leave a

Fig. 19-3

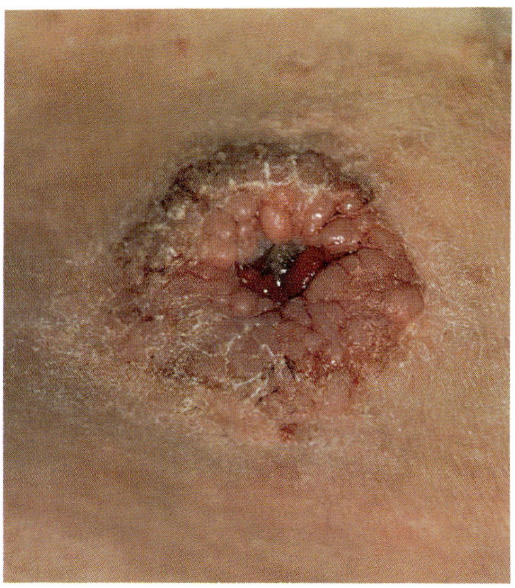

Fig. 19-4

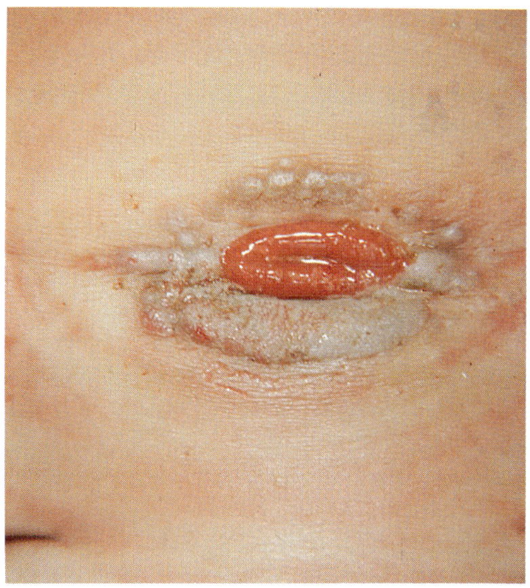

Fig. 19-3. Flush stoma surrounded by pseudoepitheliomatous hyperplasia.
Fig. 19-4. Pseudoepitheliomatous hyperplasia adjacent to an ileostomy placed in an abdominal wall skin crease. A seal between the ostomy device and the skin cannot be maintained.

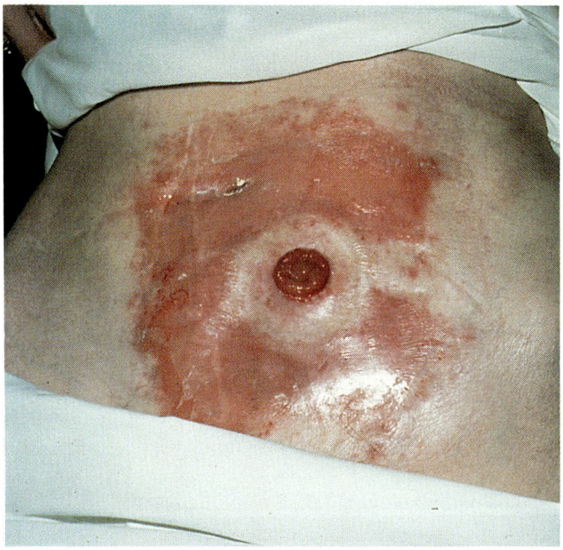

Fig. 19-5. Allergic reaction to the adhesive used with an ostomy device.

chemical residue; therefore the skin must be rinsed thoroughly with water (preferably in the shower) after such agents have been used. Glues should be applied sparingly, as a thin coat, and allowed to dry completely before the ostomy management system is placed; otherwise nonevaporated solvents can become sealed beneath the ostomy device and cause dermatitis (Fig. 19-5). Solvents used to remove adhesive glues should be rinsed thoroughly from the skin before new adhesive is applied.

Treatment

It is imperative to establish a properly fitted ostomy management system to protect the skin from chemical irritants. Unless this goal is met, other forms of treatment have little chance of success. Scars or skin creases adjacent to the stoma can be filled in with a paste to create an even surface that adheres to the skin barrier and pouch. Skin ulcers that cannot be excluded from the pouching system and treated separately can be filled with pastes, powders, or granules that do not contain alcohols or solvents. The area then can be covered with nonadherent dressings (e.g., Telfa) that fit the configuration of the ulcer. Next, a hydrocolloid barrier can be placed directly over the protected ulcer. The skin barrier should be changed and the ulcer treated until healing is complete. The frequency of treatment is determined by the severity of the skin ulcer. Inflamed skin may be treated with compresses of saline solution or 1% sodium propionate/chlorophyllin. Use of a nonfluorinated steroid cream

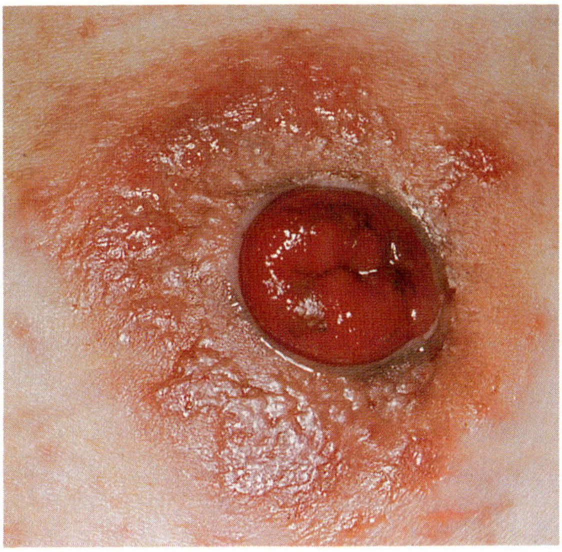

Fig. 19-6. *Candida* infection involving the peristomal skin.

may be helpful in alleviating the pruritus and burning associated with inflammation. However, topical steroids should be used sparingly because atrophy of the skin may result when they are present under an occlusive ostomy device.

The formation of urinary crystals can be prevented by acidification of the urine. This acidification usually can be accomplished by having the patient drink cranberry juice (which is metabolized to hippuric acid) or by taking vitamin C (up to 8 g/day). Urinary crystals can be treated by application of compresses of half-strength vinegar solution for 20 minutes. If the crystals have grown onto the mucosa of the stoma, the diluted vinegar can be added to the pouch and used to bathe the stoma several times a day.

Protection of the peristomal skin by following the basic principles of cleansing and selection of a proper-fitting ostomy management system will permit resolution of the skin changes of pseudoepitheliomatous hyperplasia.

INFECTION

Candida albicans (formerly *Monilia*) is the most common cause of peristomal skin infection (Fig. 19-6). This fungal infection seems especially common in patients with ileal conduits for urinary diversion. *Candida* is a component of the normal flora of the gastrointestinal tract.[5] It is likely that the overgrowth of the fungus on peristomal skin is related to the reduction of normal cutaneous protective mechanisms. Perioperative antibiotics, extensive skin cleansing, and the warm, moist environment under the ostomy device are contributing factors.

Candida infection of the skin causes itching and burning, and the clinical appearance of candidiasis is characterized by well-circumscribed erythema with satellite papules and pustules. The diagnosis may be confirmed by obtaining skin scrapings prepared with 10% potassium hydroxide and by observing the typical budding yeast for hyphae or pseudohyphae. However, a negative potassium hydroxide examination does not entirely exclude the possibility of candidiasis. If clinical suspicion is high for a fungal infection, cultures should be obtained by using Sabouraud's dextrose agar with antibiotics.[6]

A peristomal *Candida* infection is treated by dusting nystatin powder over the infected skin with each pouch change until the infection has been eradicated. Creams or ointments containing the imidazoles (ketoconazole, miconazole, clotrimazole, econazole, and sulconazole) may be effective, but these agents must be given time to absorb before the skin barrier can be applied.[7]

Recurrent infections with *Candida* may be caused by colonization of the gastrointestinal tract. In such circumstances nystatin may be given orally for 2 weeks. However, the skin infection still should be treated topically since nystatin is poorly absorbed from the gastrointestinal tract and thus has no effect on cutaneous infections.

Tinea corporis also may develop on the peristomal skin. This infestation appears as a well-circumscribed erythematous rash bordered by a layer of delicate scales. Microscopic examination of scrapings from the scaly border prepared in 10% potassium hydroxide will show septate, branching hyphae. Tinea corporis may be difficult to differentiate from candidiasis by clinical appearance. If the potassium hydroxide examination is negative, we advocate topical treatment with an imidazole cream until the diagnosis can be established by culture. Nystatin is not effective in the treatment of tinea corporis.

For serious tinea infections in which the diagnosis has been established, oral administration of griseofulvin is recommended. It must be recognized that griseofulvin is ineffective for candidiasis.[8]

Bacterial infection of the peristomal skin is relatively uncommon; probably the most common pathogen is *Staphylococcus aureus*. Gastrointestinal organisms such as *Proteus* or *Pseudomonas* may colonize ulcers caused by chemical irritation or trauma. Bacterial infection of the skin usually presents as erythematous crusty plaques. Cultures should be obtained to direct appropriate antibiotic therapy. Peristomal skin infection caused by *S. aureus* may be treated topically with mupirocin, which is applied to the affected skin three times daily. Frequent treatment of peristomal skin requires the use of a nonadherent pouch to avoid additional trauma to the skin during treatment. If a satisfactory response is not observed within 5 days, the patient should be reevaluated. Recurrent staphylococcal infections suggest that the patient may be a carrier. It is probably beneficial to treat such patients by applying mupirocin within the nares twice a day for 2 weeks.

Folliculitis may develop in the peristomal skin if hair is allowed to grow and is pulled each time the pouch is changed. Erythematous punctate lesions or pustules that occur around the hair follicles usually are caused by *S. aureus*. This problem is best prevented by cutting the hair with scissors or an electric razor. The use of razor blades should be avoided because they may cause microabrasions of the skin, producing increased susceptibility to infection. Depilatory agents seldom are recommended because of a high incidence of allergies to these substances.

ALLERGY

The number of elements to which humans can develop an allergy seems to be limitless, and the many powders, pastes, barriers, adhesives, pouches, tapes, clamps, and belts available for enterostomal therapy provide the human body with ample substrate for allergenic development.[9,10] A contact allergy commonly is manifested by cutaneous erythema and blister formation that is limited to the area of contact with the allergen. Symptoms include severe pruritus or burning of the affected skin. Identifying the offending material requires careful examination of the skin and the ostomy management system and reconstruction of each step in the process of fitting the ostomy device. A patch test may be performed by applying the suspected allergen to the skin of the back and covering the area for 2 days. A reaction to the substance confirms the diagnosis. Treatment consists of removal of the identified allergen. Affected skin may be treated with topical steroids, and oral antihistamines are useful for temporary relief of itching. Systemic steroids are indicated for severe reactions.

TRAUMA

The most common cause of trauma to the peristomal skin is repeated stripping of adhesives during changes of the ostomy device. Usually an erythematous response occurs, but the skin can be denuded and erosion and ulceration can result. It is important that an ostomy device be maintained for at least 4 days. More frequent changing is likely to cause the skin to become irritated, and in such circumstances an alternative pouching system should be devised. Skin trauma caused by pressure or friction from an improperly fitted ostomy device or from belts or faceplates secured too tightly can be diagnosed easily. Treatment involves devising a properly fitting ostomy device and educating the patient about the dangers of improperly applied belts or support straps.

The careless removal of adhesive tape from the edges of the pouching system may cause skin erythema and superficial abrasion. The amount of tape used should be limited to that needed to protect the edges of the ostomy device. The use of a skin barrier under the tape helps to minimize cutaneous trauma when the tape is removed.

DERMATOSES

Skin diseases such as psoriasis, pemphigus, and eczema may occur in patients with a stoma, and the cutaneous disease may involve the peristomal skin.[11] Meticulous care should be directed toward preventing minor trauma to the peristomal skin in these patients. Patients with psoriasis may develop the skin changes of this disease within injured skin (Köbner reaction), and this possibility is particularly likely in the peristomal area[12] (Fig. 19-7). If psoriasis should develop around the ostomy, treatments that may be beneficial include topical corticosteroids, ultraviolet radiation, retinoids, and methotrexate. During treatment of the skin disease, it may be possible to avoid the need for adhesives by using a nonadhesive karaya ring pouch with a belt.

Systemic lupus erythematosus has been reported to affect the peristomal skin. This disease may cause cutaneous bullae or maculopapular erythematous eruptions. Treatment consists of minimizing trauma to the skin, and topical or intralesional corticosteroids may be useful in this regard. Chloro-

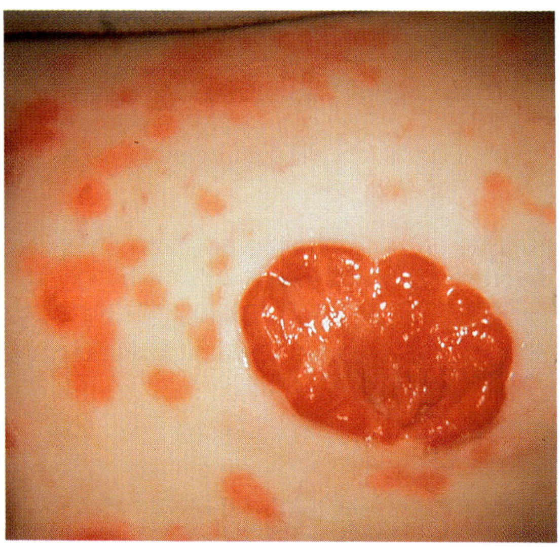

Fig. 19-7. Psoriasis occurring on the peristomal skin.

quine or hydroxychloroquine also may be of benefit in treating the skin manifestations of systemic lupus erythematosus.

MALIGNANCY

Although basal cell carcinoma and squamous cell carcinoma have been reported to arise in the peristomal skin, these malignancies seldom occur in skin that has been shielded from the sun.[13] The malignancy that occurs most commonly in this area is adenocarcinoma arising from the exteriorized bowel. Several cases of adenocarcinoma arising from an ileostomy created for ulcerative colitis more than 20 years earlier have been reported.[14] The primary treatment in such circumstances is to prove the diagnosis by biopsy and then excise the involved bowel and fashion a new stoma before extensive skin involvement occurs.

We have had one patient with metastatic colon cancer that reached the pericolostomy skin and the liver. We were able to achieve excellent palliation of the peristomal tumor with contact radiotherapy by using the instrument that we also use for endocavitary radiation of selected rectal cancers.

RADIATION

Radiation to the skin causes small-vessel damage and relative ischemia, thinning of the epidermis, and destruction of dermal elastic fibers. These changes increase the skin's vulnerability to trauma and seem to impair the normal healing process. If it is necessary to place a stoma in irradiated skin, meticulous care must be taken to avoid unnecessary trauma during the placement and changing of the ostomy device.

Occasionally a patient with a stoma will require radiation therapy. The use of high-energy radiotherapy devices (instruments that provide energy higher than 10 MeV) has dramatically decreased the incidence of skin damage associated with radiation. However, if an enterostomal device is worn during radiotherapy, the faceplate may cause radiation scatter and resultant damage to the underlying skin. This problem is diminished by using lateral ports that avoid the stoma and peristomal skin for a significant portion of the therapy. If a patient routinely changes the ostomy device approximately every week, our radiation oncologists will ask that he or she do so in their department so that the skin can be closely inspected. If peristomal erythema is observed and the stoma must be included in the radiation ports, the ostomy device is removed for each treatment. Between treatments a nonadherent karaya ring pouch with a belt may be sufficient; thus the use of adhesives is avoided until the radiation therapy has been completed.

SUMMARY

Peristomal skin problems are very common, especially in the early postoperative period, before the patient gains a satisfactory understanding of the care required to maintain the integrity of the skin. The goal is to avoid skin problems with proper use of enterostomal techniques. However, the prompt recognition and diagnosis of most skin problems should lead to appropriate treatment and satisfactory resolution.

REFERENCES

1. Lenneberg ES, Sohn N. Modern concepts in the management of patients with intestinal and urinary stomas. Clin Obstet Gynecol 15:542-579, 1972.
2. Martin AG, Leal-Khouri S. Principles of managing dermatologic and wound problems related to intestinal stomas. Semin Colon Rectal Surg 2:161-167, 1991.
3. Rothstein MS. Dermatologic considerations of stoma care. J Am Acad Dermatol 15: 411-432, 1986.
4. Bergman B, Knutson F, Lincoln K, et al. Chronic papillomatous dermatitis as a peristomal skin complication in conduit urinary diversion. Scand J Urol Nephrol 13: 201-204, 1979.
5. Montes LF, Wilborn WH. Fungus-host relationship in candidiasis: A brief review. Arch Dermatol 121:119-124, 1985.
6. Goslen JB, Kobayashi G. Candidiasis. In Jeffers JD, Scott E, White J, eds. Dermatology in General Medicine. New York: McGraw-Hill, 1987, pp 2229-2248.
7. Merk H, Mukhtar H. Azole antifungals. Clin Dermatol 7:121-126, 1989.
8. Artis WM, Odle BM, Jones HE. Griseofulvin-resistant dermatophytosis correlates with in vitro resistance. Arch Dermatol 117:16-19, 1981.
9. Camarasa JMG, Alomar A. Contact dermatitis from a karaya seal ring. Contact Dermatitis 6:139-140, 1980.
10. Beck MH, Burrows D, Fregert S, et al. Allergic contact dermatitis to epoxy resin in ostomy bags. Br J Surg 72:202-203, 1985.
11. Rodriguez DB. Treatment for three ostomy patients with systemic skin disorders: Psoriasis, pemphigus and dermatomyositis. J Enterostom Ther 8:31-32, 1981.
12. Storey VM. Persistent peristomal skin reaction: A case of psoriasis. J Enterostom Ther 9:63-64, 1982.
13. Didolkar MS, Douglass HO, Holyoke ED, et al. Basal cell carcinoma originating at the colostomy site. Dis Colon Rectum 18:399-402, 1975.
14. Roberts PL, Veidenheimer MC, Cassidy S, et al. Adenocarcinoma arising in an ileostomy. Report of two cases and review of the literature. Arch Surg 124:497-499, 1989.

20 UNUSUAL PROBLEMS IN STOMA MANAGEMENT

Donna L. Loehner and David J. Schoetz, Jr.

Challenging problems in the management of stomas vary from fairly common parastomal dermatologic conditions to unusual complications related to the stoma that represent diagnostic and therapeutic dilemmas. Three of the latter types—parastomal pyoderma gangrenosum, parastomal varices, and carcinoma arising in an ileostomy—are discussed in this chapter.

PARASTOMAL PYODERMA GANGRENOSUM

Pyoderma gangrenosum is an indolent, painful ulceration of the skin of unknown cause. In 1930 Brunsting et al.[1] described the condition now known as pyoderma gangrenosum. Since then, pyoderma gangrenosum has been considered an extraintestinal manifestation of ulcerative colitis[2,3] and Crohn's disease.[4] The estimated incidence of pyoderma gangrenosum in inflammatory bowel disease varies from 0.5% to 5% of patients with idiopathic intestinal inflammation.[5-7] Erythema nodosum,[7,8] the other serious cutaneous extraintestinal manifestation of inflammatory bowel disease, may occur in patients with pyoderma gangrenosum, although the two conditions rarely are present at the same time.[9]

Although the lesions may be found in healthy persons, most lesions are associated with an underlying systemic debilitating condition. In addition to inflammatory bowel disease, pyoderma gangrenosum has been described in association with blood dyscrasias, Hodgkin's disease, and chronic active hepatitis.[2,8]

The cause of pyoderma gangrenosum is obscure. The original description of the disease suggested a primary bacterial origin.[10] However, it is now accepted that bacterial colonization is a secondary phenomenon. Although current concepts suggest a primary immunologic mechanism,[8] it is unclear whether this mechanism is directed specifically at the skin or is part of a more generalized autoimmune response to the underlying systemic disease.

Clinically the lesion begins as a number of pustules that erupt and quickly coalesce into the classic painful ulcer with a violaceous border and undermined edge (Fig. 20-1). Most often the lesion affects the pretibial region of the lower extremities. Multiple lesions are the rule rather than the exception.[7,11,12] Associated trauma to the affected area preceding the development of pyoderma has been reported in 10% to 27% of patients.[7,11,12] Pyoderma gangrenosum also has been described in association with surgical incisions.[13]

Parallel activity of inflammatory bowel disease in pyoderma gangrenosum continues to be a source of debate, as is the response of the skin lesions to medical and surgical therapy of the underlying ulcerative colitis or Crohn's disease.[4,6,7,12] Most physicians agree that the clinical course of pyoderma gangrenosum usually correlates with the degree of intestinal inflammation; however, pyoderma gangrenosum also is seen in patients with inactive bowel disease and has been noted after surgical extirpation of ulcerative colitis. When pyoderma gangrenosum develops in a patient with inactive Crohn's disease, the intestinal tract should be reevaluated for evidence of recrudescence of disease activity. Successful medical therapy of inflammatory bowel disease has been associated with healing of pyoderma gangrenosum in approximately two thirds of patients.[12] Bowel surgery has been suggested for patients with refractory pyoderma gangrenosum. When all of the diseased bowel is removed, healing of the skin lesions often is noted. In patients with mild ulcerative colitis, prolonged delays in healing may occur, whereas in patients with severe inflammatory bowel disease, the cutaneous lesions heal

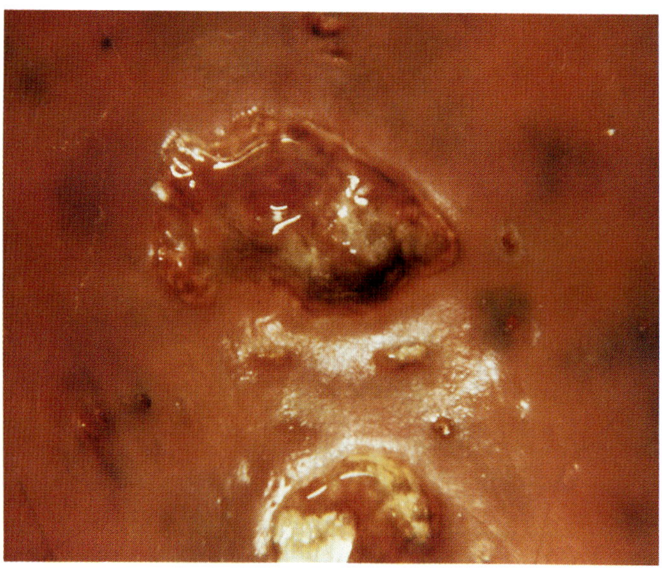

Fig. 20-1. Typical pyodermal lesion with a deep, "punched out" ulceration; undermined edges; and a violaceous border.

promptly.[6] Persistence or recurrence of pyoderma gangrenosum may be related to an operative procedure that leaves residual diseased bowel, for example, subtotal colectomy for ulcerative colitis or a bypass procedure for intestinal Crohn's disease.[7] Because healing after resection cannot be guaranteed and because pyoderma gangrenosum may appear in the postoperative period after removal of all diseased bowel, the physician should be cautious in recommending surgery solely on the basis of the presence of refractory pyoderma gangrenosum.

Surgery for inflammatory bowel disease frequently results in the creation of an ileostomy. Margoles and Wenger[14] were the first to report on the association of parastomal pyoderma gangrenosum and ulcerative colitis. McGarity et al.[15] established the association between parastomal pyoderma gangrenosum and Crohn's disease. Last et al.,[16] in a discussion of parastomal ulcers in Crohn's disease, presented a differential diagnosis of these lesions, including infected hematomas, stitch abscesses, fistulas, and reactivation of Crohn's disease. However, they did not consider pyoderma gangrenosum as a specific entity. A later series reported that half of refractory parastomal ulcers were pyoderma gangrenosum.[17]

Clinical presentation of parastomal pyoderma gangrenosum can be confusing. Fistula and abscess at the suture line may be indistinguishable from the early pustules of pyoderma gangrenosum, with a prodrome of pain, erythema, and tenderness. When the typical ulcer has formed, the diagnosis should be more apparent (Fig. 20-2).

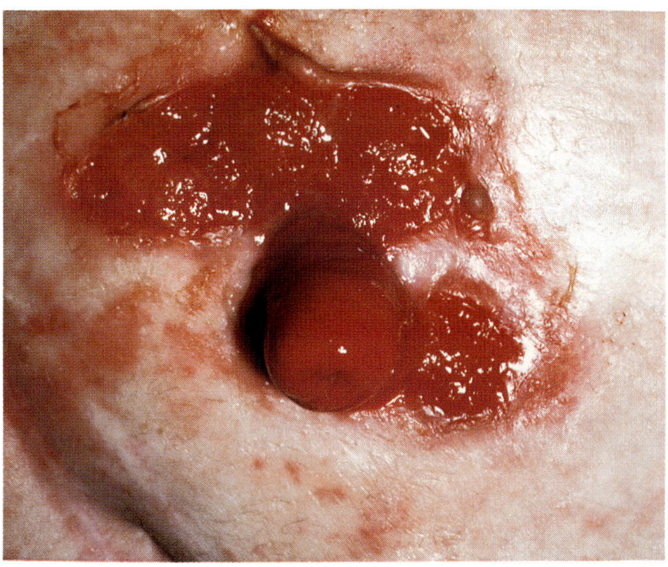

Fig. 20-2. Parastomal pyoderma gangrenosum bordering an ileostomy.

Particular problems with pyoderma gangrenosum in a parastomal location are pain under the ostomy management system and the inability to maintain a seal between the ostomy device and the skin. The goals of therapy must be to address local management of the ulcer and the underlying illness that predisposes the patient to the complication. When the ulcer is small with minimal exudate, the granulating base is covered with Telfa (Kendall Company, Boston, Mass.), and the existing pouching system is replaced. Daily changes are required to remove the exudate and to prevent undermining of the adhesive wafer.[16] Another local treatment for small ulcers includes application of Desitin ointment (Pfizer, Inc., New York, N.Y.) to the ulcer and covering it with Steri-strips (3M Company, St. Paul, Minn.); this method is preceded by wound irrigation to promote a clean granulating base.[18] Other forms of local treatment include Domeboro compresses (Miles Pharmaceutical, West Haven, Conn.), topical antibiotic ointments, and corticosteroid creams.[19]

When the ulcer is large with considerable exudate, hydroactive materials may be used to promote healing in a moist environment. Duoderm granules (E.R. Squibb & Sons, Princeton, N.J.) are applied to the ulcer to absorb moisture, and a Duoderm wafer is used to seal the ostomy device. Methods of moist wound healing combined with topical steroids have been used with some success.[19]

Topical application of disodium cromoglycate, an antiallergy medication, has been used to treat pyoderma gangrenosum in association with inflammatory bowel disease.[20,21] Although the mechanism of action is unknown, speculation regarding the ability of disodium cromoglycate to inhibit histamine release from mast cells suggests that the drug reduces the inflammatory response and permits healing to occur on that basis. In conjunction with the Section of Enterostomal Therapy and the Department of Allergy and Dermatology at the Lahey Clinical Medical Center, a protocol has been developed that includes Domeboro's compresses for the ulcer, twice-daily application of disodium cromoglycate, and topical steroids applied to the edges of the ulcer. This protocol has resulted in the most consistent healing of parastomal pyoderma gangrenosum.[9]

Intralesional injection of steroids was first successfully reported by Moschella.[22] Other authors[23] have reported success with injection of triamcinolone, usually in combination with the use of systemic or topical corticosteroids, around the periphery of the lesion. The Lahey Clinic experience with this regimen has resulted in a satisfactory response in approximately 50% of patients.[4]

Many patients with pyoderma gangrenosum are already being treated with steroids for inflammatory bowel disease. Increasing the dose may result in dramatic improvement of the pyoderma gangrenosum. Whether this improvement is the result of control of the bowel disease or is a primary effect on the skin is speculative.

When the disease is severe, the ulcer surrounds the stoma and leaves no usable skin surface for the pouch. Under these circumstances, the Perry model 51 pouch (Perry Products, Minneapolis, Minn.) is a nonadhesive collection device that can be changed frequently to permit daily wound care.[16] Protrusion of the stoma is a prerequisite for success of this system; when the stoma is flush or retracted or when local management of the ulcer with all available methods is not successful, relocation of the stoma must be considered.

Pyoderma gangrenosum of the parastomal skin requires prompt and aggressive management of the ulcerations as well as the underlying inflammatory bowel disease. Failure to control either may mandate surgical intervention. Resection of all actively involved bowel may permit healing of the pyoderma gangrenosum. Management of this condition requires close cooperation among surgeons, gastroenterologists, dermatologists, and ET therapists to resolve this unusual but debilitating stoma complication.

PARASTOMAL VARICES

Creation of a stoma in a patient with underlying liver disease can be complicated by the development of parastomal portal systemic venous shunts. Presumably these shunts are a result of anastomoses between mesenteric veins and systemic subcutaneous veins. Paracolostomy varices were first reported by Resnick et al.,[24] who noted that coincident esophageal varices did not bleed in patients with this parastomal collateral pathway. Paraileostomy varices were first noted by Eade et al.[25] in patients undergoing proctocolectomy for inflammatory bowel disease. These authors applied the term "caput medusae" to the characteristic appearance of dilated veins around the stoma (Fig. 20-3). Varices also have been described around the ileal conduits created for definitive treatment of urologic conditions.[26] The sole symptom of this rare condition is hemorrhage, which can be life-threatening.

In a review of all reported cases from 1962 to 1989, Conte et al.[27] analyzed 72 cases, of which 49 involved bleeding from an ileostomy, 15 from a colostomy, and 8 from an ileal conduit. Ulcerative colitis was the most common reason for ileostomy, whereas carcinoma of the rectum or the bladder was the most common reason for colostomy or an ileal conduit. Primary sclerosing cholangitis was the most common underlying liver disease in patients with an ileostomy, whereas metastatic liver disease was the most common cause in patients with a colostomy. Alcoholic cirrhosis was the responsible condition

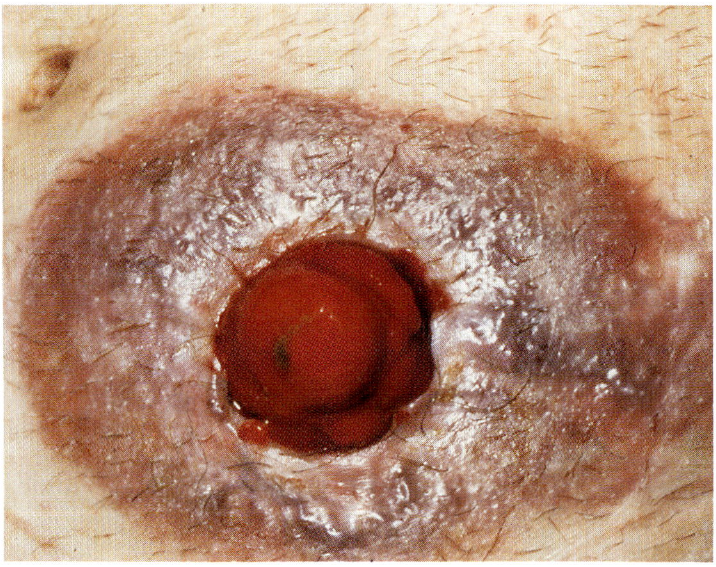

Fig. 20-3. Caput medusae surrounding an ileostomy.

in most of the other patients. The interval between creation of the stoma and the subsequent development of varices ranged from 2 months to 29 years. The clinical presentation in nearly all patients was recurrent episodes of painless gastrointestinal tract bleeding.

Early experience with management of parastomal variceal hemorrhage indicated that local pressure, sometimes with the addition of topical hemostatic agents, is the initial procedure of choice.[25] Correction of circulating blood volume and clotting abnormalities should be accomplished as expeditiously as possible. When local pressure is insufficient, suture ligatures should be placed peripheral to the mucocutaneous junction. Mucocutaneous disconnection, in which the stoma is circumferentially detached from the skin and subcutaneous tissue to the level of the fascia, with ligation of the varices, also has been successful.[28-30] When these measures are unsuccessful, relocation of the stoma may be necessary.

Because of the success of sclerotherapy in the treatment of patients with esophageal varices, sclerosing solutions have been injected into parastomal varices.[31,32] The technique involves injection of a sclerosant into the tissues peripheral to the mucocutaneous junction rather than injection into a discrete varix, which is usually not identifiable. Sclerotherapy can be repeated as necessary in an attempt to obliterate the varices and to lengthen the intervals between bleeding episodes.

Such local procedures must be implemented with careful attention given to the details of the stoma pouching procedures. Bleeding at the site of the stoma can be aggravated by a pouching system that is too small for the stoma. The ET therapist must teach the patient how to measure the stoma by using the guides provided by the manufacturers of ostomy equipment. A one-piece ostomy device that is cut ⅛ inch to ¼ inch larger than the stoma should be considered. Stomahesive paste (Convatec, Inc., Princeton, N.J.) can be used to protect visible skin when the ostomy device is cut larger than the stoma.[33] After the proper size of the equipment has been determined, the patient must discontinue the use of ostomy belts and rigid faceplates. Such products can cause friction and local trauma to the mucocutaneous junction and thus may aggravate bleeding. Patients also must be instructed in the proper gentle removal of the appliance to minimize trauma. Optimal integrity of the parastomal skin needs to be maintained to avoid further episodes of bleeding and to protect the skin from future injury. The patient also can be instructed about methods of digital local control.

Local treatment measures are designed to reduce the frequency of bleeding episodes. In a review by Conte et al.,[27] digital pressure was accompanied by rebleeding within 10 months in 98% of patients. Suture ligature, mucocutaneous disconnection, and revision of the stoma were accompanied by a rebleeding rate of 100%, necessitating further surgery in many patients. Sclerotherapy yielded similar results.

Controversy regarding the role of portosystemic shunting has existed since the original description of this approach in 1970.[34] A central splenorenal shunt was reportedly successful in three patients with paraileostomy varices, as evidenced by no recurrence of bleeding and no hepatic encephalopathy.[35] In a collected series of 72 patients, 27 were treated by portosystemic shunting.[27] Most patients had had multiple procedures before portal decompression was attempted. A central splenorenal shunt was commonly used, followed by an end-to-side portacaval shunt. A distal splenorenal shunt was successfully used to control bleeding in two of three patients in the Lahey Clinic series.[30] Rebleeding was noted infrequently after portosystemic shunt procedures, with an acceptable operative mortality rate and absence of encephalopathy. Before the use of a shunt is considered, all patients should be evaluated through biochemical testing, mesenteric arteriography, and liver biopsy when appropriate.

Despite the potential severity of recurrent bleeding from parastomal varices, few patients die as a direct result of this complication. Rather, life expectancy is determined by the nature and the severity of the underlying liver disease. Consequently, treatment planning must be based on long-term considerations of the status and function of the liver, including the possibility of hepatic transplantation. When portal hypertension is the result of metastatic liver disease or when severe benign liver disease precludes safe performance of portosystemic shunting or liver transplantation, any and all local measures must suffice. If, on the other hand, the patient is a potential candidate for transplantation with satisfactory hepatic reserve, local measures should be attempted to reach the point at which deteriorated liver function mandates liver transplantation. If this state cannot be achieved, a distal splenorenal shunt or some other peripheral shunt is preferred to a portacaval or central splenorenal shunt, which may render transplantation technically difficult or impossible.

ADENOCARCINOMA IN ILEOSTOMY

Adenocarcinoma that arises in an ileostomy is still rare enough to be described only in isolated case reports. Since the original description of this condition in 1969,[36] 11 cases have been reported.[37-45] One other case of adenocarcinoma arising in an ileostomy was thought to be secondary to residual rectal adenocarcinoma after resection of an ileorectal anastomosis and creation of an ileostomy.[46]

With one exception,[38] all reported cases of adenocarcinoma involved an ileostomy originally performed for chronic ulcerative colitis. Adenocarcinoma developed in one patient with familial adenomatous polyposis. Delay between construction of the ileostomy and subsequent carcinoma in the ileostomy varied between 9 years and 38 years, with a median of 23 years. Presenting symptoms include bleeding, parastomal ulceration, and a change in the appearance of the stoma. Pain and obstruction also have been observed.

Pathologically, the tumor is usually a well-differentiated or moderately well-differentiated mucin-producing small bowel adenocarcinoma arising at the mucocutaneous junction. Variable amounts of invasion of the skin and subcutaneous tissue have been noted. In only one patient were mesenteric nodes reported to be involved with metastatic tumor.[45] Of potential importance is the description of ileal mucosal dysplasia associated with carcinoma in five patients.[37,39-41,44]

Clinical presentation of paraileostomy carcinoma should suggest the diagnosis. Inspection of the parastomal skin reveals an ulcerated mass (Fig. 20-4). A biopsy specimen should be obtained with the patient under local anesthesia. Sampling error may result in an inaccurate diagnosis. Consequently, when the clinical suspicion is strong, further biopsies should be obtained. Definitive surgical management includes excision of the ileostomy and the distal small bowel with a wide margin of abdominal wall in continuity, translocation of the stoma to an alternative site, and closure of the primary abdominal wall defect. No reported cases have required major tissue transfer, although prosthetic mesh may be necessary for reconstruction of the abdominal wall.[45] In two series[36,41] metastatic disease to the liver was the

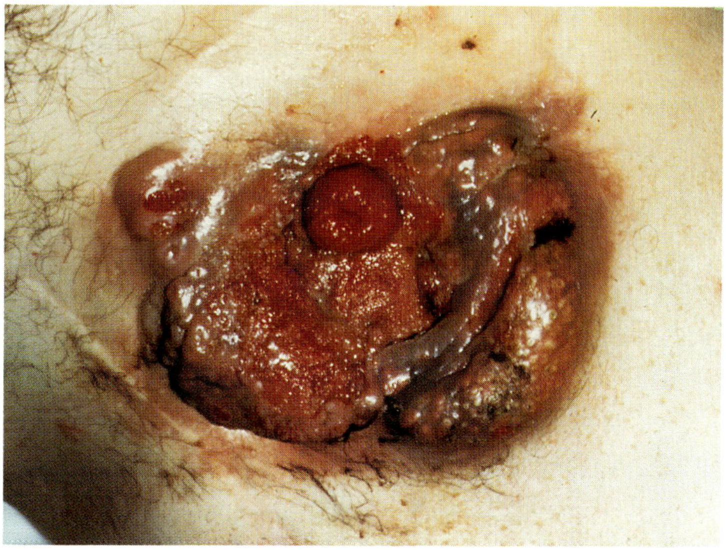

Fig. 20-4. Invasive adenocarcinoma arising in an ileostomy.

cause of death in two patients. Recurrence of disease in the abdominal wall is a consideration, but adjuvant radiotherapy has not been advocated. In one report[43] a recurrent pelvic adenocarcinoma was managed successfully by radical resection. Follow-up data are not sufficient to indicate a definitive prognosis in these patients.

Speculation regarding the cause of paraileostomy carcinoma is based on the association of backwash ileitis and dysplasia noted in many of these patients. One report suggested an association between backwash ileitis and subsequent ileal dysplasia and ileal carcinoma.[47] If this association were true, a routine surveillance program with biopsy and ileoscopy might be undertaken in all patients who have undergone construction of an ileostomy for ulcerative colitis and familial polyposis. The rarity of this clinical entity, however, may not justify such an aggressive approach. Rather, annual inspection of the stoma by a physician or an ET therapist with biopsy of any new abnormalities is probably sufficient.

REFERENCES

1. Brunsting LA, Goeckerman WH, O'Leary PA. Pyoderma (echthyma) gangrenosum: Clinical and experimental observations in five cases occurring in adults. Arch Dermatol 22:655-680, 1930.
2. Perry HO. Pyoderma gangrenosum. South Med J 62:899-908, 1969.
3. Sparberg M, Fennessy J, Kirsner JB. Ulcerative proctitis and mild ulcerative colitis: A study of 220 patients. Medicine 45:391-412, 1966.

4. Schoetz DJ Jr, Coller JA, Veidenheimer MC. Pyoderma gangrenosum and Crohn's disease: Eight cases and a review of the literature. Dis Colon Rectum 26:155-158, 1983.
5. Greenstein AJ, Janowitz HD, Sachar DB. The extra-intestinal complications of Crohn's disease and ulcerative colitis: A study of 700 patients. Medicine 55:401-412, 1976.
6. Talansky AL, Meyers S, Greenstein AJ, Janowitz HD. Does intestinal resection heal the pyoderma gangrenosum of inflammatory bowel disease? J Clin Gastroenterol 5:207-210, 1983.
7. Mir-Madjlessi SH, Taylor JS, Farmer RG. Clinical course and evolution of erythema nodosum and pyoderma gangrenosum in chronic ulcerative colitis: A study of 42 patients. Am J Gastroenterol 80:615-620, 1985.
8. Callen JP, Taylor WB. Pyoderma gangrenosum: A literature review. Cutis 21:61-64, 1978.
9. Arends T, Schoetz DJ Jr, Roberts PL. Unpublished data, 1993.
10. Basler RSW. Ulcerative colitis and the skin. Med Clin North Am 64:941-954, 1980.
11. Powell FC, Schroeter AL, Su WPD, Perry HO. Pyoderma gangrenosum: A review of 86 patients. Q J Med 55:173-186, 1985.
12. Levitt MD, Ritchie JK, Lennard-Jones JE, Phillips RKS. Pyoderma gangrenosum in inflammatory bowel disease. Br J Surg 78:676-678, 1991.
13. Klein JD, Biller JA, Leape LL, Grand RJ. Pyoderma gangrenosum occurring in multiple surgical incision sites. Gastroenterology 92:810-813, 1987.
14. Margoles JS, Wenger J. Stomal ulceration associated with pyoderma gangrenosum and chronic ulcerative colitis: Report of two cases. Gastroenterology 41:594-598, 1961.
15. McGarity WC, Robertson DB, McKeown PP, Amerson JR, Darden WA. Pyoderma gangrenosum at the parastomal site in patients with Crohn's disease. Arch Surg 119:1186-1188, 1984.
16. Last M, Fazio V, Lavery I, Jagelman D. Conservative management of paraileostomy ulcers in patients with Crohn's disease. Dis Colon Rectum 27:779-786, 1984.
17. Wolfsen HC, Brubacher LL, Ng CS, Kayne AL, Kozarek RA. Refractory parastomal ulcers: A multidisciplinary approach. J Clin Gastroenterol 12:651-655, 1990.
18. Williams S. Recognizing peristomal pyoderma gangrenosum. J Enterostom Ther 11: 77-79, 1984.
19. Cuttino C. Pyoderma gangrenosum: An innovative wound care protocol. J Enterostom Ther 14:216-219, 1987.
20. Saffouri B, Hom BM, Mertesdorf JM, Gardiner JE. Treatment of pyoderma gangrenosum with disodium cromoglycate. Dig Dis Sci 29:183-185, 1984.
21. Cave DR, Burakoff R. Pyoderma gangrenosum associated with ulcerative colitis: Treatment with disodium cromoglycate. Am J Gastroenterol 82:802-804, 1987.
22. Moschella SL. Pyoderma gangrenosum: A patient successfully treated with intralesional injections of steroid. Arch Dermatol 95:121-123, 1967.
23. Goldstein F, Krain R, Thornton JJ. Intralesional steroid therapy of pyoderma gangrenosum. J Clin Gastroenterol 7:499-501, 1985.
24. Resnick RH, Ishihara A, Chalmers TC, Schimmel EM, Boston Inter-Hospital Liver Group. A controlled trial of colon bypass in chronic hepatic encephalopathy. Gastroenterology 54:1057-1069, 1968.
25. Eade MN, Alexander Williams J, Cooke WT. Bleeding from an ileostomy caput medusae. Lancet 2:1166-1168, 1969.

26. Foulkes J, Wallace DM. Haemorrhage from stomal varices in an ileal conduit. Br J Urol 47:630, 1975.
27. Conte JV, Arcomano TA, Naficy MA, Holt RW. Treatment of bleeding stomal varices: Report of a case and review of the literature. Dis Colon Rectum 33:308-314, 1990.
28. Grundfest-Broniatowski S, Fazio V. Conservative treatment of bleeding stomal varices. Arch Surg 118:981-985, 1983.
29. Beck DE, Fazio VW, Grundfest-Broniatowski S. Surgical management of bleeding stomal varices. Dis Colon Rectum 31:343-346, 1988.
30. Roberts PL, Martin FM, Schoetz DJ Jr, Murray JJ, Coller JA, Veidenheimer MC. Bleeding stomal varices: The role of local treatment. Dis Colon Rectum 33:547-549, 1990.
31. Morgan TR, Feldshon SD, Tripp MR. Recurrent stomal variceal bleeding: Successful treatment using injection sclerotherapy. Dis Colon Rectum 29:269-270, 1986.
32. Hesterberg R, Stahlknecht CD, Röher HD. Sclerotherapy for massive enterostomy bleeding resulting from portal hypertension. Dis Colon Rectum 29:275-277, 1986.
33. Colwell JC, Dasgupta KA. Primary sclerosing cholangitis: Implications for the ET nurse. J Enterostom Ther 17:171-173, 1990.
34. Cameron AD, Fone DJ. Portal hypertension and bleeding ileal varices after colectomy and ileostomy for chronic ulcerative colitis. Gut 11:755-759, 1970.
35. Adson MA, Fulton RE. The ileal stoma and portal hypertension: An uncommon site of variceal bleeding. Arch Surg 112:501-504, 1977.
36. Sigler L, Jedd FL. Adenocarcinoma of the ileostomy occurring after colectomy for ulcerative colitis: Report of a case. Dis Colon Rectum 12:45-48, 1969.
37. Cuesta MA, Donner R. Adenocarcinoma arising at an ileostomy site: Report of a case. Cancer 37:949-952, 1976.
38. Roth JA, Logio T. Carcinoma arising in an ileostomy stoma: An unusual complication of adenomatous polyposis coli. Cancer 49:2180-2184, 1982.
39. Baciewicz F, Sparberg M, Lawrence JB, Poticha SM. Adenocarcinoma of an ileostomy site with skin invasion: A case report. Gastroenterology 84:168-170, 1983.
40. Stryker SJ. Primary stomal adenocarcinoma: An unusual complication of ileostomy. Dis Colon Rectum 26:47-49, 1983.
41. Bedetti CD, DeRisio VJ. Primary adenocarcinoma arising at an ileostomy site: An unusual complication after colectomy for ulcerative colitis. Dis Colon Rectum 29: 572-575, 1986.
42. Vasilevsky C-A, Gordon PH. Adenocarcinoma arising at the ileocutaneous junction occurring after proctocolectomy for ulcerative colitis. Br J Surg 73:378, 1986.
43. Longo WE, Stephan RN, True LD, August DA, McCullough WB. Recurrent ileal mucinous adenocarcinoma in an ileostomy. J Clin Gastroenterol 8:192-194, 1986.
44. Carter D, Choi H, Otterson M, Telford GL. Primary adenocarcinoma of the ileostomy after colectomy for ulcerative colitis. Dig Dis Sci 33:509-512, 1988.
45. Roberts PL, Veidenheimer MC, Cassidy S, Silverman ML. Adenocarcinoma arising in an ileostomy: Report of two cases and review of the literature. Arch Surg 124:497-499, 1989.
46. Johnson WR, McDermott FT, Pihl E, Hughes ESR. Adenocarcinoma of an ileostomy in a patient with ulcerative colitis. Dis Colon Rectum 23:351-352, 1980.
47. Schlippert W, Mitros F, Schulze K. Multiple adenocarcinomas and premalignant changes in "backwash" ileitis. Am J Med 66:879-882, 1979.

APPENDIXES

APPENDIX

A UNITED OSTOMY ASSOCIATION ADDRESS LIST

UNITED OSTOMY ASSOCIATION, INC., CHAPTER DIRECTORY (January 1, 1993)

Based upon information received from chapter leaders, this listing of UOA chapters is published annually. It is provided for the convenience of ostomates and professionals who need chapter services and for interchapter correspondence. Write to the UOA office for information about any new groups that may not be included here.

UOA requests that the listing not be used for general solicitation.

Chapters receiving any solicitations are advised to submit them to the UOA office before publishing the information to their members.

The following list of regions indicates the states or parts of states and provinces which are included in each of UOA's twelve regions.

Regions

CENTRAL NORTHEAST: New Brunswick, Newfoundland, New York (north of Sullivan and Duchess Counties), Nova Scotia, Ontario, Prince Edward Island, Quebec.

GREAT LAKES: Indiana, Kentucky, Michigan (south of Lakes Huron and Michigan), Ohio, Pennsylvania (west of and including Potter, Clinton, Centre, Huntington, and Fulton Counties), West Virginia.

MIDDLE ATLANTIC: Delaware, District of Columbia, Maryland, Pennsylvania (east of and including Tioga, Lycomin, Mifflin, Union, Snyder, Juniata, and Franklin Counties), Virginia.

MIDWEST: Illinois, Iowa, Kansas, Missouri, Nebraska.

NEW ENGLAND: Connecticut, Maine, Massachusetts, New Hampshire, Rhode Island, Vermont.

Compiled and published by: United Ostomy Association, Inc., 36 Executive Park, Suite 120, Irvine, CA 92714-6744, Phone (800) 826-0826, (714) 660-8624, Fax (714) 660-9262.

NEW JERSEY-METROPOLITAN NEW YORK: Bermuda, Long Island, New Jersey, New York City, New York (Sullivan, Duchess Counties and south).

NORTH CENTRAL: Manitoba, Michigan (north of Lakes Huron and Michigan), Minnesota, North Dakota, Saskatchewan, South Dakota, Wisconsin.

NORTHWEST: Alaska, Alberta, British Columbia, Idaho, Montana, Northwest Territories, Oregon, Washington, Yukon.

PACIFIC COAST: California, Guam, Hawaii, Nevada.

ROCKY MOUNTAIN: Arizona, Colorado, New Mexico, Texas (El Paso, Hudspeth, Culberson, Loving, Jeff Davis, Presidio, and Brewster Counties), Utah, Wyoming.

SOUTH CENTRAL: Arkansas, Louisiana, Mississippi, Oklahoma, Texas (except seven counties in Rocky Mountain Region).

SOUTHEAST: Alabama, Florida, Georgia, North Carolina, Puerto Rico, South Carolina, Tennessee.

UNITED STATES

Alabama

Ostomy Association of Birmingham Alabama #7
205-823-7216
Annie Jacobs
2865 B Regal Circle
Birmingham, AL 35216

Gadsden Alabama Chapter #5
205-442-8710
Grace Gramling
4101 Skylark Circle N.
Gadsden, AL 35901

Huntsville Alabama Chapter #9
205-773-2947
James Roden
Rt. 5, Box 254
Hartselle, AL 35640

Cullman Alabama Satellite #1 (Huntsville Chapter)
205-734-6917
Joseph Sisulak
712 Scenic Drive
Cullman, AL 35055

Mobile Alabama Ostomy Association #6
205-476-7563
Cheryl Johnson
710 Glenwood Street
Mobile, AL 36606

Ostomy Association of Montgomery Alabama #8
205-272-7426
Deborah Burrows
2913 Willow Lane
Montgomery, AL 36109

Morgan County Alabama Area Chapter #699
205-350-3766
James Elliott
632 Johnston Street S.E.
Decatur, AL 35601

Tuscaloosa Alabama Area Chapter #680
205-333-1619
Nell P. Hixon
11120 Lighter Drive
Northport, AL 35476-9645

Alaska

Anchorage Alaska Chapter #447
907-345-4430
Larry Disbrow
P.O. Box 110527
Anchorage, AK 99511

Fairbanks Alaska Satellite #81 (Anchorage Chapter)
907-456-5345
Sherry L. Morrison
260 Bentley Drive East
Fairbanks, AK 99701

Arizona

Cochise County Arizona Chapter #673
602-456-1227
Billy Shelton
309 2nd Street
Huachuca City, AZ 85616

Gila Valley Arizona Satellite #87 (Cochise County Chapter)
602-428-3389
Marvin Erickson
922 Stratton Drive
Safford, AZ 85546

Mesa Tri-City Arizona Ostomy Chapter #667
602-986-2178
Albert L. Mentzer
8203 E. Frito Drive
Mesa, AZ 85208

Tonto-Payson Arizona Satellite #103 (Mesa Tri-City Chapter)
602-474-2482
Margaret Sipple
1107 S. McLane, #34
Payson, AZ 85541

Scottsdale Arizona Satellite #123 (Mesa Tri-City Chapter)
602-986-2178
Albert L. Mentzer
8203 E. Frito Drive
Mesa, AZ 85208

Mission Ostomy Chapter of Tucson Arizona #12
602-749-3262 602-749-2863
Thomas B. Noble
P.O. Box 41454
Tucson, AZ 85717

Greater Phoenix Arizona Colostomy #10
602-944-4500
Ralph Schmich
1001 W. Northview
Phoenix, AZ 85021

Phoenix Arizona Ileostomy/ Urostomy #11
602-973-8981
Keith Richardson
5610 N. 38th Drive
Phoenix, AZ 85019-2107

Sun City Arizona Satellite #2 (Phoenix Ileostomy/ Urostomy Chapter)
602-974-5145
Chester Gadomski
10218 Kelso Drive
Sun City, AZ 85351

Prescott Arizona Chapter #496
602-445-6283
Kate Thompson
525 Shalimar Drive
Prescott, AZ 86303

Arkansas

Batesville Area Arkansas Chapter #644
501-698-2154
Leo Rainey
1230 Marywood Drive
Batesville, AR 72501

Central Arkansas Ostomy Association at Little Rock #314
501-982-4928
Dotty Gillis
516 Sorells Street
Jacksonville, AR 72076

El Dorado Arkansas Chapter #417
501-863-5576
Mrs. A. L. Roberson
417 W. Second Street
El Dorado, AR 71730

Fort Smith Arkansas Chapter #392
501-785-7815 501-646-1438
Mr. Cleatis Carroll
3131 Edinburgh Drive
Fort Smith, AR 72903

Hot Springs National Park Arkansas Chapter #766
501-623-7119
Jan Diggs
106 Edgewood
Hot Springs, AR 71901

Jonesboro Arkansas Chapter #455
501-932-8228
Margaret Scott
1410 Lamar Place
Jonesboro, AR 72401-4821

Northwest Arkansas Chapter #581
501-925-3825
Melissa Becton, R.N.
Rt. 1, Box 825
Rogers, AR 72756

Twin Lakes-Mountain Home Arkansas Chapter #492
501-425-9173
Margaret E. Schaefer
1109 Bluebird Lane
Mountain Home, AR
72653-3303

Bermuda

Bermuda Chapter #535
Kae Thomas
P.O. Box HM 2281
Hamilton HM JX Bermuda

California

Cascade California Chapter #13
916-223-3177
Natalie Parks
1947 Bechelli Lane
Redding, CA 96002

Redwood California Satellite #89 (Cascade Chapter)
707-839-2005
Linda Span
1350 Mill Creek Road
McKinleyville, CA 95521

Tehama County California Satellite #129 (Cascade Chapter)
916-527-1973
Amy Kerby
15 Cabernet Court, #2A
Red Bluff, CA 96080

Central Valley California Chapter #239
209-523-5559
Lloyd Ohlson
1319 Paradise Road
Modesto, CA 95351

Ostomy Association of Greater Chico California #316
916-533-0763
Marjorie Webber
58 Cottonwood Circle
Oroville, CA 95965

Contra Costa County California Chapter #541
510-682-1303
Harry Tse
3510 Torino Way
Concord, CA 94518

West Contra Costa California Satellite #5 (Contra Costa County Chapter)
510-524-6975
Arthur Copen
1659 Shasta Street
Richmond, CA 94804

Downey-Lynwood-Whittier California Chapter #515
Guy Turgeon, M.D.
P.O. Box 904
La Mirada, CA 90637

Golden Gate California Chapter #14
415-664-4443
Margaret Macko
826 Portola Drive
San Francisco, CA 94127

Hemet-San Jacinto California Chapter #558
714-927-4607
William H. Seifert
24913 Howard Drive
Hemet, CA 92544-1901

Lake Elsinore California Satellite #72 (Hemet-San Jacinto Chapter)
714-737-2989
John S. Way
1003 E. Francis Street
Corona, CA 91719

Inland Empire California Chapter #19
714-823-7201
Scott Bayless
16235 Diantlus
Fontana, CA 92335

Laguna Hills California Chapter #642
714-951-5928
Dean Lacy
25211 Stockport Drive, #267
Laguna Hills, CA 92653

Lancaster California Chapter #676
805-943-2461
Jane Minutella
P.O. Box 4271
Lancaster, CA 93539

Long Beach California Chapter #738
310-427-6323
Ruby Kosaka
P.O. Box 91872
Long Beach, CA 90809

Los Angeles California Ostomy Association #15
213-255-4681
5015 Eagle Rock Boulevard, #215
Los Angeles, CA 90041

Monterey County California Chapter #376
408-663-2317
Barbara Nelson
462 Paradise Road
Salinas, CA 93907

Napa Valley California Chapter #17
707-226-3436
Del Lorenzo
1890 Adrian Street
Napa, CA 94559

North County California Ostomy Association #682
619-726-8909 619-433-3440
Pearle Reilly
15636 High Ridge Drive
Oceanside, CA 92056

Escondido California Satellite #85 (North County Chapter)
619-745-3727
Johnie A. Watkins
1339 Taft Street
Escondido, CA 92026

Ontario-Pomona Valley California Chapter #662
714-989-6936
Susan Lycan
7221 Teak Way
Alta Loma, CA 91701

Ostomy Association of Orange County California #18
714-229-0033
Rochelle Kantor
P.O. Box 7041
Orange, CA 92613

Palm Springs-Desert California Chapter #542
619-343-0220
Edward Iarossi
74890 Conestoga
Thousand Palms, CA 92276

Riverside California Chapter #679 (Pull-through and Children)
714-683-4181
Jacquelyn Vizthum
3575 Rosewood Place
Riverside, CA 92506

Sacramento California Ostomy Association #21
916-722-9774
Bob Keller
8235 Old Ranch Road
Citrus Heights, CA 95610

Gold Country California Satellite #4 (Sacramento Chapter)
916-885-4765
Florence Matzka
P.O. Box 5773
Auburn, CA 95604

San Joaquin County California Satellite #6 (Sacramento Chapter)
209-466-2273
Judy Canepa
4111 N. West Lane
Stockton, CA 95204

San Diego California Area Chapter #22
619-223-2966
Robert Danzl
P.O. Box 81324
San Diego, CA 92138-1324

Ostomy Association of San Gabriel Valley California #235
818-791-4730
Gaye Thuen
1701 Elizabeth Street
Pasadena, CA 91104

San Luis Obispo County California Chapter #518
805-773-2896
Betty Ann Johnson
122 Paddock Avenue
Pismo Beach, CA 93449

San Mateo County California Chapter #366
415-697-8673
E.F. "Whitey" Nottke
1215 Manzanita Drive
Millbrae, CA 94030-2933

Santa Barbara California Chapter #23
805-965-4243
Fern Bueschel
10 Via Alicia
Santa Barbara, CA 93108

Santa Clara Valley California Chapter #24
408-377-3633
Ann Pedersen
P.O. Box 305
Santa Clara, CA 95052

Santa Cruz County California Chapter #272
408-662-1336
Jim Victory
245 Via Lantana
Aptos, CA 95003

Santa Maria-Lompoc California Chapter #491
805-925-2359
Raymond Dean
1207 E. Dena Way
Santa Maria, CA 93454

Sequoia/Visalia California Chapter #751
209-625-4701
Nadine Anderson
710 N. Fulgham
Visalia, CA 93291

Solano County California Chapter #564
707-643-3629
Louise Johnson
611 Valle Vista
Vallejo, CA 94590-3455

Sonoma County California Chapter #255
707-838-7079
Betty Rose
9135 Bambi Lane
Windsor, CA 95472

Southern Alameda County California Chapter #643
510-656-0468
Fred Hodsoll
42949 Homewood Street
Fremont, CA 94538

Southern California Parent Support Group #637
619-679-0575
Ruth Rook
13437 Montego Drive
Poway, CA 92064

Ventura County California Chapter #736
805-983-7666 805-485-3663
Virginia Allen
P.O. Box 5285
Oxnard, CA 93030-5285

Thousand Oaks California Satellite #96 (Ventura Chapter)
805-379-9622
Dottie Altamirano
1949 Los Feliz, #144
Thousand Oaks, CA 91362

Victorville and High Desert California Chapter #692
619-244-8697
Hasner Haase
18935 Centennial
Hesperia, CA 92343

Colorado

Metro Denver Colorado Chapter #38
303-447-5909
Richard Hanken
4145 Clay Street
Denver, CO 80211

Larimer County Colorado Chapter #355
303-667-4137
Bob Reeves
2102 Firestone Court
Loveland, CO 80537

Northern Colorado Ostomy Association #39
303-353-2686
Cecil Davis
1712 26th Avenue Court
Greeley, CO 80631

Estes Park Colorado Satellite #7 (Northern Colorado Chapter)
303-586-2575
Teddie Haines
2037 S. Saint Vrain Highway
Estes Park, CO 80517

Pike's Peak Colorado Chapter #40
719-634-2390
Ramona Malone
2010 Preuss Road
Colorado Springs, CO 80910

Valley Colorado Ostomy Association #42
303-249-2048
Dick Willard
61670 W. Popular Road
Montrose, CO 81401

Connecticut

Great Bridgeport Connecticut Area Ostomy Association #275
203-335-0595
Sal Astengo
577 Wood Avenue
Bridgeport, CT 06604

Bristol Connecticut Area Chapter #258
203-582-3962
Helena Davis
1444 Farmington Avenue, RR #1
Bristol, CT 06010

Greater Danbury Connecticut Chapter #394
203-743-1563
Jeffrey Hull
10 Park Avenue
Danbury, CT 06810

Hartford Connecticut Ostomy Association #43
203-634-0098
Ann Mozeliak
P.O. Box 2153
Meriden, CT 06450

Lower Naugatuck Connecticut Chapter #212
203-888-2498
Pauline Walsh
12 Deerfield Drive
Seymour, CT 06483

Manchester Connecticut Area Ostomy Association #44
203-429-5987
Jessie Daniels
35 Birchwood Heights
Storrs, CT 06268

Meriden-Middlesex Connecticut Chapter #349
203-342-4061
Palma Cannata
18 Victoria Road
Portland, CT 06480

New Britain Connecticut Area Chapter #614
203-223-2093
Stanley Paulauskas
2222 Stanley Street
New Britain, CT 06053

Greater New Haven Connecticut Chapter #45
203-934-2034
Francis Coyle
57 Templeton Street
West Haven, CT 06516

New London County Connecticut Chapter #262
203-448-0036
Lisa Markle
25 Greenwood Street
Groton, CT 06340

Southern Fairfield County Connecticut Chapter #46
203-762-8836
Patricia J. Childs
115 Hurlbutt Street
Wilton, CT 06897

Waterbury Connecticut Area Chapter #378
203-758-9362
Shirley Renkun-Harkins
33 Watertown Road
Middlebury, CT 06762

Delaware

Kent/Sussex Counties Delaware Chapter #438
302-697-2440
Virginia M. Dewey
RD #2, Box 289
Camden, DE 19934

Wilmington Delaware Chapter #361
302-329-5907
Frank Hough
334 Willa Drive
Hockessin, DE 19707

District of Columbia

Metropolitan Washington DC Chapter #47
301-630-9260 202-877-6019
Anastasia Johnson
110 Irving N.W.
#3102 E. Boulevard
Washington, DC 20010

Florida

Brooksville-Hernando Florida Chapter #755
904-796-2722
Charles Schwartz
977 Coachlight Lane
Brooksville, FL 34601

Broward Florida Ostomy Association #48
305-983-0620
Irving B. Kay
3340 B Simms Street
Hollywood, FL 33021

Charlotte County Florida Chapter #536
813-629-5650
Rose Antonelli
4158 Tamiami Trail, #N-8
Port Charlotte, FL 33952

Citrus Florida Ostomy Chapter #719
904-726-4706
Frank Caravetto
6101 Ann Jo Drive
Inverness, FL 32652

Clearwater Area Florida Chapter #563
813-786-3922
James Smalls
2700 Nebraska Avenue, B5 U205
Palm Harbor, FL 34684

Coral Gables Florida Chapter #252
305-235-2910
Louis H. Lashinsky
12900 S.W. 110 Avenue
Miami, FL 33176-5422

Daytona Beach Florida Chapter #421
904-738-5176
Esther Westbrook
219 N. Hill Avenue
Deland, FL 32724

Gainesville Florida Chapter #615
904-466-3110
Faye Greene
Rt. 2, Box 190
Micanopy, FL 32667

Swannee Valley Ostomy of Live Oak Florida Satellite #106 (Gainesville Chapter)
904-776-2691
Norma Greenlee
Rt. 2, Box 407-D
O'Brien, FL 32071

Highlands County Florida Chapter #591
813-655-2219
Walton Webb
6041 Thomas Terrace
Sebring, FL 33870-6496

Indian River Florida Ostomy Association #587
407-567-5939
Judith Peirce
1306 29th Avenue
Vero Beach, FL 32960

Jacksonville Florida Chapter #211
904-384-7371
John Lockhart
1002 Acosta Street
Jacksonville, FL 32204

Key West Florida Keys Chapter #725
305-296-4231
Bonita Bishop
B-31 9th Avenue
Key West, FL 33040

Lake County Florida Chapter #322
904-326-8219
Mary Jane Fischer
1211 Pear Lane
Leesburg, FL 34788

Lee County Florida Chapter #557
813-543-1906
Jean Simmonds
376 Harbor Lane
N. Fort Myers, FL 33917

Martin-St. Lucie County Florida #602
407-335-5901
Robert Otto
2874 S.E. Italy Street
Port St. Lucie, FL 33452

Miami Florida Ileostomy/Colostomy Association #49
305-861-9567
Meyer Levine
601 74th Street
Miami Beach, FL 33141

New Port Richey Florida Chapter #468
813-868-7386
Betty Hopper
12006 Vandalia Drive
Hudson, FL 34667

Ocala Florida Chapter #404
904-694-3082
Shirley Dowdy
3816 N.E. 4th Street
Ocala, FL 32670

Greater Orlando & Central Florida Chapter #51
407-282-8973
Margaret Kaye
5816 Blue Dahlia Way
Orlando, FL 32807

Osceola County Florida Chapter #767
407-892-5581
Debbie Hart
1121 Pennsylvania Avenue
St. Cloud, FL 34769

Palm Beach County Florida Ostomy Association #55
407-965-7834
Donna Gough Faquir, R.N.
6101 Woodlake Boulevard
Lake Worth, FL 33463

Panama City Area Florida Chapter #746
904-648-8559
Robert La Plante
P.O. Box 13238
Mexico Beach, FL 32410

Pensacola Florida Chapter #50
904-456-1894
Stephen Batuk
6600 Chelsea Street
Pensacola, FL 32506-4550

Okaloosa-Walton-Santa Rosa Counties Florida Satellite #93 (Pensacola Chapter)
904-678-7478
Ray H. Rudolph
262 Tennessee Avenue
Valparaiso, FL 32580-1566

Polk County Florida Chapter #53
813-853-1760
Mrs. Verne Thompson
3154 Otter Creek Court
Lakeland, FL 33809

Pompano Florida Ostomy Association #632
Stan Fraschner
2315 N.W. 114th Avenue
Coral Springs, FL 33351

Ostomy Association of Sara-Tee Florida #215
813-792-5561
Irvin S. Nance
7707 19th Avenue N.W.
Bradenton, FL 34209

South Brevard Florida Ostomy Association #656
407-733-0445
Renee Wolff
339 Markley Court
Indian Harbour Beach, FL 32937

South Hillsborough Florida Chapter #629
813-633-2386
Robert J. Hellwig
633 Masterpiece Drive
Sun City Center, FL 33573

South Palm Beach County Florida Chapter #752
407-499-0583
Robert W. Rich
14872 Wildflower Lane
Delray Beach, FL 33446

Southwest Florida Ostomy Association #52
813-774-4025
Pat Henn
5651 Rattlesnake Hammock
Naples, FL 33962

Space Coast Florida Ostomy Association #265
407-784-2830
Eve Kelly
201 St. Lucie
Cocoa Beach, FL 32931-4135

St. Augustine/Palatka Florida Chapter #758
904-471-3499
Glenn Logston
19 Oak Road
St. Augustine, FL 32084

St. Petersburg Florida Chapter #341
P.O. Box 12302
St. Petersburg, FL 33733

Tallahassee Florida Area Chapter #353
904-386-7640
Evelyn M. May
2652 Egret Lane
Tallahassee, FL 32312

Tampa Florida Chapter #54
813-681-7483
Larry Bauer
821 Chadsworth Avenue
Seffner, FL 33584

Tarpon Springs Florida Chapter #788
813-784-6651
Marky Kriete
3301 Alternate 19 N., #470
Dunedin, FL 34698

Venice Florida Area Chapter #241
813-475-7058
Donna Hargis
11241 Waterford Avenue
Englewood, FL 34224

Winter Haven Florida Chapter #697
813-324-6728 800-398-9927
Earl B. Harris
6 Lake Winterset Drive
Winter Haven, FL 33884

Georgia

Albany Georgia Chapter #323
912-436-3523
Mary Benford
602 Gable Road
Leesburg, GA 31763

Greater Atlanta Georgia Chapter #57
404-962-6040
James Parnell
P.O. Box 11
Lawrenceville, GA 30246

Kennestone Ostomy Satellite #135 (Greater Atlanta Chapter)
404-422-9803
Herschell Bottrell
1264 Rolling Oaks Drive
Kennesaw, GA 30144

Augusta Georgia Area Chapter #56
404-863-1370
Beth Bartles
P.O. Box 502
Evans, GA 30809

Aiken South Carolina Satellite #39 (Augusta Chapter)
Julie Corbett, R.N.
Aiken Community Hospital
Aiken, SC 29801

Clayton County Georgia Chapter #768
404-361-5742
Sarah Childers
4569 College Street
Forest Park, GA 30050

Coastal Georgia Chapter #243
912-927-5204
Anne Rodgers
64 Brown Pelican Drive
Savannah, GA 31419-2954

Columbus/Fort Benning Georgia Chapter #251
404-327-4771
Lula Bruce
4243 Hamilton Road
Columbus, GA 31904

Gainesville Georgia Area Chapter #606
404-867-3035
Earl Bowen
P.O. Box 464
Winder, GA 30680

Middle Georgia Ostomy Association #58
912-922-5609
Betty Futrell
508 Ivelyn Court
Warner Robins, GA 31088

Dublin Georgia Satellite #67 (Middle Georgia Chapter)
912-275-2000
Jean Holley
200 Industrial Boulevard
Dublin, GA 31021

Northeast Georgia Ostomy Association #317
404-548-2306
Andy Beck
150 Clifton Drive
Athens, GA 30606

Valdosta Georgia Area Chapter #205
912-247-0121
Marjorie Winkler
1107 McRee Drive
Valdosta, GA 31602

Guam

Guam Ostomy Association #652
671-565-2427 671-472-9451
Angel Johnson
P.O. Box 7185
Agat, GU 96928

Hawaii

Hawaii Island Ostomy Association #284
808-959-8089
Ernest A. Smith
156 Makalani Street
Hilo, HI 96720

Honolulu Hawaii Ostomy Association #59
808-734-3182
Adolph Lino
1814 Paula Drive
Honolulu, HI 96816

Maui Hawaii Ostomy Association #60
808-244-0118
Edwin H. Kokubun
2138 Kolo Place
Wailuku, Maui, HI 96793

Idaho

Boise Idaho Area Chapter #347
208-939-7292
Earl Silverstein
3096 Holl Drive
Eagle, ID 83616-2834

Idaho Falls/Upper Valley Idaho Chapter #727
Vernon D. Ricks
P.O. Box 96
Ucon, ID 83454

Lewiston-Clarkston Idaho Chapter #497
509-758-7920
Dick Barnes
1604 Highland Avenue
Clarkston, ID 99403

Pocatello Idaho Chapter #578
208-232-6481
Ralph Stephenson
137 S. 10th
Pocatello, ID 83201

Illinois

Alton Illinois Area Chapter #601
618-466-0894
Gerald McLaughlin
P.O. Box 241
Godfrey, IL 62035

Aurora Illinois Chapter #325
708-879-5295
Joseph Rundle
120 N. Washington Avenue
Batavia, IL 60510

Barrington Illinois Chapter #773
708-438-7728
John Sandberg
676 Coventry Lane
Crystal Lake, IL 60014

Bloomington/Normal Illinois Chapter #519
309-829-1577
Mary Lou Rhodes
RR #3, Box 520
Bloomington, IL 61704

Capitol Chapter Springfield Illinois #61
217-732-6234
George Dahm
1228 Rutledge Drive
Lincoln, IL 62656

Carbondale Illinois Chapter #660
618-542-2594
Loretta Barrett
915 S. Lake Drive
DuQuoin, IL 62832

Champaign-Urbana Illinois Chapter #217
217-583-3261
Duane Buhr
RR #1, Box 40A
Penfield, IL 61862

Charleston-Mattoon Illinois Chapter #363
217-235-1552
Phyllis Huckstep
3327 Moultrie
Mattoon, IL 61938

Chicago Illinois Ostomy Association #63
708-998-1515
Harriet Klemptner
1828 C Wildberry Drive
Glenview, IL 60025

Danville Illinois Chapter #336
217-446-0981
Addie Krage
43 Schultz Street
Danville, IL 61832

De Kalb County Illinois #762
815-758-5830
Steve Johnson
1718 Judy Lane
De Kalb, IL 60115

Du Page County Illinois Ostomy Association #375
708-837-5890
Cathy Tomasik
950 Bryn Mawr
Bartlett, IL 60103

Elgin Illinois Chapter #306
708-837-3762
William Milligan
513 Ridge Circle
Streamwood, IL 60107-2010

Woodstock Illinois Satellite #11 (Elgin Chapter)
815-568-7123
George J. Francicevic
625 Stanford Drive
Marengo, IL 60152

Galesburg Illinois Area Chapter #427
309-343-7389
Bob Lanier
RR #3
Galesburg, IL 61401

Illiana Illinois Chapter #218
708-720-2265
Fred Cross
87 Candlegate Circle
Matteson, IL 60443

Illinois Pull-Thru Network Chapter #778
708-665-1268
708-682-4330 (Fax)
Chris Szczap
1126 S. Grant Street
Wheaton, IL 60187

Joliet Illinois Area Chapter #64
815-723-3027
Norma Chavez
1018 Valley Street
Joliet, IL 60432

Kankakee Illinois Ostomy Association #66
815-937-0346
John Settle
146 S. Jackson
Bradley, IL 60915

Lake County Illinois Chapter #67
708-244-7028 708-360-4198
Barbara Jenkins
38285 N. Sheridan Road, #19
Beach Park, IL 60087

North Shore/Highland Park Illinois Chapter #457
708-945-0595
Karin Williams
1343 Warrington Road
Deerfield, IL 60015

North Suburban Chicago Illinois Chapter #343
708-692-3592
Richard Dorman
242 Gillick Street
Park Ridge, IL 60068-4930

Northern Du Page County Illinois Chapter #684
708-532-2948
Bill Kleiser
183 Hampshire
Elmhurst, IL 60126

Peoria Illinois Area Chapter #62
309-688-9455
Linda Blough
2929 N. Bigelow
Peoria, IL 61604

Quincy Illinois Chapter #479
314-288-5685
Harold Collins
RR 1
Canton, MO 63435

Rockford Illinois Ostomy Association #68
815-624-7263
Stan Phelps
4639 W. Rockton Road
Rockton, IL 61072

Short Circuit Illinois Chapter #69
217-422-8141
Dean Allen
252 N. Westlawn
Decatur, IL 62522-1819

Southeast Chicago Illinois Ostomy Chapter #677
312-324-0770 312-660-0563
Sylvia Copeland
7150 S. Cyril Court, #307
Chicago, IL 60649

Southern Illinois Ostomy Association #70
618-244-1812
Gene Cox
200 N. 14th Street
Mt. Vernon, IL 62864

Sterling Illinois Area Chapter #616
815-625-2625
Jeanette Wolf
312 E. 12th Street
Sterling, IL 61081

Southwest Suburban Chicago Illinois Chapter #495
708-423-2206
Cindy Orr
7512 S. Laramie
Burbank, IL 60459

West Suburban Cook County Illinois Chapter #436
708-344-6270
Robert Bruns
1733 N. 38th Avenue
Stone Park, IL 60165

Indiana

Bloomington Indiana Area Chapter #709
812-336-3793
Melissa Pardue
583 Green Road
Bloomington, IN 47401

Columbus Indiana Area Chapter #477
812-579-6553
Ralph Brown
20002 E. 200 South
Hartsville, IN 47244

Connersville Indiana Area Chapter #512
317-825-1900 317-827-7176
Don York
RR 5, Box 233
Connersville, IN 47331

Evansville Indiana Chapter #72
812-424-8570
Lawrence Trapp
320 Reis Avenue F
Evansville, IN 47711

Fort Wayne Indiana Chapter #71
219-485-8720
Mark Miller
5317 Sunnybrook Drive
Fort Wayne, IN 46835

Indianapolis Indiana Chapter #73
317-861-4606 317-274-2541
Phoebe Alfke
4816 W. Oak Drive
New Palestine, IN 46163

Kokomo Indiana Chapter #344
317-452-7113
Leslie Cook
1413 W. Walnut Street
Kokomo, IN 46901

Marion Indiana Satellite #62 (Kokomo Chapter)
317-998-2948
Janet Gutzwiller
8582 E. 300 South
Marion, IN 46953

Lafayette Indiana Chapter #74
317-474-1955
Warren Thompson
3304 S. County Line Road
50 E.
Lafayette, IN 47905

Lake & Porter County Indiana Chapter #770
219-886-4328
Faye Urello
600 Grant Street
Gary, IN 46402-6001

La Porte County Indiana Chapter #75
219-879-8759
Robert Tiedeman
213 Jackson Street
Michigan, IN 46360

Madison County Indiana Ostomy Assocation #568
317-644-6352
Dianna Benzenbower
28 S. Elma Street
Anderson, IN 46012

Muncie Indiana Area Chapter #227
219-726-4995
William Calhoun
805 W. 7th Street
Portland, IN 47371

Richmond Indiana Ostomy Association #303
317-966-9403
Henry Heath
1526 Belbrook Drive
Richmond, IN 47374

Saint Joseph County Indiana Chapter #76
219-234-8491
Barbara White
1622 E. Ewing Avenue
South Bend, IN 46613

Terre Haute Indiana Chapter #371
812-877-1482
Mary Ruth Carrico
2515 N. Stop 19th Street
Terre Haute, IN 47803

Wabash Valley Indiana Chapter #277
812-735-5615
Ruth Carnahan
RR #1
Edwardsport, IN 47528

Iowa

Ames Iowa Chapter #388
515-388-4701
Shirley Sim
RR 1, Box 75
Roland, IA 50236-9730

Burlington Iowa Area Chapter #474
319-372-1347
Arleen Matta
#9 Storms Court
Ft. Madison, IA 52627

Fairfield Iowa Satellite #110 (Burlington Chapter)
515-693-9641
Skeeter Leroy Haynes
P.O. Box 101
Libertyville, IA 52567

Des Moines Iowa Chapter #77
515-224-7182
Lloyd Pace
412 Cedar Crest Drive
West Des Moines, IA 50265

Carroll Iowa Area Satellite #79 (Des Moines Chapter)
712-792-4509
Rose Mary Lappe
1503 N. Crawford Street
Carroll, IA 51401

Fort Dodge Iowa Satellite #130 (Des Moines Chapter)
515-332-1354
Ruth Freels, R.N., E.T.
109 S. 3rd Street
Humboldt, IA 50548

Dubuque Iowa Chapter #346
319-556-1849 319-589-8053
Ruth Turnis
2203 St. Celia Street
Dubuque, IA 52001

Iowa City Iowa Area Chapter #206
319-337-2466
Marilyn Cermak
912 Brown
Iowa City, IA 52245-5903

Keokuk Iowa Chapter #592
319-524-7557
Rita Hickey
RR 2, Box 43-C
Keokuk, IA 52632

Mason City Iowa Area Chapter #79
515-797-2643
Curtis Amundson
Rt. 1, Box 70
Joice, IA 50446

Oskaloosa Iowa Area Chapter #387
515-673-6723
Gloria Eveland
RR 5, Box 64
Oskaloosa, IA 52577

Quad City Iowa Chapter #319
309-786-4752
Barbara Sheley
2021 38th Street
Rock Island, IL 61265-4634

Clinton Iowa Satellite #12 (Quad City Chapter)
James Lamb
Memorial Hospital
638 S. Bluff Boulevard
Clinton, IA 52732

Siouxland Iowa Chapter #80
712-277-1030
George A. Cole
3604 Jennings
Sioux City, IA 51104

Spencer Iowa Chapter #444
712-262-6689
Richard Hansen
118 E. 21st Street, #312
Spencer, IA 51301

Waterloo Iowa Area Chapter #381
319-578-5416
David Pries
Rt. #2, Box 21
Sumner, IA 50674

Marshalltown Iowa Satellite #112 (Waterloo Chapter)
515-366-2964
Donna Kadner
RR 1, Box 159
Conrad, IA 50621

Kansas

Dodge City Kansas Chapter #760
316-227-6638
Pat Synder
RR #2, Box 401
Dodge City, KS 67801

Emporia Kansas Chapter #443
316-342-4719
Helen Sellers
902 Lawrence
Emporia, KS 66801

Fort Scott Kansas Chapter #331
316-223-0246
Gareth D. Reed
612 S. Judson
Fort Scott, KS 66701

Hays & Northwest Kansas Chapter #448
913-628-1329 (H)
913-628-2558 (W)
Lynn Sparkman
P.O. Box 648
Hays, KS 67601

Hutchinson Kansas Area Chapter #465
316-662-2473
Jean Johnson
2501 Westminster Drive
Hutchinson, KS 67502

Greater Kansas City Area Chapter #107
816-356-7415
Ron Hauk
6217 Crisp
Raytown, MO 64133-4422

Kansas City Area Continent Ostomy Group Satellite #104 (Kansas City Chapter)
913-884-5679
Margie Reeder
19140 S. Waverly Road
Gardner, KS 66030

Leavenworth Kansas Satellite #14 (Kansas City Chapter)
913-682-3721
Eileen Welch, R.N. I.C.U.
St. John 3500 S. 4th
Leavenworth, KS 66048

Lawrence Kansas Chapter #513
913-843-8130
Carl Schaake
1719 W. 9th Street
Lawrence, KS 66044

Manhattan-Junction City Kansas Area Chapter #720
913-776-2349 (H)
913-776-2811 (W)
Janice Gustafson
6201 Cedar Creek Road, #77
Manhattan, KS 66502

Salina-North Central Kansas Chapter #409
913-667-2791
Lois Buxton
P.O. Box 83
Assaria, KS 67416

Topeka Kansas Chapter #260
913-266-6880
Howard Abernathy
55 Pepper Tree Lane
Topeka, KS 66611

Wichita Kansas Chapter #81
316-682-6783
Glenn A. Cooper
6003 E. Bayley
Wichita, KS 67218

Kentucky

Barren River/Bowling Green Kentucky Chapter #689
502-842-2225
Serena Mansfield
1625 Cave Mill Road
Bowling Green, KY 42104

Blue Grass Kentucky Chapter #83
606-885-7157
Diana Judy
1290 Clearcreek Road
Nicholasville, KY 40356

Cumberland Valley of Corbin Kentucky Chapter #650
606-549-9308
Charles White
39 N. Oak Street
Williamsburg, KY 40769

Elizabethtown Kentucky Chapter #593
502-765-7322
Susan Harned
31 Maple Lane
Elizabethtown, KY 42701

Kentuckiana Kentucky Chapter #82
502-893-6654
Stanley Frager, Ph.D.
3906 Dupont Square S.
Louisville, KY 40207

Owensboro Kentucky Area Ostomy Association #440
502-886-3050
Mary McGhee, R.N.
811 E. Parrish Avenue
Owensboro, KY 42301

Paducah Kentucky Chapter #570
502-898-6411
Faye Overby
Rt. 13, Box 330
Paducah, KY 42001

Louisiana

Acadiana Louisiana Ostomy Association #84
318-332-2358
Alfred Zeringue
4417-D Main Highway
Breaux Bridge, LA 70517

Baton Rouge Louisiana Area Ostomy Association #250
504-925-8260 (H)
504-342-5683 (W)
Thomas Austin
P.O. Box 64938
Baton Rouge, LA 70896

Calcasieu Parish Louisiana Chapter #476
504-868-3428
Debbie Duplechin
513 W. View Drive
Houma, LA 70364

Houma Louisiana Area Chapter #556
504-876-2071 504-876-1391
Arnold Pellegrin
208 Country Estate Drive
Houma, LA 70364

Greater New Orleans Louisiana Ostomy Association #85
504-626-1437
Joann Dupre
704 B Colbert Street
Mandeville, LA 70448

Covington Louisiana Satellite #66 (New Orleans Chapter)
504-626-1437
Joann Dupre
704 B Colbert Street
Mandeville, LA 70448

Marrero/Westbank Louisiana Satellite #68 (New Orleans Chapter)
Vera Becnel
2800 Ramsey Drive
Algiers, LA 70114

Rapides Parish Louisiana Chapter #484
318-443-6232
Lee Salter
2659 Betty Avenue
Pineville, LA 71360

Shreveport Louisiana Chapter #86
310-687-9146
Debbie Vaughn
P.O. Box 3956
Shreveport, LA 71103

Maine

Androscoggin Maine Chapter #254
207-782-3663
Gerald N. Bouffard
42 Bushey Circle
Lewiston, ME 04240

Aroostook Maine Chapter #259
207-435-6273 207-764-2985
Joanne Tardif
18D Dewberry Drive
Presque Isle, ME 04769

Central Maine Chapter #88
207-453-6586
Bettina Barker
26 Island Avenue
Fairfield, ME 04937-1305

Ostomy Association of Eastern Maine #89
207-945-3167
John Lane
RR #1, Box 1225
Bangor, ME 04401

Mid-Coast Maine Chapter #478
Marie Connell
67 Mechanic Street
Camden, ME 04843

Portland Maine Area Chapter #87
207-797-5125
Peter McGinn
1390 Forest Avenue, Box 1D
Portland, ME 04103

Rumford Maine Ostomy Association #90
207-364-8104
Doris M. Robbins
102 Lincoln Avenue
Rumford, ME 04276

Maryland

Anne Arundel County Maryland Chapter #295
301-766-7623
James Plott
612 Elizabeth Road
Glen Burnie, MD 21061

Baltimore Maryland Ostomy Association #91
301-484-8031 (H)
301-484-8030 (W)
Bernard Kaufman
P.O. Box 15000
Baltimore, MD 21208

Cumberland Maryland Chapter #92
301-729-6976
Mitzi Giles
1233 W. Braddock Road
La Vale, MD 21502

Delmarva Maryland Ostomy Association #270
301-289-7919
Bill Gibbs
208 N. Philadelphia Avenue
Ocean City, MD 21842

Frederick County Maryland Chapter #380
301-271-7776
Robert Stull
13015 Layman Road
Thurmont, MD 21788

Harford-Cecil Counties Maryland Chapter #522
301-676-2590
Clarence Pegram
2700 Clayton Road
Joppa, MD 21085

Cecil County, Elkton Maryland Satellite #88 (Harford-Cecil Counties Chapter)
301-398-8172
Neal A. Greer
313 Catswamp Road
Elkton, MD 21921

Metro Maryland Ostomy Association #312
301-588-8844 (AM only)
301-434-2647 (PM only)
Horace Saunders
9803 E. Light Drive
Silver Spring, MD 20903

Metro Maryland Youth Group #313
301-588-8844 (AM only)
Nerissa Dixon
11325 Amherst Avenue
Silver Spring, MD 20902

South Maryland Counties Chapter #374
301-645-5564
Margaret Goldsmith
423 Piney Church Road
Waldorf, MD 20602-3105

Washington County Maryland Chapter #308
301-733-5425
Doris Worthington
1829 Gilbert Avenue
Hagerstown, MD 21740

Massachusetts

Berkshire County Massachusetts Ostomy Association #326
413-447-2634
Jane Carmel
49 Eleanor Road
Pittsfield, MA 01201

Ostomy Association of Boston Massachusetts #93
617-734-9098
In MA: 800-952-7664
Linda Urbach
137 Sewall Avenue
Brookline, MA 02146

Boston Massachusetts Satellite #118 (Boston Chapter)
617-734-9098
Linda Urbach
137 Sewall Avenue
Brookline, MA 02146

Framingham Massachusetts Satellite #17 (Boston Chapter)
617-479-4811
Jean Clancy, R.N., E.T.
115 Lincoln Street
Framingham, MA 01701

Gay & Lesbian Satellite #121 (Boston Chapter)
508-358-6684

North Shore Massachusetts Satellite #119 (Boston Chapter)
508-774-1151
Ronald Titlebaum
12 Seneca Drive
Danvers, MA 01923

Northwest Massachusetts Satellite #18 (Boston Chapter)
617-479-4811
Donna Loehner, R.N., E.T.
41 Mall Road
Burlington, MA 01805

South Shore Satellite #120 (Boston Chapter)
508-587-0704
Irving Watnick
26 N. Ash Street
Brockton, MA 02401

Young Adults Satellite #122 (Boston Chapter)
508-473-8643
Robert McCarthy
8 Esther Drive
Milford, MA 01757

Ostomy Association of Cape Cod Massachusetts #94
508-255-7329
Helen Enochs
P.O. Box 31
Eastham, MA 02642-0031

Franklin County Massachusetts Chapter #400
413-773-8619
Carol Jones, E.T.
51 Lovers Lane
Greenfield, MA 01301

Merrimack Valley Massachusetts Chapter #280
603-893-6078
Robert Ferrier
P.O. Box 477
North Salem, NH 03073

Greater New Bedford-Fall River Massachusetts Chapter #487
508-994-3685
Arthur Thomas
104 Sutton Street
New Bedford, MA 02746

North Essex County Massachusetts Chapter #454
508-462-7855
Cecilia Lavoie
70 Turkey Hill Road
Newburyport, MA 01950

North Worcester County Massachusetts Chapter #342
508-342-0818
Norbert Beauchene
27 Fairview Street
Fitchburg, MA 01420

Ostomy Association of Springfield Massachusetts #95
413-786-2940
Ann Favreau
90 Pleasant Drive
Feeding Hills, MA 01030

Greater Taunton Massachusetts Chapter #453
617-824-6082
Leon Marchand
20 Francine Road
Raynham, MA 02767

Worcester Massachusetts Chapter #538
508-755-4511
Robert Pickett
19 White Terracc
Auburn, MA 01501

Michigan

Ann Arbor Michigan Ostomy Association Area #391
313-971-8214
Roberta Gildersleeve
3264 Williamsburg
Ann Arbor, MI 48104

Battle Creek Michigan Chapter #329
616-963-5521
Community Hospital
Jackie Sheldriek, R.N.
183 West Street
Battle Creek, MI 49017

Berrien County Michigan Chapter #613
616-925-8293
Betty Swanson
P.O. Box 363
St. Joseph, MI 49085

Coldwater Michigan Area Chapter #247
517-369-9235
Jewel Troth
1641 Matteson Lake
Bronson, MI 49028

Greater Detroit Michigan Chapter #98
313-336-0487
Michael Wilson
10038 Hazelton
Redford, MI 48239

Escanaba Michigan Chapter #481
906-786-1402
Mary Greer
E. 5079 Highway, M-35
Escanaba, MI 49829

Flint Michigan Area Chapter #96
313-732-7675
Velma Oswald
2029 Roland Avenue
Flint, MI 48532

Grand Rapids Michigan Chapter #434
616-245-9291
Kim Beck
1137 Ottilia S.E.
Grand Rapids, MI 49507

Grand Traverse Michigan Area Chapter #529
616-943-9565
Carolyn Priest
664 Highland
Traverse City, MI 49684

Greater Hurley Wisconsin-Ironwood Michigan Chapter #622
715-561-5520
Sandra Gordon
P.O. Box 247
Hurley, WI 54534

Jackson Michigan Chapter #207
517-531-3074
John Wellman
219 John Street, Box 285
Parma, MI 49269

Kalamazoo Michigan Ostomy Association #99
616-344-2326
Walter Ludwig
2950 Berry Street
Kalamazoo, MI 49001

Ostomy Association of Greater Lansing Michigan #223
517-723-6474
Thomas Lundquist
711 N. Pine Street
Owosso, MI 48867

Lenawee Michigan Area Ostomy Association #701
517-263-5272
Janet Lennard
617 Chesnut Street
Adrian, MI 49221

Macomb County Michigan Chapter #577
313-268-4829
Thomas Owen
35333 Ellsworth Drive
Sterling Heights, MI 48312

Marquette Michigan Area Chapter #696
906-249-3981
Linda Symons, E.T.
322 Lakewood Lane
Marquette, MI 49855

Mount Pleasant Michigan Chapter #624
517-875-3372
Harold Stadlberger
9510 W. Pierce Road
Sumner, MI 48889-9724

Muskegon Michigan Area Ostomy Association #224
616-724-1747
Mary Powell
2001 N. Weber
Muskegon, MI 49445

Oakland County Michigan Ostomy Association #97
313-673-2705
Mary Ann Bova
1826 Colonial Village, #1
Waterford, MI 48328

Ottawa County Michigan Chapter #385
616-392-7186
Paul Kleinheksel
438 W. 30th
Holland, MI 49423

Owosso Michigan Area Chapter #460
517-723-2078
Gerald Hudson
797 Pasadena
Owosso, MI 48867

Port Huron Michigan Chapter #498
313-982-8701
Helen Graves
3549 Holland Park Lane
Port Huron, MI 48060-1559

Southwestern Wayne County Michigan Chapter #554
313-388-2947
Helen Rariden
16153 Oceana
Allen Park, MI 48101

Straits Michigan Area Chapter #269
616-347-2225
Charlene Taylor
3094 Parkview
Petosky, MI 49770

Tri-City Michigan Area Chapter #100
517-781-2707
Judy Barckholtz
7463 Swan Creek
Saginaw, MI 48603

Minnesota

Albert Lea Minnesota Chapter #509
507-373-4038
Ray Hershey
636 E. 7th Street
Albert Lea, MN 56007

Duluth Minnesota Area Chapter #731
218-722-0762
Gerald Novack
2412 Florence Avenue
Duluth, MN 55811

Marshall Minnesota Area Ostomy Association #716
507-734-6151
Lyle Anderson
RR #1, Box 116
Balaton, MN 56115

Worthington Minnesota Area Satellite #86 (Marshall Chapter)
507-926-5261
Charlotte Engels
Box 16
Wilmont, MN 56185

Minneapolis Minnesota Chapter #101
612-378-1875 612-455-9283
Karen A. Tourdot
2965 Bruce Court
Inver Grove Heights, MN 55077

International Falls Minnesota/Fort Frances Ontario Satellite #82 (Minneapolis Chapter)
218-283-8363
Shirley DeMarchi
813 2nd Street
International Falls, MN 56649

Redstone Minnesota Area Ostomy Association #244
Walter Bushard
816 6th Street N.
New Ulm, MN 56073

Rochester Minnesota Chapter #263
507-288-0854
Mary Pat Adams
P.O. Box 6684
Rochester, MN 55903

St. Cloud Minnesota Chapter #640
612-983-2138
Bonnie Sjoberg
Rt. 4, Box 94
Milaca, MN 56353

St. Paul Minnesota Ostomy Association #103
612-698-1543
Marjorie Azzone
P.O. Box 75365
St. Paul, MN 55175

Chisago-Northern Washington Counties Minnesota Satellite #108 (St. Paul Chapter)
612-462-2151
Gayle Whipple
5613 East Viking Road, 105
Wyoming, MN 55092

Virginia Minnesota/Mesabi Chapter #763
218-229-3119
Dorothea Lesar
5023 Highway 110
Aurora, MN 55705-1622

Willmar Minnesota Area Chapter #242
612-857-2109
Ronald Schultz
P.O. Box 242
Grove City, MN 56243

Mississippi

Gulf Coast Mississippi Ostomy Association #104
601-374-5812
J. A. Hilton
P.O. Box 802
Ocean Springs, MS 39564

Hattiesburg Mississippi Chapter #635
601-268-9648
Richard Feinberg
108 Colonial Place
Hattiesburg, MS 39401

Ostomy Association of Jackson Mississippi #290
601-536-2497
Cliff Arinder
Rt. 4, Box 851
Forest, MS 39074-9802

Meridian Mississippi Satellite #132 (Jackson Chapter)
601-655-8448
Robert Bowyer
Rt. 1, Box 145
Enterprise, MS 39330

Tupelo Mississippi Area Chapter #555
205-356-9221
Edna Pauline Files
Rt. 2, Box 302 Meadow Drive
Red Bay, AL 35582

Missouri

Cape Girardeau Missouri Chapter #397
314-788-2384
Loyd Statler
Rt. 1
Oak Ridge, MO 63769

Columbia Missouri Chapter #410
314-635-3561
Betty Pavitt
P.O. Box 1601
Jefferson City, MO 65102

Pike County Missouri Satellite #128 (Columbia Chapter)
314-754-4209
Linda Ince
110 Dolbeare Drive
Louisiana, MO 63353

Randolph County Missouri Satellite #100 (Columbia Chapter)
816-277-3216
Joy Purnell
Rt. 2, Box 18
Huntsville, MO 65259

Joplin Missouri Ostomy Association #106
417-624-4275
Raymond Koch
108 N. Jackson Avenue
Joplin, MO 64801

Greater Kansas City Missouri Area Chapter #107
816-356-7415
Ron Hauk
6217 Crisp
Raytown, MO 64133-4422

Kansas City Area Continent Ostomy Group Satellite #104 (Kansas City Chapter)
913-884-5679
Margie Reeder
19140 S. Waverly Road
Gardner, KS 66030

Leavenworth Kansas Satellite #14 (Kansas City Chapter)
913-682-3721
Eileen Welch., R.N. I.C.U.
St. John 3500 S. 4th
Leavenworth, KS 66048

Poplar Bluff Missouri Chapter #771
314-785-0367
Pat Donnelson, Jr.
Rt. 6, Box 14, Oak Tree Street
Poplar Bluff, MO 63901

St. Joseph Missouri Area Chapter #357
816-232-1113
David White
2915 Penn Street
St. Joseph, MO 64507

St. Louis Missouri Area Chapter #105
314-423-4263
Jim Brogan, Jr.
4146 Wright Avenue
St. Ann, MO 63074-1936

Springfield Missouri Area Chapter #271
417-881-6853
Frank Ott
2017 E. Wayland
Springfield, MO 65804

Montana

Billings Montana Area Ostomy Association #108
406-252-9460
Connie Waggener
P.O. Box 31081
Billings, MT 59107-1081

Great Falls Montana Area Chapter #109
406-452-1052
Robert Purdy
606 6th Street S.
Great Falls, MT 59401

Missoula Montana Five Valley Ostomy Association #756
406-251-3845
Linda Buxton
2422 56th Street
Missoula, MT 59803

Northwest Montana Chapter #757
406-862-7228
Pam Stewart
321 Cougar Trail
Whitefish, MT 59937

Nebraska

Beatrice Nebraska Area Chapter #586
402-228-2787
Douglas Jorn
2109 Hoyt Street
Beatrice, NE 68310

Kearney Area Nebraska Chapter #741
308-486-2641
Horst Tobaben
P.O. Box 20
Eustis, NE 69028-0204

Lincoln Nebraska Ostomy Association #111
402-786-5393
Karen Maki
10511 N. 136th
Waverly, NE 68516

McCook Area Nebraska Chapter #744
308-345-6753
Jeannie Welborn
1525 Norris Avenue
McCook, NE 69001

Norfolk-Columbus Nebraska Chapter #482
402-371-1682
Tom Chamberlin
2400 Madison Avenue
Norfolk, NE 68701-4433

North Platte Nebraska Area Chapter #671
308-532-2178
Maxine Reynolds
3020 Cedarberry Lane
North Platte, NE 69101

Omaha Nebraska Chapter #112
402-553-9615
Fred Kudym
4661 Mason Street
Omaha, NE 68106

Shenandoah Iowa Satellite #13 (Omaha Chapter)
712-246-1230
Sharon Klein
Box 116
Farragut, IA 51639

Nevada

Reno Nevada Chapter #113
Lee Kocka
2195 Elmcrest Drive
Reno, NV 89503-3411

Southern Nevada Chapter #114
702-435-3010
Diana Roberts
351 Amalfi Street
Henderson, NV 89014-4923

Pahrump Nevada Satellite #116 (Southern Nevada Chapter)
702-727-6264
Frank Baldwin
P.O. Box 35
Pahrump, NV 89041

New Hampshire

Concord New Hampshire Chapter #116
603-224-9942
Susan Fraser
122B Smith Avenue
Pembroke, NH 03275

Greater Manchester New Hampshire Ostomy Association #115
603-624-1016
Pauline Lussier, R.N., E.T.
RD #4, 106 Village of Glen
Goffstown, NH 03045

Rochester New Hampshire Chapter #431
603-749-4480
Phyllis Daigneau
Rt. 3, 322 Toland Road
Dover, NH 03820

Sullivan-Grafton New Hampshire Chapter #666
603-542-7771
Terry Strichland
Valley Reg Hospital
Elm Street
Claremont, NH 03743

New Jersey

Audubon New Jersey Area Chapter #335
609-546-5376
Mary Dare
111 Ward Avenue
Audubon, NJ 08106

Bergen County New Jersey Chapter #377
201-772-8532
Henry Tencza
179 Banta Avenue
Garfield, NJ 07026-3632

Burlington County New Jersey Chapter #466
609-877-4520 609-273-8934
Kathy Schuler
100 N.W. Albany Road
Moorestown, NJ 08057

Cape May County New Jersey Chapter #576
609-522-7288
Bernard Wapner
117 W. Syracuse Avenue
Wildwood Crest, NJ 08260

Essex County New Jersey Chapter #123
201-403-0022
Roberta Ferrara
5 Woodland Road
West Caldwell, NJ 07006

Hudson County New Jersey Chapter #118
201-795-8200
Wendy Hanak, R.N., C.E.T.N.
176 Palisade Avenue
Jersey City, NJ 07306

Mercer County New Jersey Chapter #209
609-799-4681
Anne Daughtrey
96 Tennyson Drive
Plainsboro, NJ 08536-3007

Ostomy Association of Middlesex County New Jersey #122
201-257-5009
Robert Berg
3 Clinton Court
East Brunswick, NJ 08816

Monroe New Jersey Satellite #80 (Middlesex County Chapter)
609-655-1428
Philip Swirsky
86A Empress Plaza
Cranbury, NJ 08512

Monmouth County New Jersey Chapter #120
908-264-9462
Lowell White
12 Edgewood Drive
Holmdel, NJ 07733

Morris County New Jersey Ostomy Association #121
201-398-4208
Marie Walsh
18 Sunset Lane
Landing, NJ 07850

Ocean County New Jersey Ostomy Association #309
908-240-0431
Frank Roznoy
26 Exiter Street
Toms River, NJ 08757

Passaic County New Jersey Chapter #599
201-838-6425
Michael Sherr
190 Boonton Avenue
Butler, NJ 07405

Salem County New Jersey Chapter #382
602-299-0906
Clarence MacNeal, Jr.
18 Fenwick Drive
Carney's Point, NJ 08069

Somerset County New Jersey Chapter #124
908-281-6557
Maureen A. Mitru
47 Foxhill Lane
Hillsborough, NJ 08876

Ostomy Association of Union County New Jersey #213
201-388-1747
Robert Arkin
115 McKinley Avenue
Colonia, NJ 07067

Warren County New Jersey Ostomy Association #641
201-453-2808
Joe Sawran
P.O. Box 222
Oxford, NJ 07863

New Mexico

Ostomy Association of Albuquerque New Mexico #125
505-883-0852
Edward Brown, Jr.
5021 La Fiesta N.E.
Albuquerque, NM 87109

Carlsbad New Mexico Chapter #654
505-885-2804
James Bujac
Box 667
Carlsbad, NM 88220

Las Cruces New Mexico Area Chapter #401
505-522-3691
Mike Smith
1105 Sharon Circle
Las Cruces, NM 88001

Roswell New Mexico Chapter #446
505-623-4490
Dova Callahan, R.N., E.T.
701 La Jolla Lane
Roswell, NM 88201

New York

Albany New York Area Chapter #126
518-283-1808
Eugene Gilchrist
2 Brookside Avenue
Troy, NY 12180

Southwestern Vermont Satellite #109 (Albany Chapter)
802-375-9681
Mrs. Thelma Oventhal
RD 2, Box 1725
Arlington, VT 05250

Auburn New York Chapter #340
315-253-2158
Richard Cowell
RD 6, Box 2
Auburn, NY 13021

Ostomy Association of Brooklyn New York #127
718-692-1132
Harold Rosenblaum
612 Argyle Road, #6L
Brooklyn, NY 11230

Buffalo New York Youth Chapter #543
716-542-9680
Roseanne Yaeger
125 East Avenue
Akron, NY 14001

Chautauqua County New York Chapter #360
814-368-5597
Richard Dittman
61 Birch Street
Bradford, PA 16701

Colostomy Society of New York #130
212-982-8112
Jennifer Savary
145 4th Avenue, #17F
New York, NY 10003

Ostomy Association of Delaware County New York #132
607-865-5750
Paul Miller
Mt. Pleasant
Walton, NY 13856-9683

Fulton/Montgomery New York Chapter #411
518-842-1147
Gloria McCune
46 McClellan Avenue
Amsterdam, NY 12010

Genesee Valley New York Ostomy Association #133
716-381-8567
John Young
9 Santa Drive
Pittsford, NY 14534

Greater New York Pull-Thru Network #776
201-264-3936
Kim Weigard Casola
48 Atlantic Street
Keyport, NJ 07735

Herkimer New York Chapter #549
315-894-9560
Naomi Mursch
80 E. North Street, #409
Ilion, NY 13357

Ileostomy Association of New York, QT-NY #136
201-489-7233 (H)
212-698-7216 (W)
Jonathon Brodman
P.O. Box 1390, Gracie Station
New York, NY 10028

The Tri-State Ileoanal Pull-Through Group (NY, NJ, CT)
Help line: 212-864-1968

Jefferson County New York Chapter #389
315-482-2041
Lyle Spies
P.O. Box 27
Redwood, NY 13679-0027

Long Island New York Ileostomy Association #138
516-561-0896
Anna Pascale
374 Rockaway Parkway
Valley Stream, NY 11580

Mid-Hudson New York Chapter #139
914-691-8713
Anne Howard
247 North Road
Highland, NY 12528

Niagara County New York Chapter #588
716-625-8844
Ronald McMorris
5828 Robinson Road
Lockport, NY 14094

Niagara Frontier New York Chapter #140
716-876-3435
Albert Licata
298 Orchard Drive
Kenmore, NY 14223

Oneonta New York Chapter #141
607-432-6933
Howard Berkowitz, M.D.
181 East Street
Oneonta, NY 13820

Greater Orange New York Area Chapter #134
914-343-5612
Helen Barlow
RD 1, Box 106
Otisville, NY 10963

Orleans County New York Chapter #327
716-638-8182
Pamela Boynton
12 East Avenue
Holley, NY 14470

Queens County New York Chapter #611
718-424-3633
James Rogers
3520 Leverich Street
Jackson Heights, NY 11372

Rockland County New York Chapter #142
914-353-2683
Debbi Siddi, R.N., C.E.T.N.
86 Piermont Avenue
Nyack, NY 10960

Schenectady New York Chapter #145
518-452-5750 (H)
518-869-7562 (W)
Patricia Hurley
44 Fuller Terrace
Albany, NY 12205

Southern Tier New York Ostomy Management Association #144
607-334-9741
John Poggioli
RD 2, Box 352
Norwich, NY 13815

Staten Island New York Ostomy Association #395
718-356-5687
Thomas Sanfilippo
186 Colon Avenue
Staten Island, NY 10308

Suffolk New York Ostomy Association #264
516-567-9489
Darlena Daniels
835 10 B Broadway Avenue
Holbrook, NY 11741

Northern Brookhaven New York Satellite #107 (Suffolk Chapter)
516-473-8239
Gloria Varela
332 Sheep Pasture Road
E. Setauket, NY 11733

Smithtown New York Satellite #29 (Suffolk Chapter)
516-864-6034
Bob Goldstein
23 Winston Drive
Smithtown, NY 11787

Syracuse New York Ostomy Association #146
315-478-8603
Theresa Retunno
300 Pond Street, #221
Syracuse, NY 13208

Tompkins County New York Ostomy Association #424
607-272-4104
Reeshon Feuer
52 Woodcrest Avenue
Ithaca, NY 14850

Twin Tier New York Chapter #128
717-549-7601
Marian Sanphy
RD 3, Box 35C
Columbia Cross Roads, PA 16914

Greater Utica-Rome New York Chapter #135
315-724-9528
Anthony Abraham
2107 Highland Avenue
Utica, NY 13502

Oneida City Area New York Satellite #30 (Greater Utica-Rome Chapter)
Marlene Whaley
137 Allen Street
Sherrill, NY 13461

Westchester New York Chapter #402
914-337-5248
L. Hess
#3 Sadore Lane
Yonkers, NY 10710

North Carolina

Asheville North Carolina Ostomy Association #147
704-693-1586
Kenneth G. Clark
Rt. 1, Box 72A
Zirconia, NC 28790

Franklin North Carolina Ostomy Satellite #111 (Asheville Chapter)
704-524-9773
Howard Trevey
235 Cat Creek Road
Franklin, NC 28734

Haywood County North Carolina Satellite #101 (Asheville Chapter)
704-456-6900
Jean Hall
905 Sulfur Springs Road
Waynesville, NC 28786

Cabarrus County North Carolina Chapter #734
704-933-0884
Dennis Compton
512 Evelyn Avenue
Kannapolis, NC 28083

Charlotte North Carolina Chapter #149
704-364-0860
Jack Mulholland
6736 Rocky Falls Road
Charlotte, NC 28211

Durham/Orange County North Carolina Chapter #462
919-933-8780
Carol Siebert
B-1 Village Green
Elizabeth Street
Chapel Hill, NC 27514

Greater Fayetteville North Carolina Chapter #420
919-425-6444
Earl Aiken
Rt. #15, Box 19
Fayetteville, NC 28306

Gaston North Carolina Area Chapter #268
704-739-6275
Robert Smith
501 W. Mountain Street, #5
Kings Mountain, NC 28086

Hickory-Unifour North Carolina Chapter #419
704-397-3342
Calvin Robinson
P.O. Box 413
Hildebran, NC 28637

Iredell County North Carolina Chapter #739
704-878-6966
Pamela Harr
116 S. Patterson Street
Statesville, NC 28677

Moore County North Carolina (Sandhills) Chapter #764
919-295-6754
Leonard Skamser
350 Robin Lane
Pinehurst, NC 28374

Onslow County North Carolina Chapter #545
919-455-7292
Henry Taylor
917 Lynchburg Drive
Jacksonville, NC 28540

Piedmont North Carolina Ostomy Association #210
804-792-7760
Dale Watson
14 Glen Oak Drive
Danville, VA 24541

Asheboro/Randolph North Carolina Satellite #127 (Piedmont Chapter)
919-672-1156
Frank Lestienne
605 Ingram Drive
Asheboro, NC 27203

Raleigh North Carolina Area Chapter #148
919-515-2605 919-851-6623
Edmund Estes
412 Lochside Drive
Cary, NC 27511

Wilmington North Carolina Chapter #750
919-392-3332
Leslie Owen
P.O. Box 3614
Wilmington, NC 28403

Wilson County North Carolina Chapter #456
919-237-0954
Carolyn Whitley
Rt. 2, Box 137
Bailey, NC 27807

North Dakota

Bismarck-Mandan North Dakota Area Chapter #334
701-223-3995
Albinus Reis
2209 Avenue A
Bismarck, ND 58501

Dickinson North Dakota Area Chapter #728
701-764-5783
Kenneth Rehn
Box 178
Killdeer, ND 58640

Fargo-Moorhead North Dakota Chapter #359
701-232-3122
Laura Funouits
60 17th Avenue N.
Fargo, ND 58102

Perham Minnesota Satellite #77 (Fargo-Moorhead Chapter)
218-346-3120
Ceil Nundahl
559 5th Street S.W.
Perham, MN 56573

Grand Forks North Dakota Area Ostomy Association #324
701-780-5000 701-775-5158
Pat Guthmiller, R.N., C.E.T.N.
United Hospital Medical Park
S. Columbia Road
P.O. Box 6002
Grand Forks, ND 58206-6002

Minot North Dakota Area Chapter #261
701-338-2343
Merle Swartz
P.O. Box 22
Velva, ND 58790

Williston North Dakota Chapter #425
701-572-3396
Arvid Olson
508 12th Street W.
Williston, ND 58801

Ohio

Akron Ohio Area Chapter #154
216-773-9904 216-836-9051
Eric Floyd
2067 Penguin Drive
Akron, OH 44319

Canton Ohio Area Chapter #161
216-832-8150
John Moulos
1521 Tremont Avenue S.W.
Massillon, OH 44646-6342

Central Ohio Chapter #155
614-888-7077
Robert L. McDannold
7959 Fairway Drive
Worthington, OH 43235

Greater Cincinnati Ohio Chapter #156
513-231-7386
Doris L. Willard
7386 Gungadin Drive
Cincinnati, OH 45230-2253

Clermont County Ohio Chapter #596
513-752-0458
Phyllis Martin
780 Ohio Pike, #3, Bldg. 4
Cincinnati, OH 45245

Cleveland Ohio Ostomy Association #157
216-232-2742
Byron Koepke
135 Wandle Avenue
Bedford, OH 44146

Clinton County Ohio Chapter #708
513-685-3306
Jerry Florea
11855 SR 134 S
Martinsville, OH 45146

Darke County Ohio Ostomy Chapter #547
513-548-2918
Joanne Hughes
5803 Hartzell Road
Greenville, OH 45331

Dayton Ohio Chapter #158
513-275-4193
Nancy Eresman
1201 Larriwood Drive
Kettering, OH 45429

Findlay Ohio Area Chapter #774
419-458-5681
John Snyder
Rt. 1, Box 76
Wharton, OH 43359

Gallipolis Ohio Area Ostomy Chapter #729
614-446-5080
Phyllis Brown
Rt. 3, Box 358
Bidwell, OH 45614

Hamilton Ohio Area Chapter #723
513-892-7771
Bob Harbron
848 Louise Avenue
Fairfield, OH 45014

Lake County Ohio Chapter #687
216-256-1547 216-953-9600
Beverly Wallace
P.O. Box 348
Willoughby, OH 44094

Lima Ohio Area Chapter #742
419-738-7692
J. Ernie Gray
P.O. Box 2100
Cridersville, OH 45806

Lorain County Ohio Chapter #159
216-327-4613
Chuck & Eloise Bashak
36261 Chestnut Ridge
N. Ridgeville, OH 44039

Mansfield Ashland Ohio Chapter #561
419-756-5269
Theodore Hartman
1247 Rosedale Drive
Mansfield, OH 44906

Marion Ohio Chapter #403
614-383-3746
William Moloney
571 N. Greenwood Street
Marion, OH 43302

Miami-Shelby County Ohio Chapter #621
513-492-1737
Kay Rickey
15655 Sharp Road
Sidney, OH 45365

Middletown Ohio Chapter #712
513-988-6415
Harold Poplin
211 Johns Street
Trenton, OH 45067-1219

Mount Vernon Ohio Chapter #339
419-768-3449
Forest Noble
P.O. Box 586
Mount Vernon, OH 43050

Newark Ohio Area Chapter #647
614-344-6152
Eunice Conaway
59 N. 23rd Street
Newark, OH 43055

Portage County Ohio Chapter #740
216-274-2171
Norman Park
4495 N. High Street
Mantua, OH 44255-9404

Portsmouth Ohio Chapter #364
614-353-2556
Juanita Yuenger, R.N., E.T.
2521 Sunrise Avenue
Portsmouth, OH 45662

Ironton Area Ohio Satellite #33 (Portsmouth Chapter)
614-353-2556
Juanita Yuenger, R.N., E.T.
2521 Sunrise Avenue
Portsmouth, OH 45662

Salem Ohio Chapter #715
216-424-7674
Betty Reynolds, E.T.
7300 Lisbon Road
Lisbon, OH 44432

Sandusky Ohio Chapter #301
419-483-4196
Harold L. Fulmer
307 Albina Drive
Bellevue, OH 44811

Springfield Ohio Ostomy Association #160
513-399-7067
Dorothy Everhart
1229 Glenmore Drive
Springfield, OH 45503

Steubenville Ohio Area Chapter #517
614-264-1568
Charles Fonow
4508 Scioto Drive
Steubenville, OH 43952

Toledo Ohio Area Ostomy Association #162
419-691-5239
Mark Murphy
2744 Luverne Avenue
Oregon, OH 43616

Tuscarawas County Ohio Chapter #526
216-343-8030
Linda Gibbs
725 Fair Avenue N.E.
New Philadelphia, OH 44663

Wayne/Holmes Counties Ohio Chapter #705
216-264-8505
Dotti Shank
1449 Arthur Drive
Wooster, OH 44691

Youngstown Ohio Chapter #163
216-788-9170
Gene Payton
5008 Glenwood Avenue, #302
Youngstown, OH 44512

Zanesville Ohio Ostomy Chapter #653
614-452-1807
Forest Cale
1885 N. Dietz Road
Zanesville, OH 43701

Oklahoma

ADA Oklahoma Chapter #732
405-332-2323, Ext. 143
Lillian Penrod, R.N., E.T.
430 N. Monta Vista
Ada, OK 74820

Bartlesville Oklahoma Chapter #714
918-336-0394 (H)
918-661-0856 (W)
Sharon Lankford
2144 S. Dewey
Bartlesville, OK 74003

Lawton-Fort Sill Oklahoma Chapter #449
405-353-6908
Marcus Mullins
1906 Ash
Lawton, OK 73507

Muskogee Oklahoma Chapter #623
918-682-4684
Mildred Kerns
430 S. 13 Street
Muskogee, OK 74401

Ostomy Association of Oklahoma City Oklahoma #165
405-848-3443
Lucille Abbott
729 N.W. 90
Oklahoma City, OK 73114

McAlester Oklahoma Satellite #115 (Oklahoma City Chapter)
918-426-2843
J.E. Bob Wright
1601 S. 5th Street
McAlester, OK 74501

Stillwater Oklahoma Chapter #569
405-377-5273
Lavenia Hutchinson
1618 W. 12th Avenue
Stillwater, OK 74074

Tulsa Oklahoma Ostomy Association #232
991-842-5617
Phillip Stewart
6447 N. Victor
Tulsa, OK 74130-1324

Oregon

Astoria Oregon Chapter #582
503-325-5974
Peggy Goodenberger
1120 Irving
Astoria, OR 97107

Coos Bay Oregon Area Chapter #356
503-267-3942
Hattie Haughawout
3693 Spruce
North Bend, OR 97459

Douglas County Oregon Chapter #472
503-673-6307
Edith Hope
2071 N.E. Stephens, #12A
Roseburg, OR 97470

La Grande Oregon Chapter #690
503-963-2344
Loree Leonard
11106 S. McAlister Road
Island City, OR 97850

Lane County Oregon Chapter #216
503-344-1111
Jim Henderson
2290 Onyx Street
Eugene, OR 97403

Medford Oregon Chapter #645
503-776-7483
Carol Cullin
135 N. Ivy
Medford, OR 97501

Mid-Columbia Oregon Chapter #631
503-296-4277
Glen Mollet
719 W. 11th
The Dalles, OR 97058

Oregon Ostomy Association Metro-Portland Chapter #166
503-644-5331
Caroline Uphill
P.O. Box 40026
Portland, OR 97240

Pendleton Oregon Chapter #670
503-276-5472
Juanita Dames
1610 S.E. Court Street
Pendleton, OR 97801

Willamette Valley Oregon Chapter #238
503-364-0629
John DeVries
P.O. Box 3062
Salem, OR 97302

Pennsylvania

Armstrong County Pennsylvania Chapter #710
412-548-4382 (H)
412-543-2007 (W)
B. Albert Bertocchi
274 N. Grant Avenue
Kittanning, PA 16201

Beaver Pennsylvania Area Chapter #168
412-843-0149
Patti Smolar
774 Blackhawk Road
Beaver Falls, PA 15010

Central Pennsylvania Ostomy Society #170
Sam Mallory
405 Rt. 36 South
Duncansville, PA 16635

Chambersburg Pennsylvania Area Chapter #565
717-264-5945
Marie Kauffman
255 S. 7th Street
Chambersburg, PA 17201

Clarion County Pennsylvania Chapter #639
814-226-8239
Ruth Showers
RD #2
Clarion, PA 16214

Delaware County Pennsylvania Chapter #225
215-353-5919
Stanley Malis
328 Hastings Boulevard
Broomall, PA 19008

Dubois Pennsylvania Area Chapter #528
814-265-8066
Clair Foulks
Box 49 2nd Avenue
Brockway, PA 15851

East Stroudsburg Pennsylvania (Pocono) Chapter #721
717-476-3347
Herman Meinhart
36 Lackawanna Street
East Stroudsburg, PA 18301

Erie Pennsylvania Ostomy Association #219
814-825-2157
Linda Johnson
1133 E. 39th Street
Erie, PA 16504

Franklin/Oil City Pennsylvania Ostomy Association #396
Susan Detrich
111 E. 4th Street
Oil City, PA 16301-2467

Gettysburg Pennsylvania Area Chapter #506
717-642-6237
Jacquelyn B. Brown
3 Field Trail
Carroll Valley, PA 17320

Greensburg-Keystone Pennsylvania Chapter #220
412-836-2581
Paul A. Bizub
1104 W. Newton Road, #B
Greensburg, PA 15601

Harrisburg Pennsylvania Ostomy Association #173
717-737-9526
Mary Boob
1189 Kingsley Road
Camp Hill, PA 17011

Lewiston Pennsylvania Ostomy Outreach Satellite #37 (Harrisburg Chapter)
717-248-5165
Marilyn Burnham
107 Lombardy Circle
Lewistown, PA 17044-2528

Upper-Dauphin Pennsylvania Satellite #38 (Harrisburg Chapter)
717-896-3749
Jenny Zimmerman
117 Market Street
P.O. Box 135
Halifax, PA 17032

Indiana County Pennsylvania Chapter #713
412-459-6279
Frances Newman
Rt. 2, Box 226
Blairsville, PA 15717

Johnstown Pennsylvania Chapter #282
814-536-4581
Mabel Yoder
Joseph Johns Towers, #1002
Johnstown, PA 15901

Lackawanna County Pennsylvania Chapter #279
717-457-6949
Pamela Smith
409 Hudson Street
Moosic, PA 18507

Lancaster Pennsylvania Chapter #174
717-733-0538
Ronald Troy
127 Martin Avenue
Ephrata, PA 17522

Lawrence County Pennsylvania Chapter #525
Olive Martin
RD #3, Box 106A
Volant, PA 16156

Lebanon County Pennsylvania Chapter #489
717-949-2777
C. Eugene Wilman
RD #2, Box 310A
Myerstown, PA 17067

Lower Bucks County Pennsylvania Chapter #169
215-638-3297
Dennis Hickey, Jr.
4102 Portsmouth Court
Bensalem, PA 19020

Luzerne County Pennsylvania Chapter #176
717-824-3036
Joseph Sakaduski
659 E. Northampton Street
Wilkes-Barre, PA 18702

Meadville Pennsylvania Chapter #530
814-763-3790
Julia Clark
RD #4, Box 182
Saegertown, PA 16423

Mercer County Pennsylvania Chapter #379
412-981-3031
William Goshorn
540 Thorton Avenue
Sharon, PA 16146-3559

Philadelphia Pennsylvania Ostomy Association #172
215-483-1818 302-475-6979
Rebecca Polss
105 W. Sutton Place
Wilmington, DE 19810

Pittsburgh Pennsylvania Chapter #178
412-822-7826
Carole Delach
54 Arlington Court
Pittsburgh, PA 15223-1654

Pottstown Pennsylvania Area Chapter #406
Norman Yocom
95 W. 5th Street
Pottstown, PA 19464

Schuylkill County Pennsylvania Chapter #589
717-462-0040
Betty Piampi, R.N., E.T.
227 S. Jardin Street
Shenandoah, PA 17976-1642

Upper Central Bucks County Pennsylvania Chapter #521
215-855-4050
Donald Gehringer
301 Delaware Avenue
Lansdale, PA 19446

Warren Pennsylvania Area Chapter #464
814-757-8197
Martha Neel
13 Melody Lane
RD #1, Box 1313
Russell, PA 16345

Williamsport Pennsylvania Area Ostomy Chapter #214
717-322-6323
Fred Thomas
RR #6, 107 Tiffany Drive
Williamsport, PA 17701

Lewisburg Pennsylvania Satellite #36 (Williamsport Chapter)
717-523-2500
Barbara Ritter, R.N., C.E.T.N.
Evangelical Community Hospital
1 Hospital Drive
Lewisburg, PA 17837

York County Pennsylvania Chapter #524
717-741-1944
Lou Tracy
2727 Iron Stone Hill Road
York, PA 17403

Puerto Rico

Puerto Rico Chapter #546
Jose Vazquez
Gardenia 1701
San Francisco
Rio Piedras, PR 00927

Rhode Island

Rhode Island Chapter #179
508-336-4194
Dorothy Soczek
120 Sykes Road
Seekonk, MA 02771

South Carolina

Anderson Area South Carolina Chapter #610
803-944-2432
Jeanne Colberg, R.N., E.T.
26 Pine Garden Way
Salem, SC 29676

Charleston South Carolina Chapter #180
803-795-7394
John Wolfe
812 Farnham Road
Charleston, SC 29412-4806

Greater Columbia South Carolina Chapter #437
803-736-1418
James Campbell
7719 Exeter Lane
Columbia, SC 29223

Florence South Carolina Chapter #655
803-667-9653
William Dixon
900 Wisteria Drive
Florence, SC 29501

Greenville South Carolina Chapter #320
803-233-0018
William W. Adkins, Jr.
112 Glenn Burnie Drive
Easley, SC 29640

Horry County South Carolina Chapter #585
803-236-7829
Jaci Morgan
102 Brookgate
Myrtle Beach, SC 29577

Orangeburg South Carolina Area Chapter #609
803-536-2758
Ruth Webber
423 Hillsboro N.E.
Orangeburg, SC 29115

Spartanburg South Carolina Chapter #333
803-578-3539
George Bruce
303 Ferndale Drive
Spartanburg, SC 29303

Sumter South Carolina Area Chapter #678
803-773-8344
Louise Dossey
200 Crestwood Drive
Sumter, SC 29154

South Dakota

Mitchell South Dakota Area Chapter #691
605-946-5508
Al Lightenberg
RR 1, Box 29
Corsica, SD 57328-9707

Rapid City South Dakota Area Chapter #735
605-343-4607
Melvin Parlet
221 E. Nevada Drive
Rapid City, SD 57701

Sioux Falls South Dakota Area Ostomy Association #398
605-334-6555
Henry Dingman
4315 Locust Drive
Sioux Falls, SD 57103

Watertown South Dakota Area Chapter #634
605-625-3498
Carl Johnsen
RR 1, Box 173C
Willow Lake, SD 57278-9650

Tennessee

Chattanooga Tennessee Ostomy Association #182
615-624-0277
Paralee Davis
P.O. Box 4799
Chattanooga, TN 34705

Etowah Tennessee Area Ostomy Association #700
615-263-9694
Priscilla Cornwall
Rt. 2, Box 589
Etowah, TN 37331

Jackson Tennessee Chapter #560
901-425-6985
Hope Voegli, R.N.
General Hospital
708 W. Forest Avenue
Jackson, TN 38301

Kingsport/Johnston City/ Bristol TN/VA Chapter #733
615-542-2433
J. Ronald Winter
749 Quail Hollow Drive
Elizabethtown, TN 37643

Knoxville Tennessee Chapter #183
615-690-6069
Irene Small
141 Suffolk Drive
Knoxville, TN 37922

Memphis Tennessee Area Ostomy Group #233
901-388-9938
Ken Russell
3247 Glen Logan
Memphis, TN 38134-3121

Nashville Tennessee Ostomy Association #548
615-868-3953
Eugene Wardell
1286 Old Hickory Boulevard
Nashville, TN 37207

Rutherford County Tennessee Chapter #630
615-893-3713
Roseann Smith
1007 Elliott Drive
Murfreesboro, TN 37129

Texas

Austin Texas Chapter #248
512-339-6388
Carol Laubach, E.T.
P.O. Box 12861
Austin, TX 78711

Beaumont Texas Chapter #628
409-892-0019
Kurt Seligman
4860 Bellechase Drive
Beaumont, TX 77706-7773

Brenham Texas Chapter #769
409-836-5153 (H)
409-836-3794 (W)
Jim Tom House
404 N. Dixie
Brenham, TX 77833

Corpus Christi Texas Chapter #337
512-852-6743
James Brents
4426 Moravian
Corpus Christi, TX 78411

Dallas Texas Area Chapter #185
214-692-5876
Sharon Jackson
3716 Centenary
Dallas, TX 75225

Irving Texas Satellite #105 (Dallas Chapter)
214-579-8377
Allee Anderson, E.D.R.S.R.C.
1901 N. MacArthur Boulevard
Irving, TX 75061

El Paso Texas Chapter #285
915-772-3735
Carlos Rodriguez
8300 Maye
El Paso, TX 79925-4926

Fort Worth Texas Area Chapter #187
817-295-2375
Lester Hughes
Rt. 5, Box 860
Burleson, TX 76028-9735

Denton Texas Satellite #42 (Fort Worth Chapter)
817-565-1320
Sally Ann Davis
2111 Greenway
Denton, TX 76201

Golden Spread Texas Chapter #278
806-378-4673
Gloria Griffin, R.N., E.T.
1500 Wallace
P.O. Box 32051
Amarillo, TX 79120

Harlingen Texas Area Chapter #493
512-761-4951
Debbie Moutsos
P.O. Box 2583
South Padre Island, TX 78597

Houston Texas Chapter #186
713-894-8906
Clarice Kennedy
14239 Barrone Drive
Cypress, TX 77429

Houston Bay City Texas Satellite #114 (Houston Chapter)
409-798-8729
Barbara Carpenter
P.O. Box 1004
Brazoria, TX 77422

Houston Northwest Texas Satellite #98 (Houston Chapter)
713-376-4320
Jo England
12711 Mutineer Lane
Tomball, TX 77375-8418

Richmond/Rosenberg Texas Satellite #117 (Houston Chapter)
713-331-6079
Anita Price
P.O. Box 872
Manvel, TX 77578

Longview Texas Area Chapter #318
903-236-7953
Barbara Williams
Rt. #3, Box 182L #33
Kilgore, TX 75662

Lubbock Texas Ostomy Association #293
806-747-1408
Juanita Gililland
2129 55th Street
Lubbock, TX 79412

McAllen Texas Area Chapter #499
512-781-5460
William Hauck
1402 S. Cage, #129
Pharr, TX 78577-6230

Midland/Odessa Texas Chapter #590
915-570-8822
Elizabeth Hatfield
2517 Shell
Midland, TX 79705

Ralph Kaye/San Antonio Texas Chapter #188
512-655-6659
Arvid N. Skogerboe
8623 Starcrest, Apt. X-1
San Antonio, TX 78217-4707

New Braunfels Texas Satellite #91 (Ralph Kaye/ San Antonio Chapter)
512-899-2726
Thomas Schaffer
Rt. #4, Box 374U
Canyon Lake, TX 78133

Uvalde County Texas Satellite #84 (Ralph Kaye/ San Antonio Chapter)
512-278-4881
Sammy Romans
524 E. Oppenheimer
Uvalde, TX 78801

Sherman Texas Area Ostomy Association #289
903-893-5423
Maria Boyd
204 Kessler
Sherman, TX 75090

Texarkana Texas Area Chapter #423
903-838-0861
Leta Mae Maxey
612 Witt Lane
Texarkana, TX 75501-3162

Tyler Texas Chapter #321
903-882-4069
Jack Winn
1328 Hideaway Lane W.
Lindale, TX 75771

Lufkin/Nacogdoches Texas Satellite #126 (Tyler Chapter)
409-875-3102
Becky Womack
401 Cedaridge Drive
Lufkin, TX 75901

Victoria Texas Chapter #694
512-575-5506
Pat Goerlitz
Rt. 3, Box 38
Victoria, TX 77901

Waco Texas Chapter #300
817-547-6027
Virginia Taylor
804 Keelman
Copperas Cove, TX 76522

West Texas Ostomy Chapter #189
915-655-5053
Elmer Edgington
525 S. Bishop
San Angelo, TX 76901-4503

Wichita Falls Area Chapter #297
817-692-1060
Myrtle Bell
4610 Sierra Madre
Wichita Falls, TX 76310

Utah

Logan Utah Area Chapter #669
801-753-7874
T.O. Lemon
526 W. 200 South
Logan, UT 84321

Ogden Utah Chapter #730
801-825-9158
Edward Isler
1659 W. Camelot Drive
Layton, UT 84041-1507

Saint George Utah Chapter #473
801-628-9047
Alfreda Erikson
335 N. Donlee Drive
St. George, UT 84770-4541

Salt Lake City Utah Chapter #190
801-295-6573
Nancy Rodgers
548 South 200 East
Salt Lake City, UT 84010

Virginia

Fredericksburg Virginia Chapter #367
703-659-5234
John Tomlin
2204 Harpoon Drive
Stafford, VA 22554

Lynchburg Virginia Chapter #452
804-237-1687
Vicki Graham
308 Myrtle Lane
Lynchburg, VA 24502

Martinsville Virginia Chapter #759
703-956-2277
Martin Wheeler
859 Southland Drive
Martinsville, VA 24112

Northern Virginia Chapter #567
703-273-2008
Sid Miller
9245 Bailey Lane
Fairfax, VA 22031-1903

Peninsula Virginia Ostomy Association #192
804-898-6432
Joseph Kalista
12 Quillen Terrace
Newport News, VA 23606

Williamsburg Virginia Satellite #46 (Peninsula Chapter)
804-229-1576
Mary Nell Morris
129 Underwood Road
Williamsburg, VA 23185

Petersburg Virginia Area Chapter #787
804-862-3045
Kathy Clay
1006 Hampton Road
Petersburg, VA 23805

Richmond Virginia Ostomy Association #193
804-282-6013 (H)
804-232-2323 (W)
Robert Mosby
8005 Costin Drive
Richmond, VA 23229

Roanoke Virginia Chapter #428
703-774-4146
William G. Mason
2355 Howard Road, S.W.
Roanoke, VA 24015-3961

Rockingham County Virginia Area Chapter #743
703-984-8803
Aubey Dellinger, Jr.
Rt. 4, Box 445
Edinburg, VA 22824

Tidewater Virginia Chapter #194
804-488-2906
Janice Nyman
5 Sunset Lane
Portsmouth, VA 23701

Suffolk Virginia Satellite #45 (Tidewater Chapter)
804-539-4745
Thomas Powers
714 Turlington Road
Suffolk, VA 23434

Winchester Virginia Area Chapter #488
703-662-1617
Louise Greiner
636 Valley View Drive
Winchester, VA 22603-9802

Fauquier County Virginia Satellite #102 (Winchester Chapter)
703-752-9462
John Wilkins
P.O. Box 8
Somerville, VA 22739

Washington

Aberdeen/Grays Harbor Washington Chapter #407
206-532-3869
Sarah Ross
2524 Cherry Street
Hoquiam, WA 98550

Kitsap County Washington Ostomy Association #500
206-692-3869
Donald or Kim Moberg
12470 Gregory Lane
Silverdale, WA 98383-9505

Mount Vernon Washington Chapter #338
206-293-8124
Roseanne Bush
2003 9th Street
Anacortes, WA 98221

Whatcom Washington Satellite #31 (Mount Vernon Chapter)
206-734-5492
Anne Christensen
1200 Lincoln Street, #198
Bellingham, WA
98226-5734

Olympia Washington Chapter #608
206-491-6938
Ed Young
7624 Rich Road S.E.
Olympia, WA 98501

Lewis County Washington Satellite #63 (Olympia Chapter)
206-736-2205
Susan Krause
304 W. Roanoke
Centralia, WA 98531-3434

Pasco-Columbia Basin Washington Chapter #648
509-783-2347
Beatrice Nelson
7104 W. Arrowhead
Kennewick, WA 99336

Greater Seattle Washington Chapter #196
206-242-3222
Marion Hornsby
4028 S. 168th Street
Seattle, WA 98188

Kirkland Washington/ Eastside Satellite #48 (Seattle Chapter)
206-823-5334
Valerie Thornton
10512 N.E. 123rd Court
Kirkland, WA 98034

Snohomish County Washington Chapter #722
206-481-0896
Marilyn Adams
820 E. Cady Road, C-106
Everett, WA 98203

Olympic Peninsula (Callam-Jefferson Counties) Washington Satellite #95 (Snohomish Chapter)
206-457-8879
Sally Mowbray
1417 E. Front Street
Port Angeles, WA 98362

Tacoma Washington Chapter #292
206-531-9288
Steve Strizic
8643 Tacoma Avenue S.
Tacoma, WA 98444

Vancouver Washington Chapter #505
509-427-8001
Rhoda Kite
MPO 03 Walnut Lane
Shamania, WA 98648-9537

Walla Walla Valley Washington Chapter #703
503-938-3425
Mary Kerns
1209 Davis
Milton-Freewater, OR 97862

Greater Wenatchee Washington Chapter #486
509-663-4560
Aletha Cusick
1910 Skyline Drive
Wenatchee, WA 98801

Okanagan County Washington Satellite #49 (Wenatchee Chapter)
Viola McLeish
Box 70
Okanagan, WA 98840

West Virginia

Charleston West Virginia Ostomy Association #266
304-925-0857
Sophie Resko
4308 Lancaster Avenue S.E.
Charleston, WV 25304-2525

Wheeling West Virginia Area Chapter #358
614-633-5004
George Smith
57503 Washington Heights Boulevard
Martins Ferry, OH 43935

Wood County West Virginia Chapter #706
304-375-7620
Linda Bayles
513 Henderson Avenue
Williamstown, WV 26187

Wisconsin

Chippewa Valley Wisconsin Chapter #198
715-834-4699
Linda Lauritzen
1808 Arlene Place
Eau Claire, WI 54703

Indianhead Wisconsin Satellite #52 (Chippewa Valley Chapter)
715-924-3319
Elaine Fostvedt
Box 171
Chetek, WI 54728

St. Croix Valley Wisconsin Satellite #90 (Chippewa Valley Chapter)
715-796-2666
Ann Campbell
1280 Charlotte, #204
Hammond, WI 54015

Fond du Lac Wisconsin Ostomy Association #490
414-921-7187
Dorie Theyerl
150 E. Merrill Avenue
Fond du Lac, WI 54935

Green Bay Wisconsin Area Chapter #510
414-494-1777
Lois Valitchka
1493 Western Avenue
Green Bay, WI 54303

Greater Hurley Wisconsin-Ironwood Michigan Chapter #622
715-561-5520
Sandra Gordon
P.O. Box 247
Hurley, WI 54534

Jefferson County Wisconsin Chapter #625
414-674-3535
Emma Schulz
152 N. Main Street
Jefferson, WI 53549

Kenosha-Racine Wisconsin Ostomy Association #330
414-637-5325
Harold Lehmann
27 N. Indiana Street
Racine, WI 53405-1959

La Crosse Wisconsin Chapter #201
608-782-2386
Rosemary Hickisch
1222 Cass Street
La Crosse, WI 54601

Winona Minnesota Satellite #20 (La Crosse Chapter)
507-643-6597
Therese Albrecht
Rt. 4, Box 71 CA
Winona, MN 55987

Madison Wisconsin Ostomy Association #345
608-241-8133
Paul Syftestad
5132 Reynolds Avenue
Waunakee, WI 53597

Marshfield Wisconsin Chapter #627
715-748-2348
Marvin Lang
205 W. Allman Street
Medford, WI 54451

Marshfield Wisconsin Ileal-Anal Support Group #133 (Marshfield Chapter)
715-387-4113
Carol Hamus
M634 Elm Street
Marshfield, WI 54449

Milwaukee Wisconsin Chapter #199
414-782-3821
Adam Janicsek
12840 Winthrop Court
Brookfield, WI 53005

Oshkosh Wisconsin Chapter #717
414-231-3725
David Schwartz
1125 W. Linwood Avenue
Oshkosh, WI 54901

Rock County Wisconsin Chapter #246
608-365-9719
Penny Govert
2117 Huebbe Parkway
Beloit, WI 53511

Sheboygan Wisconsin Ostomy Chapter #595
414-458-1747
Lorraine Gerhartz
1234 Alabama Avenue
Sheboygan, WI 53081

Minocqua-Woodruff Wisconsin Satellite #53 (Sheboygan Chapter)
Sandra Gordon
P.O. Box 247
Hurley, WI 54534

Washington County Wisconsin Satellite #54 (Sheboygan Chapter)
414-338-4462
Marjo Lloyd
528 S. Second Street
West Bend, WI 53095

Wyoming

Central Wyoming Chapter #202
307-265-4579
Leo Sanchez
818 Sally Lane
Casper, WY 82609

Cheyenne Wyoming Chapter #686
307-635-3003 307-775-7984
Kathy Morrell
10507 E. Polo Plate
Cheyenne, WY 82009

Laramie Wyoming Satellite #55 (Cheyenne Chapter)
307-322-3614
Darlene Palmer
711 Tunnel Road
Garrett Rt.
Rock River, WY 82083

CANADA

Alberta

Calgary Alberta Chapter #25
403-281-7629
Linda Joechle
36 Woodfield Road S.W.
Calgary, AB T2W 4G7

Edmonton Alberta Ostomy Association #365
403-476-8313
Sheelah Zapf
6315-152 A Avenue
Edmonton, AB T5A 1X9

Grande Prairie/Peace District Alberta Chapter #619
403-532-8622
Dianne Lowe
1-207, 7201 Poplar Drive
Grande Prairie, AB TV8 6C5

Lethbridge Alberta Chapter #675
403-327-0118
Thomas Hacker
1702 - 6 Avenue N.
Lethbridge, AB T1H 0T3

Medicine Hat Alberta Chapter #257
403-529-8826 403-527-0858
Phyllis Pudwell
2179 19th Avenue S.E.
Medicine Hat, AB T1A 3X3

British Columbia

Nanaimo British Columbia Chapter #665
Margo Baldassi
Site N, C-17, RR #1
Nanaimo, BC V9R 5K1

North Vancouver Island British Columbia Chapter #646
604-338-9535
Yves Bernard
282 Nim Nim Place
Courtenay, BC V9N 8A5

Okanagan Mainline British Columbia Chapter #33
604-549-2263
Leslie Davis
RR 1, Site 3, Comp 98
Vernon, BC V1T 6L4

Trail British Columbia Satellite #113 (Okanagan Mainline Chapter)
604-866-5790
Louise Hodgins
RR 4, Site 15, Box 9
Wynndel, BC V0B 2N0

Prince George British Columbia Chapter #516
604-963-3437
Fran Willman
RR 8, Site 5, Comp 1-A-9
Prince George, BC V2N 4M6

Surrey British Columbia Chapter #520
604-599-6938
Jim Singleton
6514 152nd Street
Surrey, BC V3S 3L1

Vancouver British Columbia Chapter #36
604-430-1522
Beverly Ewoniak
6291 Burns Street
Burnaby, BC V5H 1X3

Victoria British Columbia Chapter #29
604-477-9173 604-387-4791
Nancy Cuthbert
2600 Sinclair Road
Victoria, BC V8N 1B9

Manitoba

Brandon-Westman Manitoba Chapter #445
204-728-4743
Don Rose
1226 4th Street
Brandon, MB R7A 3J6

Winnipeg Manitoba Ostomy Association #37
204-837-4405
Norm Fossheim
7 Sellwood Avenue
Winnipeg, MB R3R 2P7

New Brunswick

Bathurst New Brunswick Chapter #668
506-546-2141
Bette Melanson
1496 Keith Avenue
Bathurst, NB E2A 1M3

Campbellton & Area New Brunswick Chapter #748
506-759-8109
Miss Carmel Roy
17 Malcolm Avenue, Apt. 2
Campbellton, NB E3N 2S7

Fredericton New Brunswick Chapter #414
506-459-7088
Judy Wilkie
24 Bradford Street
Fredericton, NB E3B 5H7

Moncton New Brunswick Chapter #573
506-386-7276
Susan Kydd-Haynes
31 Craig Court
Riverview, NB E1B 4M4

Saint John New Brunswick Chapter #226
506-696-2325
Janice Bridgeport
47 Creighton Avenue
Saint John, NB E2J 3G8

Newfoundland

Saint John's Newfoundland Chapter #604
709-753-1160
Dorothy Dick
167 Blackmarsh Road
St. John's, NF A1E 1T1

Nova Scotia

Antigonish Nova Scotia Chapter #559
902-863-0145
Francis Dhooge
82 St. Ninian Street, #53
Antigonish, NS B2G 1Y8

Cape Breton Nova Scotia Chapter #415
902-849-5059
Anna Currie
59 Lake Road
Glace Bay, NS B1A 2H2

Metro Halifax Nova Scotia Chapter #32
902-889-3184
Patrick Horne
RR 1
Musquodoboit Harbour, NS
B0J 2L0

Middleton & Valley Nova Scotia Area Satellite #56 (Metro Halifax Chapter)
902-825-3207
Hazel Dauphinee
RR 3
Middleton, NS B0S 1P0

Pictou County Nova Scotia Chapter #661
902-755-6706
Caroline Jardine
P.O. Box 519
Tenton, NS B0K 1X0

Southwest Nova Scotia Chapter #459
902-761-2756
Roseanne Deveau
Carleton
Yarmouth, NS B0W 1L0

Truro Nova Scotia Chapter #552
902-895-3055
Tony Nickerson
36 Robertson Crescent
Truro, NS B2N 5P6

Ontario

Belleville-Trenton Ontario Chapter #299
613-967-1007
George Palmer
35 Janlyn Crescent
Belleville, ON K8N 1L1

Brantford Ontario Chapter #287
519-753-6846
Emmy Merz
RR 7
Brantford, ON N3T 5L9

Halton-Peel Counties Ontario Chapter #711
416-338-3749
Glenn Waterston
1360 White Oaks Boulevard
#306
Oakville, ON L6H 2R7

Hamilton & District Ontario Ostomy Association #28
416-627-3273
Henry Gardiner
18 Glenmorris Drive
Dundas, ON L9H 1S4

Kitchener-Waterloo Ontario Chapter #441
519-743-7446
Clare Swan
36 Sherwood Avenue
Kitchener, ON N2B 1J9

Lindsay/Kawartha Ontario Chapter #737
705-738-4228
Ken Duncan
149 Port Colony Road
Bobcaygeon, ON K0M 1A0

London & District Ontario Chapter #30
519-660-4346
John Delaney
124 Grenfell Crescent
London, ON N5X 2R9

Sarnia-Lambton Ontario Satellite #124 (London & District Chapter)
519-660-4346
Stephen Lambley
1102-11 Derby Lane
Sarnia, ON N7T 7V2

Niagara Ontario Chapter #208
416-834-7216
Don Fenmore
109 Hampton Avenue
Port Colbourne, ON L3K 5R9

Norfolk & District Ontario Ostomy Association #761
519-426-9733
Peter Cleland
88 Oakwood Avenue
Simcoe, ON N3Y 1H6

North Bay Ontario Chapter #514
705-474-0362
Phyllis Arsenault
135 Worthington Street W., 809
North Bay, ON P1B 8M6

Oshawa District Ontario Chapter #305
416-576-9516
Blanche Alward
393 Rossland Road E.
Oshawa, ON L1G 2X2

Ottawa Ontario Chapter #27
613-722-4314
Fred Tait
493 Highcroft Street
Ottawa, ON K1Z 5J3

Brockville & Area Ontario Satellite #131 (Ottawa Chapter)
613-345-1712
John Addison
114 Front Avenue W.
Brockville, ON K6V 4K1

Oxford Ontario Chapter #765
519-537-7551
Mae Fleming
1074 Cree Avenue
Woodstock, ON N4T 1A2

Sault Ste. Marie Ontario Chapter #523
705-759-4940
Carole Parton
715 Fourth Line E.
Sault Ste. Marie, ON P6A 5K9

Stratford & District Ontario Chapter #707
519-393-5316
Raymond Rynor
RR 5
Stratford, ON N5A 6S6

Toronto Ontario Chapter #26
416-742-3605
Lorne Aronson
53 Riverdale Drive
Rexdale, ON M9V 2T5

Windsor District Ontario Chapter #695
519-255-1850
Lorna Gardner
1651 Pelissier Street
Windsor, ON N8X 1N1

York-Simcoe Aurora District Ontario Chapter #775
416-898-6035
Diane Heath
168 Glenwary Circle
Newmarket, ON L3Y 7S5

Prince Edward Island

Prince Edward Island Chapter #501
902-894-7231
Linda Harding
82 Wescomb Crescent, #1
Charlottetown, PE C1C 1B4

Quebec

Association des stomises de l'Estrie Quebec #298
819-752-7473
Mme Georges Herbert
199 Notre Dame Ouest
Victoriaville, PQ G6P 1R8

Association des stomises de la Mauricie, Trois Rivières #902
819-379-1679
Jeannine Ferron
763 St. Maurice, AP #2
Trois Rivières, PQ G9A 3P5

Ileostomy/Colostomy Association of Montreal Quebec #31
514-645-4023
Jean Pierre LaPointe
949 Pierre Lacroix
Montreal, PQC H1B 3C7

Association des stomises de Quebec #901
155, 13E Rue
Quebec, PQ G1L 2K4

West Montreal Quebec Chapter #779
514-630-3802
Peter Connolly
4 LeGault Place
Beaconsfield, QUE H9W 5A2

Saskatchewan

Regina Saskatchewan Chapter #274
306-545-2528
Sheila McKendrick
222 Wells Street
Regina, SK S4R 5Z8

Moose Jaw Saskatchewan Satellite #60 (Regina Chapter)
306-693-4730
Annette Geisler
947 Hall Street W.
Moose Jaw, SK S6H 2S3

Saskatoon Saskatchewan Chapter #229
306-242-8346
Bev Fry
238 Russell Road
Saskatoon, SK S7K 5T2

Prince Albert Saskatchewan Satellite #61 (Saskatoon Chapter)
Herman Knoke
510 16th Street
W. Prince Albert, SK
26V 3V8

INTERNATIONAL OSTOMY ASSOCIATION ADDRESS LIST

EUROPE

Austria

Österreichische ILCO
Obere Augartenstrasse 26-28
A-1020 Vienna
Phone 02 22-3 56 87 72

Belgium

Stoma ILCO Belgie
Dalialaan, 8
B-3191 Boortmeerbeek
Phone 0 15-61 48 60

Stoma Club Antwerpen
Van Notenstraat 123
B-2100 Deurne
Phone 3-3 21 57 00

Stoma Club Liège
34, Rue Victor Carpentier
B-4020 Liège-Bessoux

Bulgaria

Bul-ILCO c/o Union of Invalids
Christo Beltscher Str. 21, IV/48
Sofia 1000
Phone 9 02-65 84 71
Fax 9 02-57 66 43

Czechoslovakia

ILCO Czechoslovakia
c/o Mrs. Jitka Zemanova
Hospital Bulovka 180 81
Prague 8
Phone 818-2257/818-8575

Denmark

COPA
c/o Mrs. Merete Moeller
Aertebjergvej 28
4660 Store-Heddinge
Phone 53 70 85 65

Finland

FINNILCO Ry.
c/o Osmo Lindroos
PL 2 42
SF-33101 Tampere
Phone 9 31-14 09 80

France

Fédération des stomises de France
76 Rue Balard
F-75015 Paris
Phone 1 45.57.40.02

I.A.S. - France (Fédération française des Associations l'Information et l'Aide aus Stomises)
Hôtel-Dieu
1 Place de l'Hôpital
F-69288 Lyon Cedex 02
Phone 78.92.20.43

Germany

Deutsche ILCO
Kepserstrasse 50, Postfach 12.65
D-8050 Freising
Phone 0 81 61-8 49 09/8 49 11
Fax 0 81 61-8 55 21

Great Britain

British Colostomy Association
15 Station Road
Reading Berkshire RG1 1LG
Phone 07 34-39 15 37
Fax 07 34-56 90 95

Ileostomy Association of Great Britain and Ireland
Amblehurst House
Black Scotch Lane
Mansfield, Notts NG18 4PF
Phone 06 23-2 80 99

Urostomy Association
c/o Mrs. Angela Cooke
"Buckland" Beaumont Park
Danbury, Essex CM3 4DE
Phone 024-541-4294

Greece

ILCO Greece
c/o Hellenic Anticancer Institute
171 Alexandras Avenue
603 Athens 115-22
Phone (01) 6 40 93 91
Fax 1-6 42 01 46

Hungary

Magyar ILCO Szovetseg
Pf. 93, H-7401 Kaposvar
Phone 0 82-1 27 23

Iceland

ISILCO
Skogarhlid 8
IS-101 Reykjavik

Israel

Israel Ostomy Association
c/o Israel Cancer Association
P.O. Box 4 37
Givalaim 53104
Phone 03-5 71 72 34
Fax 03-5 71 05 78

Italy

A.I. Stom
Via Venezian 1
I-20133 Milano Italia
Phone 02-2 36 02 74
Fax 02-2 39 05 08

Luxemburg

ILCOLUX
c/o Justine Jacque
51 Rue de Centre
L-3960 Ehlange/Mess

Netherlands

Nederlandse Stomavereniging
"Harry Bacon"
Wilhelminastraat 45
NL-3621 VG Breukelen
Phone 03462-62286

Norway

NORILCO
Fr. Nansens VEI 12
Postboks 5327
Majorstua
0304 Oslo 3 Norway
Phone 02-46 10 10
Fax 02-60 69 80

Poland

POL-ILKO
c/o Mrs. Ewa
Degorskaszewczyk
Zawiszy 13/35, 91-829 Lodz

Portugal

Associacao Portuguesa de Ostomizados
Av. Joao Paulo II
Zona J. de Chelas
Lote 552 - 2.B
P-1900 Lissabon
Phone 01.85.60.54

Russia

Soviet Ostomy Association Asstom
c/o Dr. Willen Y. Klour
Box 19, 195176
St. Petersburg
Phone 2 72 24 03
Fax 2 79 62 11

Spain

Asociación Española de Ostomizados
c/ Gral. Martínez
Campos
42 DPDO, 4
28010 Madrid
Phone 01-3 08 41 86

Sweden

ILCO-Forbundet
P.O. Box 2004
S-291 02 Kristianstad
Phone 044/125594

ILCO Schweiz
c/o Mr. Heinz Striffeler
Schermenweg 129
CH-3006 Bern

Ukraine

Transkerpatia Ostomy Association
c/o Dr. Vitaly Tsubar
Bauman St. 2, Uzgorod
294014
Phone 2 62 27

AFRICA

Algeria

ILCO Algérie
c/o Mr. Rachid Rezgui
Cité des 145 Logts. Bt. D
Local No. 7 Nouvelle Ville
Tizi-Ouzou - 15000
Phone (03) 21.79.60

South Africa

South African Ostomy Association
139 Smit Street, Braamfontein
P.O. Box 2000
Johannesburg
Phone 0 11-4 03-28 25
Fax 0 11-4 03-19 46

Zimbabwe

Ostomy Association of Zimbabwe
P.O. Box 3881, Harare
Phone 70 55 22

NORTH & CENTRAL AMERICA

Canada

UOA Canada
c/o Mr. Allan M. Porter
5 Hamilton Avenue
Hamilton, ON L8V 2S3
Phone 416-389-8822

Costa Rica

Asociación pro Ayuda al Ostomizado
P.O. Box 148
Belen, 4005 Heredia

Mexico

Ostomex
Alfonso Esparza Oted
139/12 Col. Guadalupe Inn
Mexico D.F. 01020
Phone 5-48-84-47/5-66-12-81

USA

United Ostomy Association
36 Executive Park, Suite 120
Irvine, CA 92714-6744
Phone 800-826-0826
714-660-8624
Fax 714-660-9262

SOUTH AMERICA

Argentina

Asociación Argentina de Ostomizados
c/o Señor Gualterio Rossmaier
Casilla de Correo 2477
1000 Buenos Aires
Phone 90-14 10

Bolivia

Asociación Boliviana de Ostomizados
c/o Señora Elsa Velarde Vesarano
Murillo 247
P.O. Box 310, Santa Cruz
Phone 33-46 30

Brazil

Sociedade Brasileira dos Ostomizados
c/o Señora Candida Carvalheira
Rua do Acre, 47 Sala 613
Centro CEP 20.081, Rio de Janeiro
Phone (021) 233-5068

Chile

Corporación Chileña de Ostomizados
c/o Señor José Levia
Irarrazabal 4849
Santiago de Chile
Phone 2 25 68 22

Colombia

Asociación Colombiana de Ostomizados
c/o Señora Leonora de Acosta
Carrera 22 #54-A-23
Bogota

Ecuador

Asociación Ecuatoriana de Ostomizados
c/o Señor Dr. Reinaldo Burgos
P.O. Box 09.04.202, Guyaquil
Phone 28 02 38

Peru

Asociación de Ostomizados del Peru
c/o Señor Dr. Gerado Galvan
Scipion Llona 180
Miraflores Lima 18 Peru
Phone 45 35 40

Uruguay

Asociación Uruguaya de Ostomizados
c/o Mrs. Elena Fosman
Rambla Mahatma Gandhi 667/601
11300 Montevideo
Phone 70 21 53
Fax 5 98-2 94 72 40

Venezuela

Asociación Venezolana de Ostomizados
c/o Señora Lic. Nelida Moreno
P.O. Box 62.268
Chacao, Caracas 1060

ASIA

China

Ostomy Association of China
c/o Mr. Yu De-Hong, M.D.
Chang Hai Hospital
174 Chang Hai Road
Shanghai
Phone 48 87 06-4 25 20

Hong Kong

Hong Kong Stoma Association Ltd.
G.P.O. Box 10984 Central
Hong Kong
Phone 5-1 12 86 89

India

Ostomy Association of India
74 Jerbai Wadia Road
Parel Bombay 400 012
Phone 412.8087

Japan

Japan Ostomy Association
1-1-6-204, Hamamatsu-cho
Minato-ku
Tokyo 105 Japan
Phone 03-4 59-63 90

Korea

Korea Ostomy Association
c/o E. H. Whang
CPO Box 5216
102 Ho Daedo Bld. 44-2
Juja Dong Chung Gu Seoul
Phone 5 98-2 94 72 40

Singapore

Singapore Ostomy Society
15 Enggor Street, #06-30 & 04
Realty Centre
Singapore 0207
Phone 2219577

AUSTRALIA/ NEW ZEALAND

Australia

Australian Council of Stoma Associations
P.O. Box 363
Strathfield 2135 N.S.W.
Phone (02)-7 47-66 19/57 20
Fax (02)-7 45-42 84

New Zealand

Federation of New Zealand Ostomy Societies
P.O. Box 96024
Balmoral, Auckland 3
Phone 04-5 28 35 43
Fax 06-3 42 88 08

OTHER KNOWN ASSOCIATIONS

Benin

Université Nationale du Benin
Abomey-Calavy BP 526
Contonou, Republic of Benin

Botswana

Department of Medicine
University College of Botswana
P.O. Box 0022, Gaborone

Jamaica

Ostomy Welfare Group of Jamaica
St. Joseph's Hospital
Kingston 3

Sri Lanka

Noboru Yabatu
12 Melbourne Avenue,
P.O. Box 596
Colombo 4

Taiwan

Ostomy Service Center
Chuen Kwang Ko, President
No. 36 Fu-Heng 1st Road
Kaohsiung, Taiwan R.O.C.

APPENDIX

B CROHN'S & COLITIS FOUNDATION ADDRESS LIST

CROHN'S & COLITIS FOUNDATION OF AMERICA, INC., CHAPTER DIRECTORY

NATIONAL HEADQUARTERS

444 Park Avenue South
11th Floor
New York, NY 10016-7374
(800) 932-2423
(212) 685-3440
Fax: (212) 779-4098

REGIONAL OFFICES

Northeast Regional Office
94 Church Street, Suite 302
New Brunswick, NJ 08901
(908) 937-9100

Mid-Atlantic Regional Office
1314 Bedford Avenue
Suite 114
Baltimore, MD 21208
(301) 486-9511

Midwest Regional Office
395 East Dundee Road
Suite 450
Wheeling, IL 60090
(708) 459-6342

South/Southwest Regional Office
One Davis Boulevard
Suite 707
Tampa, FL 33606
(813) 251-2191

Southern California Regional Office
4201 Wilshire Boulevard
Suite 624
Los Angeles, CA 90010
(213) 935-4673

Western Regional Office
9740 Washington Boulevard
Culver City, CA 90232
(310) 559-8667

NORTHEAST REGION

Connecticut

Fairfield/Westchester Chapter
22 West Putnam Avenue
Greenwich, CT 06830

Greater Hartford Chapter
P.O. Box 230466
Old State House Station
Hartford, CT 06123-0466

New Haven Regional Satellite
Contact Northeast Regional Office

New London Regional Satellite
Contact Northeast Regional Office

Waterbury Satellite
Contact Northeast Regional Office

Delaware

Contact Philadelphia/Delaware Valley Chapter

Massachusetts

Greater Boston Chapter
280 Hillside Avenue
Needham, MA 02194

New Jersey

Greater New Jersey Chapter
300 Somerset Street
New Brunswick, NJ 08901

New York

Capital District (Albany) Chapter
4 Normanskill Boulevard
Delmar, NY 12054

Central New York Chapter
P.O. Box 6675 Teal Avenue
Syracuse, NY 13217

Fairfield/Westchester Chapter
22 West Putnam Avenue
Greenwich, CT 06830

Greater New York Chapter
444 Park Avenue South
2nd Floor
New York, NY 10016-7374

Long Island Chapter
Bennett Building, Suite 212
45 North Station Plaza
Great Neck, NY 11021-5011

Rochester Chapter
1279 Chili Avenue
Rochester, NY 14624

Southern Tier (Binghamton) Chapter
1159 Vestal Avenue
Binghamton, NY 13903

Western New York Chapter
P.O. Box 224
Williamsville, NY 14221

Pennsylvania

(See also Mid-Atlantic Region.)

Central Pennsylvania Chapter
P.O. Box 6162
Reading, PA 19610

Philadelphia/Delaware Valley Chapter
7718 Castor Avenue
Philadelphia, PA 19152

Rhode Island

Rhode Island Chapter
P.O. Box 6771
Providence, RI 02940

Vermont

Vermont Chapter
P.O. Box 275
Jericho, VT 05465

MID-ATLANTIC REGION

District of Columbia

Washington, D.C. Area Chapter
Contact Mid-Atlantic Regional Office

Kentucky

Kentucky Chapter
P.O. Box 36051
Louisville, KY 40233-6051

Maryland

Maryland Chapter
1314 Bedford Avenue
Suite 114
Baltimore, MD 21208

Michigan

Michigan Chapter
20300 Civic Center Drive
Suite 302
Southfield, MI 48076

North Carolina

Charlotte Regional Satellite
Contact Mid-Atlantic Regional Office

North Carolina Triad Chapter
P.O. Box 10714
Greensboro, NC 27404

North Carolina Triangle Chapter
P.O. Box 177
Graham, NC 27253-0177

Ohio

Northeastern Ohio Chapter
23366 Commerce Park Drive
Suite 203
Beachwood, OH 44122

Pennsylvania

Greater Pittsburgh Chapter
580 South Aiken Avenue
Suite 427
Pittsburgh, PA 15232

South Carolina

South Carolina Chapter
134 McSwain Drive
West Columbia, SC 29169

Virginia

Tidewater Regional Satellite
Contact Mid-Atlantic Regional Office

Virginia Chapter
P.O. Box 29211
Richmond, VA 23242-00211

MIDWEST REGION

Illinois

Greater Chicago Carol Fisher Chapter
395 East Dundee Road
Suite 450
Wheeling, IL 60090

Indiana

Indiana Regional Satellite
Contact Midwest Regional Office

Iowa

Iowa Chapter
2012 Western Road
Iowa City, IA 52240

Kansas

Kansas City Chapter
8900 State Line
Suite 354
Leawood, KS 66206

Minnesota

Minnesota Chapter
Midway Hospital
1700 University Avenue West
St. Paul, MN 55104

Missouri

St. Louis Chapter
8420 Delmar, Suite 503
St. Louis, MO 63124

Nebraska

Nebraska Regional Satellite
Contact Midwest Regional Office

Wisconsin

Wisconsin Chapter
Sinai Samaritan Medical Center
950 North 12th Street
P.O. Box 342
Milwaukee, WI 53201-0342

SOUTH/SOUTHWEST REGION

Alabama

Birmingham Chapter
6 Office Park Circle
Suite 202A
Birmingham, AL 35201

Arkansas

Arkansas Regional Satellite
Contact South/Southwest
Regional Office

Florida

Gold Coast Chapter
900 North Federal Highway
#230
Boca Raton, FL 33432

South Florida/Ann Gorlitz Chapter
1600 South Federal Highway
2nd Floor
Hollywood, FL 33020

West Coast/Tampa Chapter
One Davis Boulevard
Suite 707
Tampa, FL 33606

Georgia

Georgia Chapter
2531 Briar Cliff Road
Suite 216
Atlanta, GA 30002

Louisiana

Louisiana Regional Satellite
Contact South/Southwest
Regional Office

Mississippi

Mississippi Chapter
P.O. Box 4736
Jackson, MS 39296

Oklahoma

Oklahoma Chapter
3150 East 41st Street
Suite 106
Tulsa, OK 74105

Tennessee

Chattanooga Chapter
P.O. Box 80054
Chattanooga, TN 37411

Texas

Austin Regional Satellite
Contact South/Southwest
Regional Office

Dallas Chapter
6007 Twin Coves
Dallas, TX 75248

Houston/Gulfcoast Chapter
2650 Fountainview, Suite 122
Houston, TX 77057

San Antonio Regional Satellite
Contact South/Southwest
Regional Office

Tarrant County Regional Satellite
Contact South/Southwest
Regional Office

SOUTHERN CALIFORNIA REGION

Beverly Hills/Westside Chapter
P.O. Box 5852
Sherman Oaks, CA 91403

Long Beach Chapter
Long Beach Memorial
Medical Center
2801 Atlantic Avenue
5th Floor
Long Beach, CA 90801-1428

Greater Los Angeles Chapter
Contact Southern California
Regional Office

Orange County Chapter
16478 Beach Boulevard, #319
Westminster, CA 92683

Greater San Diego/Inland Empire Chapter
411 Thorn Street, Suite C
San Diego, CA 92103

San Fernando Valley Chapter
P.O. Box 1305
Woodland Hills, CA 91364

WESTERN REGION

Arizona

Phoenix Chapter
P.O. Box 5497
Scottsdale, AZ 85261-5497

Southern Arizona Chapter
P.O. Box 32706-105
Tucson, AZ 85751-2706

California

(See also Southern California Region.)

Sacramento Valley Chapter
P.O. Box 19465
Sacramento, CA 95819

San Francisco Bay Area Chapter
2166 Hayes Street, Suite 204
San Francisco, CA 94117

Colorado

Rocky Mountain (Denver) Chapter
7720 S. Broadway, Suite G20
Littleton, CO 80122

Hawaii

Hawaii Regional Satellite
Contact Western Regional
Office

Nevada

Las Vegas Chapter
2255-A Renaissance Drive, #35
Las Vegas, NV 89119

Reno Regional Satellite
Contact Western Regional
Office

Oregon

Oregon Satellite
Contact Western Regional
Office

Washington

Puget Sound Chapter
Box 31381
Seattle, WA 98103

Spokane Regional Satellite
Contact Western Regional
Office

INDEX

D

E

J

V

W

X

Z